Cognitive–behavioral Therapy with Adults

A Guide to Empirically-Informed Assessment and Intervention

Cognitive–behavioral Therapy with Adults

A Guide to Empirically-Informed Assessment and Intervention

Edited by

Stefan G. Hofmann

and

Mark A. Reinecke

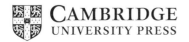

CAMBRIDGE UNIVERSITY PRESS
Cambridge, New York, Melbourne, Madrid, Cape Town, Singapore,
São Paulo, Delhi, Dubai, Tokyo, Mexico City

Cambridge University Press
The Edinburgh Building, Cambridge CB2 8RU, UK

Published in the United States of America by Cambridge University Press, New York

www.cambridge.org
Information on this title: www.cambridge.org/9780521896337

© Cambridge University Press 2010

First published 2010

Printed in the United Kingdom at the University Press, Cambridge

A catalog record for this publication is available from the British Library

ISBN 978-0-521-89633-7 Hardback
ISBN 978-0-521-72089-2 Paperback

Contents

Contributors

Martin M. Antony
Department of Psychology
Ryerson University
Toronto, Ontario, Canada

Elise Beeger
Massachusetts General Hospital
OCD and Related Disorders Program
Boston, MA, USA

Peter J. Bieling
Department of Psychology
St. Joseph's Healthcare
Hamilton, Canada

Sandra Bucci
University of Manchester
Manchester, UK

Amanda W. Calkins
Department of Psychology
Boston University
Boston, MA, USA

Zafra Cooper
University of Oxford
Department of Psychiatry
Warneford Hospital
Oxford, UK

Michelle G. Craske
Department of Psychology
UCLA
Los Angeles, CA, USA

Cynthia Cushman
South County Psychiatric and Psychotherapy
Center
Great Barrington, MA, USA

David J. A. Dozois
Department of Psychology
University of Western Ontario
London, Canada

Christopher G. Fairburn
University of Oxford
Department of Psychiatry
Warneford Hospital
Oxford, UK

Peter Fisher
Division of Clinical Psychology
University of Liverpool
Liverpool, UK

Tiffany Fuse
Behavioral Science Division
National Center for Post-traumatic
Stress Disorder
Boston, MA, USA

Jennifer L. Greenberg
Massachusetts General Hospital
OCD and Related Disorders Program
Boston, MA, USA

Bridget A. Hearon
Department of Psychology
Boston University
Boston, MA, USA

Richard G. Heimberg
Department of Psychology
Temple University
Philadelphia, PA, USA

Stefan G. Hofmann
Department of Psychology
Boston University
Boston, MA, USA

Tejal A. Jakatdar
Department of Psychology
Temple University
Philadelphia, PA, USA

Naomi Koerner
Department of Psychology
Ryerson University
Toronto, Ontario, Canada

Brett T. Litz
Behavioral Science Division
National Center for Post-traumatic Stress Disorder
Boston, MA, USA

Lawrence D. Needleman
Department of Psychiatry
Ohio State University
Columbus, OH, USA

Michael W. Otto
Centre for Anxiety and Related Disorders
Boston University
Boston, MA, USA

Jason M. Prenoveau
Department of Psychology
Loyola University Maryland
Baltimore, MD, USA

Jennifer Ragan
Massachusetts General Hospital
OCD and Related Disorders Program
Boston, MA, USA

Mark A. Reinecke
Division of Psychology
Northwestern University
Chicago, IL, USA

Melisa Robichaud
Department of Psychiatry
University of British Columbia
Vancouver, Canada

Jenny Rogojanski
Department of Psychology
Ryerson University
Toronto, Ontario, Canada

Madeline Sedovic
Massachusetts General Hospital
OCD and Related Disorders Program
Boston, MA, USA

Kristalyn Salters-Pedneault
Behavioral Science Division
National Center for Post-traumatic
Stress Disorder
Boston, MA, USA

Nicholas Tarrier
University of Manchester
Manchester, UK

Adrian Wells
University of Manchester
Manchester Royal Infirmary
Manchester, UK

Maureen L. Whittal
Department of Psychiatry
University of British Columbia
Vancouver, Canada

Sabine Wilhelm
Massachusetts General Hospital
OCD and Related Disorders Program
Boston, MA, USA

Foreword

David M Clark
Professor of Psychology
Kings College London, UK

In the last 35 years very considerable progress has been made in devcloping effective psychological treatments for mental health problems. Several schools of psychotherapy have contributed to these advances. However, the contribution of the cognitive-behavioral school has been particularly prominent, partly because it is the only school that has developed treatments for a wide range of different disorders, each of which has been shown to be effective in well-conducted, randomized controlled trials. Reflecting this substantial evidence base, governmental and professional guidelines in many countries now include the cognitive-behavior therapies among their list of first-choice treatments. This book provides an excellent introduction to these treatments in action.

There is, of course, no single cognitive-behavior therapy. Instead, researchers and clinicians have developed highly specialized interventions that target the specific psychological processes that underlie different pathological conditions, while at the same time taking into account the unique way in which people with different conditions present in treatment, and the challenges this poses for the nature of the therapeutic relationship. Stefan Hofmann and Mark Reinecke have been leading figures in the development of the field. Drawing on their broad knowledge, they have assembled for this book a stellar list of contributors, each of whom has a well-deserved reputation for their expertise in the treatment of the particular disorders that are the focus of each chapter. For each disorder, key clinical features are described, an overview of treatment is provided, and relevant evidence supporting for the effectiveness of the treatment, as well as the theoretical model on which it is based, is presented.

Introduction

Stefan G. Hofmann and Mark A. Reinecke

Cognitive–behavioral therapy (CBT) is one of the big success stories of contemporary psychology. The most recent development in the United Kingdom (UK) is a very clear example of the enormous influence CBT has gained. In October 2007, the UK Health Secretary announced that the UK will spend £300 million ($600 million) to initiate a six-year program with the goal of providing people with psychological problems, such as anxiety disorders and depression, with better access to empirically supported therapies, especially CBT. The plan is to train a total of 8,000 new therapists in these evidence-based interventions for depression and anxiety disorders. This change in healthcare delivery was based on economic data showing that provision of CBT for common mental disorders is more cost efficient than pharmacotherapy or other interventions (for more information, see [1]). Similarly, the Australian government recommended in 1996 the provision of CBT and introduced a plan to provide better access to these services.

Although impressive in magnitude, the recent developments in the UK and other countries are not surprising to us. This appears to be a logical next step from the clear scientific evidence for CBT efficacy and effectiveness to its dissemination [2, 3]. Unfortunately, the United States, Canada, and other developed countries are still lagging behind other nations, such as the UK and Australia, in necessary efforts to disseminate CBT. Therefore, wider efforts to disseminate CBT in the United States and other countries should be a priority for future research.

The CBT paradigm

Cognitive–behavioral therapy is sometimes criticized as a treatment that substitutes negative thoughts with positive thoughts. This is a misperception. Cognitive–behavioral therapy techniques do not ask patients to think positively but rather more adaptively. This central idea might be best explained by the following example provided by Beck [4]:

> A housewife hears a door slam. Several hypotheses occur to her: "It may be Sally returning from school." "It might be a burglar." "It might be the wind that blew the door shut." The favored hypothesis should depend on her taking into account all the relevant circumstances. The logical process of hypothesis testing may be disrupted, however, by the housewife's psychological set. If her thinking is dominated by the concept of danger, she might jump to the conclusion, "It is a burglar." She makes an arbitrary inference. Although such an inference is not necessarily incorrect, it is based primarily on internal cognitive processes rather than actual information. If she then runs and hides, she postpones or forfeits the opportunity to disprove (or confirm) the hypothesis.
>
> (Beck 1979, pp. 234–5 [4])

Thus, the same initial event (hearing the slamming of the door) elicits very different emotional responses, depending on how a person interprets this event. The door slam itself does not elicit any emotions one way or the other. But when the housewife believes that the door slam suggests that there is a burglar in the house, she experiences fear. She might jump to this conclusion more readily if she is somehow primed after having read about burglaries in the paper, or if she has the core belief (schema) that the world is a dangerous place and that it is only a matter of time until a burglar will enter her house. Her behavior, of course, would be very different if she felt fear than if she thought that the event had no significant meaning. This is what the Greek Stoic philosopher Epictetus meant when he said that "men are not moved by things, but the view they take of them."

In more general terms, CBT is based on the notion that behavioral and emotional responses are strongly moderated and influenced by cognitions and the perception of events. The word *cognitive* in CBT implies that treatment focuses a great deal on thought processes. However, therapy is not limited to cognitive modification. Effective CBT has to target all aspects of an emotional disorder, including cognitions, emotional experience, and behavior. Accordingly, Beck distinguishes among the intellectual, the experiential, and the behavioral approaches [4], all of which are considered important aspects of therapy. As part of the intellectual approach, patients learn to identify their misconceptions, test the validity of their thoughts, and substitute them with more appropriate concepts; the experiential approach encourages patients to experience their emotional states in more adaptive ways; and the central element of the behavioral approach is to encourage the development of specific forms of behavior that lead to more general changes in the way patients view themselves and the world. Therefore, situational exposure techniques are consistent with the behavioral approach, whereas mindfulness strategies are compatible with the experiential approach of CBT.

As we have discussed elsewhere [5], targeting the way one thinks about emotion-eliciting situations and experiences is different from approaches that attempt to regulate emotion through reduction of experiential avoidance (e.g., by embracing anxiety or pain). These latter strategies are characteristic of those employed by acceptance and commitment therapy (ACT) practitioners [6]; however, they are not incompatible with a CBT approach. Indeed, there is evidence to suggest that individuals habitually employ either cognitive reappraisal or suppression to regulate emotion [7], and that flexibility in emotional expression is important to long-term emotional adjustment [8].

The therapeutic process

The general therapeutic process of CBT is divided into various steps, with an emphasis on a number of specific therapeutic mechanisms that are outlined below. The CBT process is assumed to include all of these mechanisms to varying degrees at any given point in time.

Establishing a collaborative therapeutic relationship

Positive therapist–patient interactions flow from a collaborative relationship. In general, therapists' behavior should be honest and warm. Patients are not considered to be helpless and passive but, rather, experts about their own problems. Therefore, patients are actively involved in treatment. For example, they are encouraged to formulate and test certain hypotheses in order to get a better understanding of the real world and their own problems. The emphasis during therapy is placed on solving problems. The therapist's role is to work with the patient to find adaptive solutions to solvable problems. Every step in therapy is transparent and clearly reasoned. Patients are encouraged to ask questions to make sure that they understand and agree with the treatment approach.

The initial role of CBT therapists is very active, as they educate patients about the underlying principles of this treatment approach. In addition, therapists often find that patients need a great deal of guidance in the beginning stages of therapy in order to help them successfully identify their misconceptions and associated automatic thoughts. As treatment progresses, patients are expected to become increasingly active in their own treatment. A masterful CBT therapist reinforces his or her patients' independence while at the same time being aware of the need for continued support and education as patients first begin to apply the concepts of CBT to their difficulties.

Problem focus

Cognitive–behavioral therapy is a problem-solving process. This process includes clarifying the status of the presenting problem, defining the desired goal, and finding the means to reach that goal. Therefore, the therapist and patient discuss the goals of therapy at the beginning of treatment, including identifying the type of interventions that are to be used to reach these goals and delineating concrete observable outcomes that indicate that each goal has been achieved. Cognitive–behavioral therapy case formulation can facilitate this step. The goal of formulation-based assessment is to identify core beliefs that underlie misconceptions and associated automatic thoughts in order to intervene effectively during treatment. Through the process of problem reduction, therapist and patient then identify problems with similar causes and group them together. Once the major problem is identified, the therapist typically breaks it up into component problems to be attacked in a given case. Therapists frequently elicit feedback from the patient throughout treatment to ensure that problem-solving efforts are on target with identified goals.

Identifying and eliminating maintaining factors

Once patients define their problems and goals for treatment, CBT therapists encourage them to become aware of the processes that maintain these problems. The reason that a psychological problem develops in the first place is usually not the same as the reason the problem is maintained. The distinction between initiating factors and maintaining factors is a crucial distinction that encourages patients to focus on the here and now rather than the past.

Maladaptive cognitive processes are common maintaining factors when applying the CBT model. Cognitions are generally classified into negative automatic thoughts and maladaptive beliefs. Negative automatic thoughts are thoughts or images that occur in specific situations when an individual feels threatened in some way. Maladaptive beliefs, on the other hand, are assumptions that individuals have about the world, the future, and themselves. These more global, overarching beliefs provide a schema that determines how a person may interpret a specific situation. Just as with automatic thoughts, therapists can identify maladaptive beliefs through the process of guided questioning.

By treating thoughts as hypotheses, patients are put into the role of observers – scientists or detectives – rather than victims of their concerns. In order to challenge these thoughts, therapist and patient discuss the evidence for and against a particular assumption. This can be done in a variety of ways, most typically by using information from patients' past experiences, empirically evaluating a situation, evaluating the outcome of a situation, and by giving patients the opportunity to test their hypotheses by exposing them to feared and/or avoided activities or situations.

Once these maintaining factors are identified, patients are encouraged to modify and eliminate them. For example, the individual may be confronted with stimuli (e.g., situations, bodily sensations, images, activities) that provoke negative emotions (e.g., anxiety, embarrassment, guilt), in order to find more adaptive ways to respond to these stimuli.

Efficacy of CBT

A review of the efficacy of CBT for mental disorders would easily fill a separate textbook. A recent review of 16 meta-analytic studies found large controlled effect sizes for CBT for unipolar depression, generalized anxiety disorder, panic disorder with or without agoraphobia, social phobia (i.e., social anxiety disorder), PTSD, and childhood depressive and anxiety disorders; and medium controlled effect sizes for CBT for chronic pain, childhood somatic disorders, marital distress, and anger [2]. Furthermore, large uncontrolled effect sizes were found for bulimia nervosa and schizophrenia. Similarly, a recent review of methodologically rigorous, randomized placebo-controlled studies of anxiety disorders indicated that CBT yielded medium to large effect sizes over placebo [3]. Large effect sizes were observed for obsessive–compulsive disorder and acute stress disorder. Moreover, the various CBT treatment protocols showed clear disorder-specificity, because depression changed to a significantly lesser degree than the targeted anxiety disorder. In sum, CBT is clearly an effective treatment for a range of psychopathology. The effects of CBT have been replicated many times in well controlled studies. As a result, many CBT protocols have been classified as empirically supported treatments as defined by the American Psychological Association (APA) Division 12 Task Force in 1995 [9].

Relationship to the medical model and its diagnostic system

Many contemporary CBT models of psychopathology are aligned with medical classification systems of mental disorders, such as those provided by the *Diagnostic and Statistical Manual of Mental Disorders*, 4th edition, text revision (DSM-IV-TR; [10]) and the International Classification of Diseases-10 (ICD-10; [11, 12]). Cognitive–behavioral therapy researchers and clinicians have taken advantage of the semblance of order that these atheoretical classification systems offer to the field of psychopathology and, from that order, have developed models for a wide range of conditions. These models most often focus on understanding and explaining psychopathology reflected by specific DSM/ICD diagnostic categories (e.g., social anxiety disorder, generalized anxiety disorder, major depressive disorder), although there are some exceptions. Cognitive–behavioral therapy models of health anxiety diverge from a criteria-based categorical conceptualization, viewing the cognitive and behavioral features of conditions characterized by severe health anxiety as occurring along a continuum ranging from adaptive to maladaptive. Likewise, CBT models of chronic pain behavior are rooted neither in the traditional biomedical model of pain nor DSM-defined pain disorder. They are, instead, integrative models that account for complex interplay between biological, psychological, and sociocultural mechanisms (see, for example [13]). All CBT models of psychopathology – whether based on DSM/ICD diagnostic categories, dimensional conceptualization, mechanistic conceptualization, or some other system – serve to guide, and are informed by, research and development of treatment techniques. The development and refinement of CBT models for the various DSM-IV-TR/ICD-10 diagnoses has permitted application of specific treatment techniques across a diverse range of psychopathologies for which outcomes have been favorable. Moreover, another benefit of this alignment is evidenced in the development of novel ways for combining CBT with pharmacotherapy. Approaches such as these have substantial potential for further increasing the effectiveness of the treatments available for various forms of psychopathology.

The family of CBTs

Cognitive–behavioral therapy is not a single treatment protocol, and it is inappropriate to talk about *the* cognitive therapy or *the* cognitive model. The specific model and treatment techniques depend on the symptoms that are targeted. Thus, CBT describes a family of interventions that share the same basic elements of the CBT model that focus on the importance of cognitive processes for emotion regulation. We do not consider this to be a weakness of CBT. Instead, it is a sign that CBT is a maturing scientific discipline rather than an assembly of specific treatment techniques. The reason for this is the strong commitment to the scientific enterprise and openness to translating and integrating new empirical findings of the psychopathology of a disorder into a working CBT model of the disorder. This is an ongoing and iterative process; for example, CBT for social anxiety disorder ten years ago looked very different from CBT for social anxiety disorder today (e.g., [14]). Although the core assumptions of CBT have remained unchanged, the specific treatment techniques have certainly changed and will continue to change as basic research on psychopathology progresses. The present book will provide a review of the contemporary CBT approaches for psychiatric disorders in adults.

We were extremely fortunate to recruit the foremost experts in CBT for all major mental disorders. In Chapter 1, David J. A. Dozois and Peter J. Bieling discuss CBT for depression and in Chapter 2, Amanda W. Calkins, Bridget A. Hearon, and Michael W. Otto give an overview of CBT for bipolar disorder. These two chapters on mood disorders are followed by chapters on all major anxiety disorders, including generalized anxiety disorders (Chapter 3 by Adrian Wells and Peter Fisher), social anxiety disorder (Chapter 4 by Tejal A. Jakatdar and Richard G. Heimberg), specific phobia (Chapter 5 by Naomi Koerner, Jenny Rogojanski, and Martin M. Antony), panic disorder and agoraphobia (Chapter 6 by Jason M. Prenoveau and Michelle G. Craske), obsessive–compulsive disorder (Chapter 7 by Maureen L. Whittal and Melisa Robichaud), and post-traumatic stress disorder (Chapter 8 by Tiffany Fuse, Kristalyn Salters-Pedneault, and Brett T. Litz). Chapter 9 will provide an overview of CBT for eating disorders (Zafra Cooper and Christopher G. Fairburn), Chapter 10 for schizophrenia and psychotic disorders (Sandra Bucci and Nicholas Tarrier), and Chapter 11 for body dysmorphic disorder (Jennifer Ragan, Jennifer L. Greenberg, Elise Beeger, Madeline Sedovic, and Sabine Wilhelm). The final chapter of the book is a review of mindfulness-based CBT (by Lawrence Needleman and Cynthia Cushman), an emerging new development in CBT. We hope the readers are as excited about this book as we are, and we hope that it will provide clinicians with a guide for the assessment, conceptualization, and intervention of adult disorders.

References

1. Rachman S, Wilson GT. Expansion in the provision of psychological treatment in the United Kingdom. *Behav Res Ther* 2008; **46**: 293–5.

2. Butler AC, Chapman JE, Forman EM, Beck AT. The empirical status of cognitive-behavioral therapy: a review of meta-analyses. *Clin Psychol Rev* 2006; **26**: 17–31.

3. Hofmann SG, Smits JAJ. Cognitive-Behavioral Therapy for adult anxiety disorders: a meta-analysis of randomized placebo-controlled trials. *J Clin Psychiatry* 2008; **69**: 621–32.

4. Beck AT. *Cognitive Therapy for Emotional Disorders*. New York: Meridian, 1979.

5. Hofmann SG, Asmundson GJ. Acceptance and mindfulness-based therapy: new wave or old hat? *Clin Psychol Rev* 2008; **28**: 1–16.

6. Hayes SC, Masuda A, Bissett R, Luoma J, Geurrro LF. DBT, FAP and ACT: how empirically oriented are the new behavior therapy technologies? *Behav Ther* 2004; **35**: 35–54.

7. Gross JJ, John OP. Individual differences in two emotion regulation processes: implications for affect, relationships, and well-being. *J Pers Soc Psychol* 2003; **85**: 348–62.

8. Bonnanno GA, Papa A, Lalande K, Westphal M, Coifman K. The importance of being flexible: the ability to both enhance and suppress emotional expression predicts long-term adjustment. *Psychol Sci* 2004; **15**: 482–7.

9. Chambless DL, Baker MJ, Baucom DH, *et al.* Update on empirically validated therapies, II. *The Clinical Psychologist* 1998; **51**: 3–16.

10. American Psychiatric Association. *Diagnostic and Statistical Manual of Mental Disorders*, 4th edn., text revision. Washington, DC: APA, 2000.

11. World Health Organization. *The ICD-10 Classification of Mental and Behavioural Disorders: Clinical Descriptions and Diagnostic Guidelines*. Geneva: World Health Organization, 1992.

12. World Health Organization. *The ICD-10 Classification of Mental and Behavioural Disorders: Diagnostic Criteria for Research*. Geneva: World Health Organization, 1993.

13. Asmundson GJG, Wright KD. The biopsychosocial model of pain. In Hadjistavropoulos T, Craig KD eds. *Pain: Psychological Perspectives*. New Jersey: Erlbaum. 2004, pp. 35–57.

14. Hofmann SG. Cognitive factors that maintain social anxiety disorder: a comprehensive model and its treatment implications. *Cogn Behav Ther* 2007; **36**: 195–209.

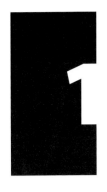

Cognitive therapy for depression

David J. A. Dozois and Peter J. Bieling

The nature of the disorder

Depression is a heterogeneous phenomenon that ranges from a mild and relatively transient negative mood state (dysphoria or despondency), often associated with a sense of loss, disappointment, or hopelessness, to a debilitating cluster of symptoms that impair most aspects of social or occupational functioning. In its clinical state, major depression refers to a constellation of symptoms that is associated with significant cognitive, emotional, behavioral, physiological, and interpersonal impairment (American Psychiatric Association [APA]) [1].

As defined by the *Diagnostic and Statistical Manual of Mental Disorders* (DSM-IV-TR; [1]), an individual must minimally experience five out of nine symptoms nearly every day for at least two weeks to meet diagnostic criteria for a major depressive episode. Unfortunately, the duration of a depressive episode often extends over a much longer period of time than is required diagnostically. One of these symptoms must be either sadness or loss of interest/anhedonia. Additional symptoms include changes in appetite or weight (increase or decrease), disturbed sleep (insomnia or hypersomnia), psychomotor retardation or agitation, loss of energy or fatigue, worthlessness, self-blame or excessive guilt, impaired concentration or ability to make decisions, and suicidal ideation, attempted suicide, or recurrent thoughts of death [1]. Exclusionary criteria include the physiological effects of a substance or general medical condition that fully accounts for the symptom profile, and short-term (i.e., up to two months) bereavement that is not characterized by worthlessness, suicidality, psychotic symptomatology, or psychomotor retardation [1]. Major depression is often characterized as an episodic condition with a distinct onset and offset.

A first episode is termed a major depressive episode whereas the diagnosis of recurrent depression is major depressive disorder (MDD).

A number of large-scale epidemiological studies have been conducted to assess the prevalence of depression in the general population. These studies indicate that depression is among the most common of psychiatric problems. The latest estimates stem from the National Comorbidity Survey – Replication (NCS-R), a nationally representative survey of 9,282 participants in the United States. Twelve-month prevalence rates were 9.5% for any mood disorder and 6.7% for MDD [2]. Lifetime estimates for any mood disorder and MDD were 21% and 17%, respectively [3].

A depressive episode can occur at any time during the lifespan, but mid to late adolescence and early adulthood represent the periods of life most commonly associated with increased risk [4]. Approximately 25% of adults with unipolar mood disorders report an onset prior to young adulthood with 50% by age 30 years [3] (also see [4]). Adolescence is also a time when the female preponderance of depression emerges [5]; thereafter, females are consistently two times more likely than males to experience depression.

Without treatment, MDD usually lasts between four months and one year [1, 6, 7]. Most individuals (65 to 70%) recover within a year [8, 9], but many do not, and some individuals do not experience remission even after five years [8]. Enduring or fluctuating periods of residual symptoms persist for months to years in 20 to 30% of cases. This partial remission is associated with increased risk of relapse [7, 10, 11]. Within treated samples, the rate of recovery is approximately 40% within three months, 60% within six months, and 80% within one year [12]. Notwithstanding these rates, a substantial proportion

Cognitive–behavioral Therapy with Adults: A Guide to Empirically Informed Assessment and Intervention,
ed. Stefan G. Hofmann and Mark A. Reinecke. © Cambridge University Press 2010.

of individuals continue on a course that is more chronic. The rate of chronicity in treated samples is 20% at two years, and between 7% and 12% after five to ten years of follow-up [13].

Depression is characterized by relapse and recurrence. Between 50% and 85% of depressed patients experience multiple subsequent episodes [14]. The risk of future episodes also increases [8, 15], and the time for an episode to recur decreases with each episode [13]. Solomon *et al.* followed 318 individuals with MDD over a period of ten years and reported that 64% of the sample suffered from at least one recurrence [16]. The number of lifetime episodes was significantly associated with the probability of recurrence, with a 16% increase in risk with each additional episode.

Earlier episodes of depression are "thought to be more susceptible to environmental stress triggers, whereas later episodes are thought to be more autonomous" [8: p. 31]. Consistent with this hypothesis, some researchers have suggested that depressed individuals may become more sensitized the longer they experience depression or the more frequently their episodes recur [17, 18]. Interpersonal phenomena may also account for the risk of relapse. Joiner [19], for instance, advanced an interpersonal model in which multiple interpersonal variables (e.g., stress generation, negative feedback seeking, excessive reassurance seeking, interpersonal conflict avoidance) interact in reciprocal ways to maintain the depressive process and increase vulnerability for the recurrence of depressive episodes (also see [20]).

Depression co-occurs with a number of psychiatric disorders and medical conditions. Particularly high rates of comorbidity have been noted between depression and anxiety, substance abuse, schizophrenia and eating disorders [8]. Most striking is the comorbidity between depression and anxiety, which often exceeds 50% [21]. Depression and anxiety also share a number of modifiable risk factors (cf. [22]), which suggests that the use of transdiagnostic interventions may be warranted (e.g., [23]). Depression also frequently co-occurs with Parkinson's disease, multiple sclerosis, temporal lobe epilepsy, Alzheimer's disease, cardiovascular illnesses, cancer, endocrine disorders, and metabolic disturbances [24, 25, 26]. Notwithstanding the importance of differential diagnosis, this overlap may complicate the evaluation of treatment efficacy for depression in these populations. For example, treating a patient for depression who is also diagnosed with Parkinson's disease will not likely result in many changes in the neurovegetative symptoms of depression.

To summarize, depression is highly prevalent and characterized by relapse and recurrence. As such, the burden of depression is substantial not only in terms of personal suffering but also with respect to its costs to society [11, 27]. Clearly there is a need for treatments that not only ameliorate the acute episode but also reduce the risk of relapse and recurrence. As we discuss subsequently, cognitive therapy is ideally suited to meet this need.

Cognitive models of depression

Cognitive theories of depression share the idea that individual differences in maladaptive thinking and negative appraisals of life stress account for the disorder (e.g., [28, 29, 30]). These theories are essentially diathesis-stress models because maladaptive cognition is believed to contribute to the onset of depression in the context of stressful life circumstances. Most contemporary cognitive models of depression have involved refinements and expansions of Beck's original theory [29, 31].

Beck proposed that a taxonomy of cognition exists, ranging from "deeper" cognitive structures to more surface-level cognitions [32, 33]: (1) schemas; (2) information processing and intermediate beliefs; and (3) automatic thoughts. Schemas may be defined as stable internal structures of stored information, including core beliefs about self. According to this model a negative self-schema develops in childhood and remains inactive until it is triggered later in life by negative circumstances (see [31]). Insecure attachment experiences and other adverse events (e.g., childhood maltreatment) are some of the early predictors of the development of a negative or maladaptive belief system [34, 35]. Once schemas are activated, they are believed to affect the manner in which information is processed and interpreted. For example, an individual vulnerable to depression may have underlying core beliefs that he or she is fundamentally incompetent or unlovable. As long as this belief system remains inactive, depression is not likely. Once this schema is kindled by life stress (e.g., a failure or rejection experience), however, the individual is more likely to engage in information processing biases (e.g., attentional or memory biases toward negative content) and to experience cognitive errors and negative automatic thoughts associated with themes of loss, failure, worthlessness, defectiveness, incompetence, and inadequacy [31, 32]. Automatic thoughts are more superficial and proximal to a given situation than are other levels of cognition but are functionally related to one's deeper beliefs and schemas. Automatic thoughts refer to the constant flow of positive and negative thoughts that run through an individual's mind and which are not accompanied by direct conscious appraisal. In the context of depression, automatic thoughts often focus on what Beck called the "cognitive triad," a negative view of oneself, the world, and the future [29].

The empirical literature has generally supported Beck's cognitive theory of depression. Numerous studies have demonstrated that depressed individuals exhibit problems with negative automatic thoughts, dysfunctional attitudes, hopelessness, worthlessness, negative explanatory styles, irrational beliefs, and negatively biased memory and attention (see [36]). The notion of a temporally stable "depressive schema" has also received empirical support [37]). Dozois and Dobson [38], for example, measured the self-representation of clinically depressed women using a computerized task. Participants were retested six months later when half of the sample had remained depressed and the other half had improved. The organization of negative adjective content remained stable across time even among individuals who no longer met diagnostic criteria for major depression (see also [39]).

Given that studies of remitted samples do not elucidate mechanisms related to the onset of depression, cognitive vulnerability has also been studied in individuals who are considered vulnerable but who are not currently depressed. Children of depressed mothers, for instance, tend to show depressotypic information processing, negative explanatory styles, greater hopelessness, and lower self-worth than do children of non-psychiatric mothers [40, 41]. Longitudinal studies have also supported Beck's theory, demonstrating that the interaction of cognitive vulnerability (e.g., dysfunctional attitudes) and life stress predicts depression [42, 43, 44].

Although cognition represents the main focus in Beck's theory and therapy, his model acknowledges that cognitions, emotions, behaviors, and biological processes are interrelated. As outlined above, Beck's conceptualization is that depression involves a top–down process – the self-schema influences information processing, which, in turn, impacts negative automatic thoughts. Cognitive therapy, however, tends to work as a bottom–up endeavor – therapists begin to target surface level cognitions (automatic thoughts) and eventually proceed to modify deeper schemas and core beliefs.

Cognitive therapy aims to help individuals shift their cognitive appraisals from ones that are unhealthy and maladaptive to ones that are more evidence based and adaptive. Patients learn to treat their thoughts as hypotheses rather than as facts. Framing a belief as a hypothesis, provides an opportunity to test its validity, affords patients the ability to consider alternative explanations, and permits them to gain distance from a thought to allow for more objective scrutiny [45].

Cognitive therapy is highly collaborative and involves designing specific learning experiences to help patients monitor their automatic thoughts, understand the relationships among cognition, affect, and behavior, examine the validity of automatic thoughts, develop more realistic and adaptive cognitions, and alter underlying beliefs, assumptions, and schemas.

Empirical evidence for cognitive therapy for depression

Cognitive therapy for depression has received considerable research attention and empirical support (see [45] for review). More than 75 clinical trials have been published on cognitive therapy for MDD since 1977 [46]. For treating an acute episode of depression, cognitive therapy is comparable to behavior therapy [47], other bona fide psychological treatments [48], and antidepressant medication, with these treatments each producing superior results than placebo control conditions [49, 50, 51]. Recent studies have also demonstrated that cognitive therapy and pharmacotherapy are equally effective for severe depression ([52, 53, 54]; but see [55]).

A particular benefit of cognitive therapy relative to antidepressant medication is that fewer patients (i.e., approximately half) relapse [56]. In their meta-analysis of the efficacy of cognitive therapy for depression, Gloaguen *et al.* reported that the average risk of relapse (based on follow-up periods of one to two years) was 25% after cognitive therapy, compared to 60% following antidepressant medication [56]. Some research data also suggest that patients who receive cognitive therapy alone are no more likely to relapse after treatment than are those individuals who continue to receive medication [51, 57]. Cognitive therapy has also been compared to antidepressant treatment (selective serotonin reuptake inhibitors, SSRIs) for severe depression [52, 53]. Both interventions resulted in equal outcomes of remission in the acute phase of treatment, but the risk of relapse at one-year follow up was favorable for individuals treated with cognitive therapy even compared to those treated with continuance medication [53].

As some researchers have argued, antidepressants may be "symptom suppressive rather than curative" [52, p. 709]. In other words, cognitive therapy and antidepressant medication may be equivalent in their modification of more surface-level cognitions (e.g., negative automatic thoughts and dysfunctional attitudes), but may differ in their ability to modify "deeper" cognitive structures. Consistent with this idea, Segal, Gemar, and Williams administered the Dysfunctional Attitude Scale (DAS) to patients who had successfully completed either a trial of cognitive therapy or pharmacotherapy [58]. The DAS was administered before and after a negative mood induction procedure in which participants were to think about a time in their lives when they felt sad. While in a neutral mood state, there were no significant between-group differences on the DAS. Following the mood induction, however, those individuals successfully treated with antidepressants exhibited an increase in dysfunctional attitudes, an effect that was not evident in those treated with cognitive therapy.

Also consistent with the notion that cognitive therapy may produce deeper cognitive change than medication are the findings from a trial that compared the combination of cognitive therapy and pharmacotherapy (CT+PT) to pharmacotherapy (PT) alone [59]. Both groups showed significant and equivalent shifts in depressive symptoms and proximal cognitions (e.g., negative automatic thoughts, dysfunctional attitudes). However, patients treated with CT+PT demonstrated significantly greater cognitive organization (interconnectedness of adjective content) of positive interpersonal content and less well connected negative interpersonal content than did those treated with medication alone. In addition, patients in the CT+PT group showed significant pre-post differences on positive and negative cognitive organization, an effect that was not evident in the antidepressant group. Although these results need to be replicated and extended, they suggest that cognitive therapy may alter conceptually deeper cognitive structures than antidepressant medication.

Introduction to a clinical case

Diane was a 59-year-old woman who presented to a specialty cognitive–behavioral therapy (CBT) clinic for the treatment of longstanding depressed mood. She had two grown daughters and her husband had recently retired from a civil service job. She had been employed for many years as a copy-editor for a publishing company, but had been struggling to keep up with the normal demands of that work. Her first clinical episode had been a post-partum depression, with approximately four or five further episodes that were often related to periods of stress or transition, including the discovery of her husband's extra-marital affair ten years earlier. Over the years she had also periodically over-used alcohol, likely meeting criteria for abuse, with the worst point occurring after knowledge of the affair. In retrospect, her drinking behavior had usually been a sign of increasing depression, and had caused some strain with her husband and family. She indicated that her marriage was now reasonably happy, but felt that in some ways she and her husband were merely cohabitating and had fairly independent lives. She described herself as quite lonely, having not had much recent contact with friends and other family. The current episode of depression was likely triggered by work-related stress – a new supervisor had been hired and she was changing a number of work procedures. Diane described her relationship with her supervisor as difficult. There was to be a new regimen of performance management in their department, and Diane had been given feedback that she ought to be more open to change.

Diane was interviewed using the Structured Clinical Interview for DSM-IV (SCID) and met criteria for both major depressive disorder, recurrent, moderate and substance abuse in sustained full remission. She also endorsed a number of symptoms related to worry about the future and social concerns, but these symptoms were not sufficient to meet diagnostic criteria. She tended to be most anxious and avoidant of others when her depression symptoms became more severe, and these worries and fears abated when the depression symptoms improved. The current episode of depression had been going on for about six months, and was marked by both sadness and loss of pleasure. Concerns about work, particularly communication with her supervisor, were daily issues and caused rumination for several hours per day. Her sleep was quite disturbed; she described having almost no restful sleep and experienced early morning awakening during which she had long crying spells, eventually resulting in her dragging herself out of bed and to work. It was at these points that she felt the worst, when she woke up early she felt like she was "the only person in the whole world." In addition to non-restorative and poor sleep, her appetite was poor and friends had begun to tell her she was looking gaunt.

Diane denied having active thoughts of suicide; she put this option "off-limits" because of her two daughters and a grandchild. She did admit that she was hopeless about the future and that the thought of no longer being alive sometimes brought her a certain amount of relief and peace. There were no signs of frank cognitive impairment, though she did describe not being as "sharp" as she was when she was not depressed. In part because of this she sometimes found it difficult to keep up at work with technological and software advances; every supposed improvement at the business seemed to her a new kind of mountain to climb.

Diane had been prescribed antidepressants and benzodiazepines when she first became depressed in her twenties. She indicated that in the past she had been diagnosed with both anxiety and depression, not surprising given the combination of anxious and depressive symptoms found during the SCID interview. She had not considered psychotherapy as an option for most of her life but had been able to overcome the substance abuse by attending Alcoholics Anonymous (AA) meetings. Alcoholics Anonymous had helped her to understand that problems could be solved by sharing, talking, and learning.

After the stress at work triggered the current episode, her family doctor had prescribed an SSRI. She had some relief from this, but associated taking medication with use of substances and was more than willing to explore alternatives. Near the end of the consultation and intake process, she also admitted that she was most concerned about starting to use alcohol again. She had contemplated doing so on a number of occasions but had managed not to by attending several AA meetings. She had an intense fear that if she began drinking again, she might well lose herself in the alcohol.

Overview of the treatment protocol

General structure of sessions

The effectiveness of CBT is based on the extent to which patients learn to use the skills conveyed in

therapy outside of the actual session. The emphasis on education, in addition to building a therapeutic alliance and the therapist's contributions to developing new behaviors and cognitions, informs the flow of each session as well as the sequence of sessions. The therapist needs to ensure that the important skills and principles of CBT are covered during each session. Therapy exercises within and between sessions allow patients to apply the skills to their own experiences, those "real life" moments when they are beginning to feel more down or depressed. At the same time, the exact way in which the skills are used by patients and the kinds of emotions, thoughts, and behaviors that are targeted is usually left up to patients, or decided on collaboratively. For example, the therapist may use a didactic approach to explain the concept "cognitive distortion" and discuss types of distortions from a list provided. The discovery aspect of the session would follow, and involve exploring some examples from the patient's life where a distortion may have been present. The "real world" examples can neither be pre-planned nor scripted, and this is what makes them powerful teaching tools. The result is "guided discovery," a term that describes both the directive and explorative nature of CBT for depression and other conditions.

Symptoms may fluctuate from session to session; therefore, it is useful before each session to have some kind of formal scale completed that gives an overview of current severity. Large changes from one week to the next in either direction often foreshadow agenda items; something "good" may have happened resulting in a positive change or something may have gone wrong that is important to focus on in the session. It is also common to briefly review the previous week's session to consolidate learning before giving a brief overview of what the next steps would be. This is followed by setting the session agenda, an important aspect of working with people who are depressed. Taking a few minutes to prioritize with the patient what needs to be discussed can prevent a session from becoming a meandering discussion of various "depressing" topics and, early in the session, sets a more productive and goal-oriented tone.

A structured approach to starting off each session is also consistent with the goal-focused, targeted approach of CBT more generally. Patients and therapists work together in the assessment and early sessions to create a list of goals to be achieved. The diagnostic/consultation process helped Diane to focus on her most troubling symptoms, and these were then translated into two goals: (1) coming to terms with the work situation, particularly untangling the situation with the new supervisor and work routines; and (2) being more productive at work and then enjoying "off" time more.

Following the agenda and moving through the content of the session can be challenging in CBT for depression. Some degree of "time-keeping" is necessary at certain points so that all of the items on the agenda can be discussed. Pacing the session, which involves determining how much time to spend on one topic before moving to the next, is important for that reason. Sometimes it is easy to stay too long with an example, especially when the example is rich and seems to tap an important area. Deviating from the agenda by spending excessive time on certain topics is almost inevitable in at least some sessions with someone who is moderately or severely depressed. However, not following the agenda can be problematic as important new material may not be covered and one can easy run out of time. At the same time, the patient's current affect needs to be attended to, and sometimes sticking to the agenda can feel artificial and forced. A useful question when considering a deviation from the agenda might be "Is the deviation I am exploring likely to be as helpful for this patient in the long run as the material we planned to cover would be?" If the answer is "yes" then a deviation is likely warranted.

The final and critical portion of the session is homework assignment. Ideally, the homework is planned based on the content of the session and the examples that emerged from the patient's life. That is, a good homework assignment blends the concepts learned in therapy with the problems experienced by the patient that need to be resolved. It is important that sufficient time be left in the session for creating homework, rather than having homework as an afterthought.

In the case of Diane, the therapist also thought it useful to have a companion manual, and *Mind over Mood* was deemed the best fit to the case [60]. The goals and the diagnostic formulation in Diane's case called for a combination of behavioral activation in early sessions, to thought-based strategies in the middle sessions, with belief work and relapse prevention in closing sessions. It was expected that about three sessions would be spent on behavioral activation, around four sessions on cognitive strategies, and a

further four sessions on beliefs, with five further sessions at somewhat longer intervals to focus on wellness and relapse prevention. This total of 16 sessions seemed warranted in light of the complexity and chronicity of this case, but is still in the range of the usual 12 to 16 sessions in typical CBT for depression trials.

The therapeutic relationship

A full review of the therapeutic alliance in CBT for depression is beyond the scope of this chapter, though this literature continues to grow and contains a number of interesting nuances. However, it seems fair to state that both the connection between patient and therapist as well as their agreement on the work of therapy may be important in facilitating change, while symptom change in turn helps to foster a strong bond between client and therapist [61]. A therapeutic stance that is understanding, empathic, and offers unconditional positive regard is a pre-requisite for working with a depressed client using CBT. Getting to this point requires two distinct perspectives to be in positive synchrony, the patient's view of the therapist and the therapist's view of the patient.

With regard to how the patient might view the therapist, one of the challenges is that negative affect, sadness, and hopelessness often pervade the presentation of people with moderate to severe depression and colors the way they see the world. Some patients will react rather strongly to therapists who seem, at least to them, to be "cheerleading" and overly positive. When the therapist appears overly positive, depressed patients are likely to conclude that the therapist is so different from them that whatever the therapist offers will provide nothing of value. The therapist needs to maintain a stance of optimism and positive expectation while, at the same time, doing so in such a way as to "join" with the patient and demonstrate understanding. It is critical to validate the patient's struggles; to admit that the work ahead may be challenging, but that the yield will be positive if followed through.

In a healthy therapeutic alliance in CBT for depression the typical pattern in sessions is one of empathy, acknowledging, supporting and then offering a change strategy to "try out." To an objective observer, it ought to appear as if both the patient and therapist are working at about the same level, in terms of talking time, offering examples, and coming up with suggestions. To the extent that one or the other party (typically the therapist) is doing more of the work there are likely to be issues in the therapeutic alliance, the patient's motivation, or the therapist's abilities with the techniques.

Strategies and techniques

Behavioral activation techniques

One of the most notable characteristics of the depressed patient is the manner in which his or her life is devoid of gratification and sense of accomplishment. As a result of loss of reinforcement from usual activities, the depressed person withdraws from many activities. Even those activities that are completed (in Diane's case, work or conversations with family) are viewed as a chore and are not enjoyable. At the outset of treatment, depressed individuals may not have enough energy to begin to examine their thoughts – they will appear sad, their rate of speech may be slow and the expression of affect impoverished. Behavioral activation can increase the person's energy level and set the stage for cognitive strategies.

Because of this behavioral profile, CBT for depression usually begins with strategies related to activation. A usual starting point for behavioral activation involves having patients monitor, or record, their daily activities and rating their mood for each waking hour of the day. This activity log provides an accurate and comprehensive "snapshot" of the person's day-to-day life and enhances understanding that variations in mood might be related to the kinds of routines the person has. Diane's monitoring revealed several interesting nuances that were not readily apparent from her self-report. Much to her own surprise, her mood seemed to be better, overall, during work times than it was on weekends. When her mood was low at work it was usually related to the supervisor situation (emails from her boss bothered her particularly and she disclosed that she would often write emotion-laden replies but delete them rather than sending them, which often made her feel worse). Her lowest mood ratings, however, were on weekends. She tended to be home alone and would ruminate about events of the past week or worry about what was to come.

Important questions related to the activity log include: How withdrawn is the patient from usual activities of daily living? Are there adequate exposures to potentially reinforcing situations? Is there a balance of pleasurable events and events that lead to a sense of accomplishment or mastery? Answers to these questions usually result in the consideration of adding activities, and sometimes finding ways to limit activities that induce a low mood. Through this process, the patient begins to understand the intimate connection between feelings and activities. It is also important to explain the concept of mastery and pleasure (or work and play), to be sure that, when consideration is given to trying on new behaviors, the core concept is to provide more of a balance of activities that are nourishing or rewarding in multiple ways. For Diane, considerable time was spent discussing basic issues that were not being attended to related to sleep hygiene, exercise, and nutrition. Central in this case, however, was the way she was spending time at work, specifically parsing the emails of her boss and then "responding" knowing there was no chance of her sending that response (and recognizing that doing so would not have been helpful). The weekends also became a priority for planning events that would pull her away from the usual rumination/anticipation cycle. With some trepidation, Diane agreed to get a group of her friends together for a program of walking on weekend mornings followed by breakfast with the group. She also asked her husband to walk with her on some evenings after work and found that, once they were out and walking, this quite naturally led to more conversation than they would have had at home. Diane found that the exercise and social activities were quite rewarding right away, but it took more concentrated effort from the therapist before she agreed to spend less time on the communications from her boss. When she did not respond to these messages she found that she was happier and could move on much quicker and refocus on the work she had to complete.

Scheduling activities (also known as graded task assignments) has benefits on two fronts. Most concretely, these activities raise the patient's energy level and are likely to lead to better concentration and less fatigue. Second, the patient begins to experience a sense of accomplishment and starts to see him/herself as more competent. Thus, such assignments are likely to produce both functional and cognitive benefits. Spending less time on those activities that decrease mood is another main focus of behavioral activation. This area is sometimes even more challenging since, at least on the surface, many patients believe that such activities (e.g., Diane venting her feelings into unsent emails) serve a function and may be associated with certain kinds of rewards. Careful scrutiny of mood patterns and a functional analysis will often be necessary for the patient to discover that the costs to these behaviors often outweigh their benefits. Over time, Diane began to contain the reading of her supervisors' emails to a segment of time at the end of the day, and responded (if strictly necessary) only the next day. This change alone resulted in a major efficiency gain and resulted in her feeling much more in control and more productive.

Cognitive techniques for automatic thoughts in depression

As therapy begins to transition from behavioral activation to cognitive work, patients begin to monitor cognitions and learn to recognize the relationship between their thoughts and their mood. For Diane, this occurred in session 4 through discussion of her weekly activities. She had noted a large change in her mood during a training program at work. As with most patients, Diane had not ever considered sharing her internal dialogue with anyone, but did acknowledge that in this situation she had doubted her abilities and was berating herself for being too slow to learn.

This process, of recording situations that produce strong affect and concomitant automatic thoughts, will usually be done on something that resembles the daily record of dysfunctional thoughts (or DRDT). Many different and specific forms of the DRDT exist, some with five columns and some with more. However, almost all will have columns to represent the situation encountered, the emotion or symptoms experienced, and associated thoughts. Like any skill learned in CBT, it may require several examples before patients are able to identify the thoughts in a given situation that really drive the strong emotion. Early in this process, the thoughts recorded are often related to the situation in a non-emotional way. For example, Diane recalled thinking many questions (e.g., "why are they moving to this new system?") and observations (e.g., "this instructor seems to speak a different language from me"). Only through Socratic questioning did Diane acknowledge that a thought, such as "I'm too stupid to learn this," was actually present and driving her negative emotions.

Once patients are more reliably able to identify their painful automatic thoughts, the process of answering back to these thoughts (or putting them on trial) can begin. This is the phase of therapy in

which Socratic dialogue becomes critical. *Socratic dialogue*, a series of interconnected questions to reach a more logical, objective conclusion about one's inner experiences, is a common theme for all cognitive techniques [45]. In fact, asking open-ended and open-minded questions is probably one of the most critical and distinguishing features of CBT. Four basic steps in this questioning process have been described: (1) characterizing the problem specifically and accurately, (2) identifying the associated thoughts, beliefs, and interpretations; (3) understanding the meanings of the thoughts for the patient; and (4) assessing the consequences of thoughts and their basis in evidence [62]. Socratic questions should neither lead nor trap the patient into agreeing with the therapist's view (which is of course also inevitably biased) and are intended to stimulate consideration of alternative perspectives and uncover information that was not previously considered.

Employing a Socratic approach, Diane learned to question thoughts along the lines of, "I'm too stupid to keep up." This was achieved by asking many informational questions and then synthesizing questions that helped her to bring that information to bear on the situation that had triggered the original negative thought. Critical questions in this process typically involve having the person think about his or her experience from another perspective, considering factors that he or she did not at first consider, and pointing out any logical leaps that might not be warranted by the actual facts. It is important to emphasize that testing beliefs and evidence gathering does not represent "positive thinking;" nor should questions be used to trap patients or invalidate their thoughts. Instead, the questions enable the patient to look at the situation objectively and non-defensively. Broadly defined, questions that gather evidence against the automatic thought are usually: (1) ascertaining all the situational parameters related to a negative thought, especially those outside of the patient's control or responsibility; (2) asking the patient to shift perspective on the situation by having him or her perceive the situation through the lens of another person; and (3) having the patient focus on information that is incomplete or unsubstantiated. Once a more complete picture of the situation emerges, the patient is asked to formulate a "balanced" thought that takes into account all of the evidence from the questioning process.

For Diane, the Socratic process helped her to discover, or perhaps rediscover, many instances in which she was able to learn something new, manage challenging relationships, and actively cope to solve problems. She found that, beyond work, this theme of not being capable came up in a variety of contexts ranging from casual social settings to caring for her grandchild. It was also helpful to her to consider other peoples' perspectives. For example, she was able to gather information from others that demonstrated that she was not the only person who felt undermined by or upset with her new boss. By sharing her own experiences with others, she learned that some of her colleagues experienced worse interactions than she did; she also benefited by hearing about some of the ways that others dealt with this negativity. This was a significant step forward in helping to contain her thinking and rumination; she continued to see the situation as troubling, but not devastating.

Systematic errors in cognitive processing, or *cognitive distortions* [31], are often the basis for negative thoughts. Various lists of cognitive distortions exist, and different distortions are seen in different kinds of disorders. In Diane's case, she tended to engage in *arbitrary inference* (drawing a specific conclusion without supporting evidence) and *personalization* (attributing external events to oneself without evidence supporting a causal connection). For example, when Diane could not respond to every request made of her at work, she thought "I'm a horrible employee." The work situation, with her supervisor, also became highly personalized for Diane. She viewed the situation as a private battle between herself and her boss when in fact the supervisor seemed to be sparing of nobody. Teaching patients about cognitive distortions (e.g., all-or-nothing thinking, catastrophizing, jumping to conclusions) in conjunction with evidence gathering is useful because patients can quickly tackle their own cognitive errors once these concepts are understood. Once patients have identified their "usual" cognitive errors, they are able to correct their thinking more efficiently.

Aside from identifying a distortion and becoming aware of the evidence, a DRDT may also point to a lack of information or leave the individual with unanswered questions about the meaning of a situation. In such instances, patients are encouraged to conduct an *experiment*, essentially a plan to gather the information they need to reach a conclusion about the accuracy of a negative thought. The experiment in cognitive therapy embodies collaborative empiricism and asking questions in an open-minded manner.

Many experiments involve some form of [...] to the situation and gathering more informa[...] the essence of any experiment is to form a hyp[...] and determine a way to test that hypothesis.

Cognitive techniques for core beliefs and assumptions

The cognitive model of depression suggests that deeply held core beliefs lead to other levels of cognition, including automatic thoughts [32]. Some amount of psychoeducation is typically conducted to explain the connection between the readily observable thoughts, early life events, and deep levels of cognition. For most patients, problematic situations and thoughts occur repeatedly, and certain "cognitive themes" emerge over the course of many thought records. Such themes are indicative of patients' more deeply held beliefs about themselves, others, and the world. These beliefs (variously called core beliefs or schemas) are believed to be rooted in early life events and learning [36, 63]. The process of understanding early learning and how it leads to the patient's beliefs and current problems is a more fluid and open-ended process compared to the DRDT. Helping patients to understand their underlying beliefs, however, helps them to change the factors that give rise to many of their troubling automatic thoughts and provides alternatives to self-defeating coping strategies.

One of the most common strategies for identifying beliefs is the downward arrow [60]. This approach begins with an automatic thought and, rather than disputing that thought with evidence gathering, the patient is encouraged to deepen his or her level of affect and explore the thought with questions such as "what would it mean if this thought were true?" This typically leads to the emergence of an underlying conditional assumption, a level of cognition that typically takes the form of "if ... then" statements. These "rules" typically specify a circumstance and an emotional consequence that is dysfunctional. For example, Diane's thought records reflected themes of being inadequate and she had rules that took the form of "I must be able to do something after seeing it done once" and "if I am not completely competent, then I am not worthwhile."

Largely, these rules exist at a level of awareness such that the patient has rarely been able to reflect on them. In these instances, it is often the therapist who picks up on a kind of emotional rule that seems to reoccur in the patient's difficulties. A number of situations may share some features and cause similar

en, this means that similar
oss these situations. The
alize this rule, and a col-
e to modify the specific
sumption. Other times
conditional beliefs and
at seem to govern their
oral responses to situations.
to conditional rules, core beliefs repre-
extreme, one-sided views of self, other, and the
world that give rise both to the conditional assumptions and automatic thoughts. Core beliefs are
assumed to be primitive, extreme views that are
formed as a result of early experiences [36]. Content
for these beliefs varies for each individual, but it is
important to emphasize that core beliefs are ways
of understanding the world and were "rational" in
those circumstances under which they originally
formed. The most important precursor to identifying
core beliefs is to explain these concepts in therapy.
Patients are encouraged to see their automatic
thoughts as outgrowths of something that is deeper
and profoundly impacts their interpretations of
events over time. The rationale (early learning) should
also be provided, as it is important for the patient
to understand that his/her negative core beliefs are
not accidental or random, but rather understandable
outcomes of previous experiences (e.g., that which
was functional and rational early in life may no longer
serve the same purpose or be grounded in evidence
given different circumstances). Core beliefs often
take on the form of an absolute statement such as
"I'm a failure," "I am unlovable," or "I am in constant
danger." Patients usually experience considerable
affect when exposed to their core beliefs; they can
often become tearful, sad, or very anxious. This is
usually a sign that a highly salient type of processing
has been tapped. For Diane, the theme of inadequacy
was a powerful one, and this seemed rooted in early
experiences with a demanding and distant father.
The notion of "not being good enough" had been
present starting with the post-partum depression in
which she had felt she could not be a good enough
mother and again after her husband's affair, which
seemed to confirm that she was "not enough."

Many of the techniques used for changing automatic thoughts (e.g., examining distortions, evidence
gathering) can be applied to working with deeper
levels of cognition, although changing beliefs will
take longer and requires more effort than altering a

negative automatic thought. In addition to these techniques, are three other processes that help to change
core beliefs. First, patients need to have some narrative
concerning the development of these beliefs. Second,
patients need to view these experiences more objectively and sympathetically, acknowledging that they
learned something negative and potentially damaging.
Third, it is important to engender hope that these
kinds of beliefs can be "relearned" with the help of
the strategies taught in therapy. Once patients have
acknowledged the need to change core beliefs, they
can be encouraged to create an alternative core belief,
just as they worked on alternatives to their automatic
thoughts and conditional assumptions. Once the
alternative belief is identified, the patient is encouraged to gather evidence for the old core belief and
the more adaptive alternative core belief. This encourages the patient to view subsequent experiences
through a new filter and assess which of the two beliefs
is a better fit to his or her current reality.

Sessions focused on deep cognition are typically
less structured than are earlier sessions, in part
because they cover more areas of the lifespan and
do not have the thought record as a unifying theme.
Discussions may involve reflections on early life
events, focusing on the rigidity of certain conditional
assumptions, or exploring a core belief, but also
moves fluidly between these points. At the same
time, therapists need to attend to opportunities to
implement various worksheets and exercises including downward arrow, a positive events log, and core
belief worksheet [63]. For Diane, all of these techniques came into play during the middle phase of
therapy. Like many patients, Diane did not immediately reject beliefs about her own inadequacy. She
did, however, acknowledge that these beliefs were
rigid and harsh, and she certainly did endorse them
as unhealthy for anyone else. She was also willing to
consider that she might simply begin to accept herself
as she was, and this theme emerged again during the
end phase of therapy and discussions of long-term
recovery and wellness.

Relapse prevention

The final sessions, often spaced at longer intervals as
a partial check on the stability of improvement, are
used to discuss relapse, readying the patient for times
when his/her mood, or stress levels, become worse.
It is important to emphasize that some negative affect
is a part of living, particularly in response to stressors.

When educating the patient about the course of depression, the therapist can normalize fluctuations in mood, both during therapy and after therapy has ended. Thus, if the patient later experiences depressed mood or a bad day, he or she will have realistic expectations regarding the meaning of these events.

Emerging evidence suggests that mindfulness-based cognitive therapy (MBCT) [17], can be added to CBT to assist with relapse prevention and symptom reduction during acute treatment [64]. Mindfulness-based cognitive therapy aims to help recovered patients with a history of depression detach and decenter from their thoughts, allowing them to observe their thought processes rather than getting caught up in them. Mindfulness involves "paying attention in a particular way – on purpose, in the present moment, and non-judgmentally" [65: p. 4]. Participants are encouraged to adopt the attitudes of non-judging, patience, non-striving, acceptance and letting go, and a number of these strategies can be adapted to relapse prevention in individual therapy. Non-judging involves witnessing, but not evaluating, one's own experience. Patience and non-striving emphasize being with an experience instead of working toward a specific goal. Acceptance involves letting an experience be what it may. For example, in relation to depression, acceptance would mean being understanding about the presence of unwanted or negative thoughts. Finally, letting go involves having an experience rather than thinking about having an experience. The more a person thinks about how he or she is interacting with others, for instance, the more stilted and awkward an encounter may be. A conversation is more likely to flow if an individual is able to focus less on what he or she is doing and more on the experience itself. The overall theme of these techniques is to create a wider field of awareness and experience, and reduce the chances of a patient getting caught up in more usual ruminative cycles. Finally, MBCT includes a focus on looking after oneself and making and maintaining healthy lifestyle modifications similar to those that are part of behavioral activation including sleep hygiene, exercise, and balanced, rewarding daily routines.

In Diane's case, acceptance strategies struck a particular chord. She recognized, for example, that there was little she could ultimately change or do about her supervisor or other changes implemented in her workplace. She also found that focusing on the present, moment-to-moment experiences deepened the pleasure of being with her grandda[...] resulted in much less rumination. Diane ag[...] monitoring her level of sadness, as well as a[...] for alcohol, could serve as important guidepos[...] signal a relapse and decided to keep a file of mater[...] she had created in therapy to consult if she felt herse[...] "slipping." About a year after completing treatment, Diane elected to complete the clinic's MBCT program because she had continued to do well and was interested in exploring whether, through regular practice of mindfulness, she could discontinue her antidepressant medication.

Difficulties encountered during treatment

Ambivalence about change and homework non-compliance

Homework is a vital component of CBT and the research literature provides strong support for the relationship between homework completion and psychotherapy outcome [66]. The therapeutic hour constitutes only a small proportion of the time that an individual with depression spends in a given week and homework assignments "provide a means to enhance mastery of newly learned coping strategies, facilitate generalization of skills to novel situations, increase self-efficacy, and ultimately reduce vulnerability to relapse" [67]. Notwithstanding the importance of extra-therapy tasks, compliance varies and clinicians report problems in approximately 50% of their cases [68]. The very symptomatology of depression may represent an obstacle to the completion of homework assignments. Individuals with depression typically lack motivation and energy to engage in extra-therapy assignments, and procrastination and avoidance are common behavioral responses to their mood state. Such individuals may also be pessimistic about the benefits of homework assignments ("This won't work for me") and have difficulty completing tasks, both of which can undermine their willingness to try new strategies [67, 69].

A number of strategies have been proposed to improve the likelihood that a patient will engage in treatment and maximally utilize homework. When non-compliance is evident, it can be handled through psychoeducation, by revisiting the treatment rationale, breaking tasks down into manageable units, discussing

ng of a session to reinforce
ork, framing homework as
 than evaluation, evaluat-
 dysfunctional attitudes
ce, and evaluating the
'].

ategies, it may also be
ze that not all individuals are at
adiness where they are willing or able to
ly engage in treatment. According to Prochaska
[72], fewer than 20% of individuals with a health or
mental health problem are in a stage of change where
they are prepared to take action on the problem at
hand. In such instances, it may be helpful to step back
from the therapist's change agenda and simply
explore, understand, and validate a patient's ambivalence regarding change – by doing so, patients themselves may begin to engage in change talk and their
motivation for change and acceptance of change
strategies will be enhanced. Outcome studies, for
instance, have demonstrated that motivational interviewing may enhance expectancy for change and
homework compliance in CBT for anxiety [73, 74],
and may be usefully applied to depression [75].

Limited (or perceived lack of) progress

There are times within the treatment of depression
when the therapy techniques do not appear to be
working despite conscientious efforts on the patient's
part to comply with homework assignments. At
other times, the patient does not appear to be gaining
traction and is instead seemingly spinning his or her
wheels. In such instances, it is important to remember
that people progress at different rates and that
improvement may simply be slower for some individuals than others. Sometimes, the apparent lack of
progress may reflect biases on the part of the therapist
or patient rather than a veridical perception of
treatment change. Depressed individuals, for example,
frequently distort information in a negatively biased
fashion and this may be true of their perspective of
treatment response.

We suggest that clinicians choose at least one
symptom-based measure (and one or more theoretically relevant instrument) to regularly monitor the
effects of their intervention [76]. Sometimes patients
might question the extent to which therapy is helping
to alleviate depression. Having weekly symptom data
on hand can facilitate discussion with a patient and

demonstrate that change is taking place even though
his or her symptoms have not remitted entirely.
Assuming a linear rate of change, for instance, one
could predict the number of sessions that would be
necessary for complete remission. In such an
instance, the therapist could emphasize the fact that
change has taken place and stress the idea that
larger goals are attained by reaching a series of
smaller goals [77]. In addition to assessing the efficacy of their approach, monitoring change over time
can help clinicians to be more cognizant of potential
problems in therapy, determine their cause (e.g.,
poor administration of treatment, case conceptualization, low patient motivation/compliance), and
address these issues early in the course of treatment.

Periodically, lack of treatment change may be
influenced by hopelessness. Expectation for change
is important in therapy outcome (cf. [78]). Therapists
can also help to uncover an individual's assumptions
and beliefs that serve to exacerbate or maintain hopelessness. There are a host of other variables that may
contribute to limited progress in CBT for depression
(e.g., insufficient dosing of strategies, pragmatic difficulties with implementing techniques or behavioral
experiments, focusing on a more peripheral target
for change, confusion on the part of the patient).
A collaborative case conceptualization provides an
important framework with which to explore various
factors that might explain a lack of response and for
suggesting alternative routes to change [79].

Clinical decision making: integrating science and practice

Cognitive–behavioral therapy has demonstrated efficacy in a number of randomized controlled trials
(RCTs) and is listed among the empirically supported
therapies for depression [80]. Considering RCTs as
the gold standard of empirical support has been met
with criticism (e.g., [81]). Some researchers contend
that this research does not address the complexity of
clinical care. One common argument, for instance,
is that the clinical reality is one of comorbidity,
whereas patients with comorbid conditions are often
excluded from controlled trials. Another frequent
criticism levied against this research is that patients
in clinical trials are often less severe than are those
commonly seen in practice. As mentioned earlier,
however, research has attested to the power of CBT
even for severe depression [52, 53].

Given these issues, clinicians are sometimes faced with difficult decisions in their attempt to implement evidence-based practice (EBP). If there is a comorbid anxiety disorder, for instance, which disorder does one target first or might a transdiagnostic approach be more suitable [23]? Unfortunately, few guidelines exist and the decision often has to be made on a case-by-case basis utilizing a case-formulation approach [79], ensuring that treatment matches a patient's expectations and fits with his or her theory of change, and takes into account the functional link between anxiety and depression in a particular case [82].

To provide another example, what should the clinician do if a patient's demographic profile deviates from what is found in the research literature? Should one opt not to use an empirically supported treatment or should one modify it in some way? It may be tempting to disregard outcome trials because the study sample is different from the individual case a clinician is working with. We contend, however, that adopting strategies that have been shown to be effective for individuals with similar problems is better than providing a treatment that does not demonstrate empirical support. Research has consistently "demonstrated that clinical judgment is not nearly as good as we believe it is, is unrelated to the confidence we feel or to the amount of training or experience that we receive, and is almost always inferior to data-driven actuarial approaches to decision making" [83: p. 147].

Clinicians need to be aware of what research evidence there is for different psychological problems. In addition to being a good consumer of research, by reading and synthesizing the results of RCTs, clinicians can also pay attention to various clinical guidelines that have been developed, for example, by the American Psychological Association (Division 12) and the National Institute for Health and Clinical Excellence. These guidelines provide up-to-date information about treatments that work for particular problems.

Although modifying or customizing an empirically supported treatment may be appropriate in certain circumstances (e.g., if a patient does not accept the rationale; lack of readiness for change; lack of progress) we encourage clinicians to make these decisions cautiously and using a case-conceptualization approach. Supported treatment protocols may, for example, be altered in ways that actually diminish their benefit or may be disregarded when they may, in fact, be helpful. Consistent with the recommendations of Ruscio and Holohan [83], we suggest that, in the absence of clear evidence to the contrary, clinicians proceed with using the treatment protocols that have been supported by the research literature.

Conclusion

In this chapter, we have described the nature of depression and noted that this disorder is not only highly prevalent in the population but also is characterized by relapse and recurrence. Cognitive–behavioral therapy is well supported for the treatment of an acute episode of depression and serves as a prophylaxis against subsequent episodes. This form of treatment stems from a coherent etiological theory of depression (e.g., [29]) that emphasizes the development of depressive schemas that originate from early experiences and later impact one's intermediate beliefs, information processing, and automatic thoughts when triggered by life stress. Cognitive–behavioral therapy for depression begins with modifications of behavioral activity (which also begins to alter negative cognitions) and then shifts toward other more explicit cognitive change strategies (beginning with automatic thoughts and moving eventually to the alteration of core beliefs and schemas). The therapist works collaboratively with patients to help them to become scientists of their own thinking, to learn to treat a thought as a hypothesis rather than a fact, and to process information in a more evidence-based manner. By doing so, patients' mood improves and they learn strategies that decrease the probability of future episodes.

Suggested readings

Beck AT, Alford BA. *Depression: Causes and Treatment*, 2nd edn. Philadelphia: University of Pennsylvania Press, 2009.

Beck AT, Rush AJ, Shaw BF, Emery G. *Cognitive Therapy of Depression*. New York: Guilford Press, 1979.

Clark DA, Beck AT, Alford BA. *Scientific Foundations of Cognitive Theory and Therapy of Depression*. Philadelphia: Wiley, 1999.

Dobson D, Dobson KS. *Evidence-based Practice of Cognitive-behavioral Therapy*. New York: Guilford Press, 2009.

Dozois DJA, Beck AT. Cognitive schemas, beliefs and assumptions. In Dobson KS, Dozois DJA, eds. *Risk Factors in Depression*. Oxford, England: Elsevier/Academic. 2008, pp. 121–43.

Young JE, Rygh JL, Weinberger AD, Beck AT. Cognitive therapy for depression. In Barlow DH, ed. *Clinical*

Handbook of Psychological Disorders: A Step-by-step Treatment Manual, 4th edn. New York: Guilford Press. 2008, pp. 250–305.

Client resources

Bieling PJ, Antony MM. *Ending the Depression Cycle: A Step-by-step Guide for Preventing Relapse*. Oakland, CA: New Harbinger, 2003.

Greenberger D, Pasesky CA. *Mind Over Mood: Change How You Feel by Changing the Way You Think*. New York: Guilford Press, 1995.

Online resources

Academy of Cognitive Therapy www.academyofct.org

Association for Behavioral and Cognitive Therapies www.abct.org

Beck Institute for Cognitive Therapy and Research www.beckinstitute.org

National Institute for Health and Clinical Excellence www.nice.org.uk (see depression treatment guidelines)

National Alliance for Research on Schizophrenia and Depression www.narsad.org

References

1. American Psychiatric Association. *Diagnostic and Statistical Manual of Mental Disorders*, 4th edn. text revision. Washington, DC: APA, 2000.

2. Kessler RC, Chiu WT, Demler O, Walters EE. Prevalence, severity, and comorbidity of 12-month DSM-IV disorders in the National Comorbidity Survey Replication. *Arch Gen Psychiatry* 2005; **62**: 617–27.

3. Kessler RC, Berglund P, Demler O, *et al.* Lifetime prevalence and age-of-onset distributions of DSM-IV disorders in the National Comorbidity Survey Replication. *Arch Gen Psychiatry* 2005; **62**: 593–602.

4. Avenevoli S, Knight E, Kessler RC, Merikangas KR. Epidemiology of depression in children and adolescents. In Abela JRZ, Hankin BL, eds. *Handbook of Depression in Children and Adolescents*. New York: Guilford. 2008, pp. 6–32.

5. Hankin BL, Abramson LY, Moffitt TE, *et al.* Development of depression from preadolescence to young adulthood: emerging gender differences in a 10-year longitudinal study. *J Abnor Psychol* 1998; **107**: 128–40.

6. Rohde P, Beevers CG, Stice E, O'Neil K. Major and minor depression in female adolescents: onset, course, symptom presentation, and demographic associations. *J Clin Psychol* 2009; **65**: 1339–49.

7. Yiend J, Paykel E, Merritt R, *et al.* Long term outcome of primary care depression. *J Affect Disord* 2009; **118**: 79–86.

8. Boland RJ, Keller MB. Course and outcome of depression. In Gotlib IH, Hammen CL, eds. *Handbook of Depression*, 2nd edn. New York: Guilford. 2009, pp. 23–43.

9. Rhebergen D, Beekman ATF, de Graaf R, *et al.* The three-year naturalistic course of major depressive disorder, dysthymic disorder and double depression. *J Affect Disord* 2009; **115**: 450–9.

10. Gotlib IH, Lewinsohn PM, Seeley JR. Symptoms versus a diagnosis of depression: differences in psychosocial functioning. *J Consult Clin Psychol* 1995; **63**: 90–100.

11. Judd LL, Akiskal HS, Zeller PJ, *et al.* Psychosocial disability during the long-term course of unipolar major depressive disorder. *Arch Gen Psychiatry* 2000; **57**: 375–80.

12. Coryell W, Akiskal HS, Leon AC, *et al.* The time course of nonchronic major depressive disorder: uniformity across episodes and samples. *Arch Gen Psychiatry* 1994; **51**: 405–10.

13. Keller MB, Boland RJ. Implications of failing to achieve successful long-term maintenance treatment of recurrent unipolar major depression. *Biol Psychiatry* 1998; **44**: 348–60.

14. Coyne JC, Pepper CM, Flynn H. Significance of prior episodes of depression in two patient populations. *J Consult Clin Psychol* 1999; **67**: 76–81.

15. Kessing L. Recurrence in affective disorder: II. Effect of age and gender. *Br J Psychiatry* 1998; **172**: 29–34.

16. Solomon DA, Keller MB, Leon AC, *et al.* Multiple recurrences of major depressive disorder. *Am J Psychiatry* 2000; **157**: 229–33.

17. Segal ZV, Williams JM, Teasdale JD. *Mindfulness-based Cognitive Therapy for Depression: a New Approach to Preventing Relapse*. New York: Guilford Press, 2002.

18. Segal ZV, Williams JM, Teasdale JD, Gemar M. A cognitive science perspective on kindling and episode sensitization in recurrent affective disorder. *Psychol Med* 1996; **26**: 371–80.

19. Joiner TE Jr. Depression's vicious scree: self-propagating and erosive processes in depression chronicity. *Clin Psychol Sci Pract* 2000; **7**: 203–18.

20. Timmons KA, Joiner TE Jr. Reassurance seeking and negative feedback seeking. In Dobson KS, Dozois DJA, eds. *Risk Factors in Depression*. San Diego: Elsevier Academic Press. 2008, pp. 429–46.

21. Barlow DH. *Anxiety and its Disorders: the Nature and Treatment of Anxiety and Panic*, 2nd edn. New York: Guilford, 2002.

22. Dozois DJA, Seeds PM, Collins KA. Transdiagnostic approaches to the prevention of depression and anxiety. *J Cogn Psychother* 2009; **23**: 44–59.

23. Allen LB, McHugh RK, Barlow DH. Emotional disorders: a unified protocol. In Barlow DH, ed. *Clinical Handbook of Psychological Disorders: A Step-by-step Treatment Manual.* New York: Guilford Press. 2008, pp. 216–49.

24. Benton T, Staab J, Evans DL. Medical comorbidity in depressive disorders. *Ann Clin Psychiatry* 2007; **19**: 289–303.

25. Fenton WS, Stover ES. Mood disorders: cardiovascular and diabetes comorbidity. *Curr Opin Psychiatry* 2006; **19**: 421–7.

26. Freedland KE, Carney RM. Depression and medical illness. In Gotlib IH, Hammen CL, eds. *Handbook of Depression*, 2nd edn. New York: Guilford Press. 2008, pp. 113–41.

27. Greenberg PE, Sisitsky T, Kessler RC, *et al.* The economic burden of anxiety disorders in the 1990s. *J Clin Psychiatry* 1999; **60**: 427–35.

28. Abramson LY, Alloy LB, Hankin BL, *et al.* Cognitive vulnerability-stress models of depression in a self-regulatory and psychobiological context. In Gotlib IH, Hammen CL, eds. *Handbook of Depression*. New York: Guilford Press. 2002, pp. 268–94.

29. Beck AT. *Depression: Causes and Treatment.* Philadelphia: University of Pennsylvania Press, 1967.

30. Ingram RE, Miranda J, Segal ZV. *Cognitive Vulnerability to Depression.* New York: Guilford Press, 1998.

31. Beck AT, Rush AJ, Shaw BF, Emery G. *Cognitive Therapy of Depression.* New York: Guilford Press, 1979.

32. Dozois DJA, Beck AT. Cognitive schemas, beliefs and assumptions. In Dobson KS, Dozois DJA, eds. *Risk Factors in Depression*. Oxford, England: Elsevier/Academic Press. 2008, pp. 121–43.

33. Garratt G, Ingram RE, Rand KL, Sawalani G. Cognitive processes in cognitive therapy: evaluation of the mechanisms of change in the treatment of depression. *Clin Psychol Sci Pract* 2007; **14**: 224–39.

34. Lumley MN, Harkness KL. Childhood maltreatment and depressotypic cognitive organization. *Cognit Ther Res* 2009; **33**: 511–22.

35. Gibb BE, Abramson LY, Alloy LB. Emotional maltreatment from parents, verbal victimization, and cognitive vulnerability to depression. *Cognit Ther Res* 2004; **28**: 1–21.

36. Clark DA, Beck AT, Alford BA. *Scientific Foundations of Cognitive Theory and Therapy of Depression.* New York: Wiley, 1999.

37. Scher CD, Ingram RE, Segal ZV. Cognitive reactivity and vulnerability: empirical evaluation of construct activation and cognitive diatheses in unipolar depression. *Clin Psychol Rev* 2005; **25**: 487–510.

38. Dozois DJA, Dobson KS. A longitudinal investigation of information processing and cognitive organization in clinical depression: stability of schematic interconnectedness. *J Consult Clin Psychol* 2001; **69**: 914–25.

39. Dozois DJA. Stability of negative self-structures: a longitudinal comparison of depressed, remitted, and nonpsychiatric controls. *J Clin Psychol* 2007; **63**: 319–38.

40. Garber J, Flynn C. Predictors of depressive cognitions in young adolescents. *Cogn Ther Res* 2001; **25**: 353–76.

41. Taylor L, Ingram RE. Cognitive reactivity and depressotypic information processing in children of depressed mothers. *J Abnorm Psychol* 1999; **108**: 202–10.

42. Alloy LB, Abramson LY, Safford SM, Gibb BE. The cognitive vulnerability to depression (CVD) project: current findings and future directions. In Alloy LB, Riskind JH, eds. *Cognitive Vulnerability to Emotional Disorders*. Mahwah, NJ: Erlbaum. 2006, pp. 33–61.

43. Joiner TE Jr, Metalsky GI, Lew A, Klocek J. Testing the causal mediation component of Beck's theory of depression: evidence for specific mediation. *Cogn Ther Res* 1999; **23**: 401–12.

44. Lewinsohn PM, Joiner TE, Rohde P. Evaluation of cognitive diathesis-stress models in predicting major depressive disorder in adolescents. *J Abnorm Psychol* 2001; **110**: 203–15.

45. DeRubeis RJ, Webb CA, Tang TZ, Beck AT. Cognitive therapy. In Dobson KS, ed. *Handbook of Cognitive-behavioral Therapies*, 3rd edn. New York: Guilford Press. 2010, pp. 277–316.

46. Butler AC, Chapman JE, Forman EM, Beck AT. The empirical status of cognitive-behavioral therapy: a review of meta-analyses. *Clin Psychol Rev* 2006; **26**: 17–31.

47. Mazzucchelli T, Kane R, Rees C. Behavioral activation treatments for depression in adults: a meta-analysis and review. *Clin Psychol Sci Pract* 2009; **16**: 383–411.

48. Wampold BE, Minami T, Baskin TW, Tierney SC. A meta-(re)analysis of the effects of cognitive therapy versus 'other therapies' for depression. *J Affect Disord* 2002; **68**: 159–65.

49. Epp A, Dobson KS. The evidence base for cognitive-behavioral therapy. In Dobson KS, ed. *Handbook of Cognitive-Behavioral Therapies*, 3rd edn. New York: Guilford Press. 2010, pp. 39–73.

50. Hollon SD, Dimidjian S. Cognitive and behavioral treatment of depression. In Gotlib IH, Hammen CL, eds. *Handbook of Depression*, 2nd edn. New York: Guilford Press. 2009, pp. 586–603.

51. Hollon SD, Thase ME, Markowitz JC. Treatment and prevention of depression. *Psychological Science in the Public Interest* 2002; **3**: 39–77.

52. DeRubeis RJ, Siegle GJ, Hollon SD. Cognitive therapy versus medication for depressions: treatment outcomes and neural mechanisms. *Nat Rev Neurosci* 2008; **9**: 788–90.

53. Hollon SD, DeRubeis RJ, Shelton RC, *et al*. Prevention of relapse following cognitive therapy vs. medications in moderate to severe depression. *Arch Gen Psychiatry* 2005; **62**: 417–22.

54. DeRubeis RJ, Gelfand LA, Tang TZ, Simons AD. Medications versus cognitive behavior therapy for severely depressed outpatients: mega-analysis of four randomized comparisons. *Am J Psychiatry* 1999; **156**: 1007–13.

55. Dimidjian S, Hollon SD, Dobson KS, *et al*. Randomized trial of behavioral activation, cognitive therapy, and antidepressant medication in the acute treatment of adults with major depression. *J Consult Clin Psychol* 2006; **74**: 658–70.

56. Gloaguen, V., Cottraux, J., Cucherat, M, Blackburn, I. A meta-analysis of the effects of cognitive therapy in depression. *J Affect Disord* 1998; **49**: 59–72.

57. Dobson D, Dobson KS. *Evidence-based Practice of Cognitive Behavioral Therapy*. New York: Guilford Press, 2009.

58. Segal ZV, Gemar M, Williams S. Differential cognitive response to a mood challenge following successful cognitive therapy or pharmacotherapy for unipolar depression. *J Abnorm Psychol* 1999; **108**: 3–10.

59. Dozois DJA, Bieling PJ, Patelis-Siotis I, *et al*. Changes in self-schema structure in cognitive therapy for major depressive disorder: a randomized clinical trial. *J Consult Clin Psychol* 2009; **77**: 1078–88.

60. Greenberger D, Padesky CA. *Mind Over Mood: Change How You Feel by Changing the Way You Think*. New York: Guilford Press, 1995.

61. Bieling PJ, McCabe RE, Antony MM. *Cognitive Behavioral Therapy Groups: Structure and Process*. New York: Guilford Press, 2006.

62. Beck AT, Weishaar ME. Cognitive therapy. In Corsini RJ, Wedding D, eds. *Current Psychotherapies*, 8th edn. Belmont, CA: Thomson. 2008, pp. 263–94.

63. Beck JS. *Cognitive Therapy: Basics and Beyond*. New York: Guilford Press, 1995.

64. Hofmann SG, Sawyer AT, Witt AA, Oh D. The effect of mindfulness-based therapy on anxiety and depression: a meta-analytic review. *J Consult Clin Psychol* 2010; **78**:169–83.

65. Kabat-Zinn J. *Full Catastrophe Living: Using the Wisdom of Your Body and Mind to Face Stress, Pain, and Illness*. New York: Dell Publishing, 1990.

66. Kazantzis N, Whittington C, Dattilio F. Meta-analysis of homework effects in cognitive and behavioral therapy: a replication and extension. *Clin Psychol Sci Pract* 2010; **17**: 144–56.

67. Thase ME, Callan JA. The role of homework in cognitive behavior therapy of depression. *J Psychother Integr* 2006; **16**: 162–77.

68. Helbig S, Fehm L. Problems with homework in CBT: rare exception or rather frequent? *Behav Cogn Psychother* 2004; **32**: 291–301.

69. Garland A, Scott J. The obstacle is the path: overcoming blocks to homework assignments in a complex presentation of depression. *Cogn Behav Pract* 2007; **14**: 278–88.

70. Beck JS. *Cognitive Therapy for Challenging Problems: What to Do When the Basics Don't Work*. New York: Guilford Press, 2005.

71. Leahy RL. *Overcoming Resistance in Cognitive Therapy*. New York: Guilford Press, 2001.

72. Prochaska JO. Change at differing stages. In Snyder CR, Ingram RE, eds. *Handbook of Psychological Change: Psychotherapy Processes and Practices for the 21st Century*. New York: Wiley. 2000, pp. 109–27.

73. Westra HA, Dozois DJA. Preparing clients for cognitive behavioral therapy: a randomized pilot study of motivational interviewing for anxiety. *Cogn Ther Res* 2006; **30**: 481–98.

74. Westra, HA, Dozois DJA, Marcus M. Early improvement, expectancy for change, homework compliance, and outcome in cognitive behavioral therapy for anxiety. *J Consult Clin Psychol* 2007; **75**: 363–73.

75. Arkowitz H, Westra HA, Miller WR, Rollnick S (eds.) *Motivational Interviewing in the Treatment of Psychological Problems*. New York: Guilford Press, 2008.

76. Dozois DJA, Dobson KS. Depression. In Antony MM, Barlow DH, eds. *Handbook of Assessment and Treatment Planning for Psychological Disorders, 2nd edn*. New York: Guilford Press, 2010.

77. Young JE, Rygh JL, Weinberger AD, Beck AT. Cognitive therapy for depression. In Barlow DH, ed. *Clinical Handbook of Psychological Disorders: A Step-by-step Treatment Manual*, 4th edn. New York: Guilford Press. 2008, pp. 250–305.

78. Dozois DJA, Westra HA. The development of the Anxiety Change Expectancy Scale (ACES) and

validation in college, community, and clinical samples. *Behav Res Ther* 2005; **43**: 1655–72.

79. Kuyken W, Padesky CA, Dudley R. *Collaborative Case Conceptualization: Working Effectively With Clients in Cognitive-behavioral Therapy*. New York: Guilford Press, 2009.

80. Chambless DL, Ollendick TH. Empirically supported psychological interventions: controversies and evidence. *Ann Rev Psychol* 2001; **52**: 685–716.

81. Westen D, Novotny CM, Thompson-Brenner H. The empirical status of empirically supported psychotherapies: assumptions, findings, and reporting in controlled clinical trials. *Psychol Bull* 2004; **130**: 631–63.

82. Otto MW, Powers MB, Stathopoulou G, Hofmann SG. Panic disorder and social phobia. In Whisman MA, ed. *Adapting Cognitive Therapy for Depression: Managing Complexity and Comorbidity*. New York: Guilford Press. 2008, pp. 185–208.

83. Ruscio AM, Holohan DR. Applying empirically supported treatments to complex cases: ethical, empirical, and practical considerations. *Clin Psychol Sci Pract* 2006; **13**: 146–62.

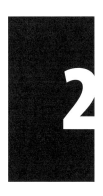

2 Bipolar disorder

Amanda W. Calkins, Bridget A. Hearon, and Michael W. Otto

Psychosocial treatments for bipolar disorder

Bipolar disorder is a prevalent and chronic condition, which affects 1% to 3% of the population [1, 2], and is associated with high rates of suicidality and significant functional and social impairment. Bipolar disorder is characterized by the occurrence of one or more manic, hypomanic, or mixed episodes and is typified by periods of mood instability. The bipolar I subtype of bipolar disorder is defined by at least one full manic episode, whereas the bipolar II subtype is defined by at least one hypomanic, but not full manic, episode and one or more depressive episodes. Although (hypo) manic episodes are necessary for bipolar diagnosis, the disorder is most frequently characterized by repeated episodes of depression. A full manic episode is defined by a period of one week or longer (which can be shorter if the episode is interrupted by treatment change or other mediating factors) of feeling euphoric, irritable, or high, along with three or more of the following symptoms: extreme feelings of self-importance, racing thoughts, distractibility, decreased need for sleep, pressured speech, and risky behavior [3]. Hypomanic episodes are similar to manic episodes, except that they are shorter in duration (lasting for four days or longer in order to meet criteria) and are less severe and impairing. A mixed episode is characterized by a one-week period during which the criteria for both a manic and major depressive episode are met. Depressive episode criteria requires at least five symptoms, present for a minimum of two weeks, with at least one of the core symptoms (1) depressed mood and/or (2) loss of interest in activity included. The additional symptoms of depression are: significant weight or appetite change, insomnia or hypersomnia, psychomotor agitation or retardation, fatigue, feelings of worthlessness, trouble concentrating or thoughts of death or suicide.

Most commonly, bipolar patients experience several episodes of depression before the emergence of an initial manic episode, and patients have been found to be 3.5 times more likely to be experiencing depressive symptoms (in bipolar I, and 37 times in bipolar II) than (hypo)manic symptoms [4–8]. However, there is significant variation in the pattern of episodes, and recent research indicates that manic symptoms occur frequently within the context of depressive episodes [9]. For example, Goldberg *et al.* [9] found that two thirds of bipolar patients in depressive episodes had manic symptoms, most commonly: distractibility, flight of ideas or racing thoughts, and psychomotor agitation. There is evidence that those who initially present with a manic episode are more likely to be male than female [5].

Episode recurrence is central to the long-term course of bipolar disorder, and studies indicate that three-quarters of patients can be expected to relapse within four to five years, with half of these relapses occurring in the first year and first relapse occurring in an average of eight months following first episode [10–13]. Even during periods of remission, continued impairment in role functioning and symptoms of bipolar disorder are common [14, 15].

Bipolar disorder and bipolar spectrum disorders are estimated to affect between 1% and 5% of the population and over 10 million individuals in the United States [16, 17]. The average age of onset for bipolar disorder is in the mid-teens, with evidence of a worse long-term course for individuals with an earlier age of onset [18, 13]. Bipolar disorder occurs equally as frequently in women and men [16], although sex differences have been found for the rapid cycling course (i.e., four or more mood episodes

Cognitive–behavioral Therapy with Adults: A Guide to Empirically Informed Assessment and Intervention,
ed. Stefan G. Hofmann and Mark A. Reinecke. © Cambridge University Press 2010.

a year), with more women meeting criteria for a rapid-cycling subtype [19] as well as an earlier age of onset of the disorder [20].

An increased likelihood of recurrence of mood episodes is associated with psychosocial factors such as stress, social environment, and psychiatric comorbidity. Stressful life events are linked with both mood episode recurrence [21–23] as well as delayed recovery [24, 25]. Moreover, stressful family environments with high levels of expressed emotion and/or negative interactional patterns have been linked to higher relapse rates [26, 27]. Greater anxiety and substance use disorder comorbidities have also been linked with poorer long-term outcome [28–30]. In addition to these psychosocial factors, early age of onset of bipolar disorder is also associated with a more chronic course of the disorder, with fewer periods of recovery, more psychotic features, and greater suicidal ideation and role disruption [18, 20].

Pharmacologic treatment

Traditionally, the core treatment for bipolar disorder has been pharmacotherapy, with a primary intervention of ongoing treatment with one or more mood stabilizer medications prescribed singly or in combination with other agents such as atypical antipsychotic or antidepressant medications. Lithium (brand names Eskalith, Lithobid) has been used as a mood stabilizer for 30 years in the United States to improve episodes of both mania and depression and prevent the risk of cycling into another mood state. Anticonvulsants, such as divalproex (brand name Depakote), carbamazepine (brand name Tegretol), and lamotrigine (brand name Lamictal), and some atypical antipsychotic medications, such as aripiprazole (Abilify), olanzapine (Zyprexa), quetiapine (Seroquel), risperidone (Risperdal), and ziprasidone (Geodon) also provide elements of mood stabilization and, in some cases, depression treatment [31–34]. Antidepressants have also been frequently used to treat bipolar disorder; however, recent studies have raised serious questions about the efficacy of this approach [35, 36]. In addition, there is a more longstanding concern that the addition of an antidepressant will promote a manic episode [37], although this risk appears to be less apparent for some of the more selectively serotonergic versus noradrenergic antidepressants (i.e., tricyclic antidepressants) [38, 39]. Benzodiazepines have also been used to calm hypomanic symptoms, manage sleep and overactivity, and treat comorbid anxiety disorders; however, there is little evidence of the efficacy of this approach for managing the emergence or length of bipolar episodes [40–42].

Pharmacologic treatment of bipolar disorder is associated with significant problems of medication adherence [43, 44, 14]. This may be due, in part, to the side-effect profiles associated with the mood stabilizers, which include: weight gain with risk of diabetes, cognitive slowing, somnolence, and extrapyramidal symptoms. These side effects are common to at least some of the atypical antipsychotics [45–48], as well as for anticonvulsant and lithium treatment [49–51]. In addition, long-term use of these medications may also be a daunting prospect for some patients aside from the challenging side-effect profiles. Regardless of the reason for non-compliance, approximately half of samples of patients have discontinued their mood stabilizer medications within two months of starting them [43, 44, 14, 52]. Discontinuation of a mood stabilizer brings with it the risk of relapse [53]. Furthermore, despite the advances in pharmacotherapy for bipolar disorder, the disorder remains chronic with recurrences of mood episodes even with the use of medication [54, 10]. For all of these reasons, consideration of alternatives to medication, such as psychosocial treatment, is important.

The role of cognitive–behavioral therapy in bipolar disorder

Psychosocial treatments

Although once thought to be secondary to medication treatments, or to serve only as medication adherence aides, psychosocial treatment strategies have emerged as a new and important force for the management of bipolar disorder in the last 15 years [55–57]. This emergence of structured psychosocial treatments has been triggered both by the limits in efficacy of pharmacotherapy alone, and by research indicating that therapy may play a significant role in alleviating psychosocial stress, interpersonal issues, and social, family, and occupational dysfunction in addition to altering the course of bipolar disorder [15, 55]. Finally, bipolar disorder is a costly illness and psychosocial treatments may reduce those costs by improving outcomes [58].

The new structured and focused treatments that have emerged were derived from very different theoretical orientations; however, they are similar in the techniques they employ in order to treat bipolar disorder [59]. Cognitive–behavioral therapy (CBT), family-focused therapy (FFT), interpersonal and social rhythm therapy (IPSRT), have all been empirically researched for the treatment of bipolar disorder. In recent randomized controlled trials of CBT, FFT, IPSRT, and a comprehensive group-treatment approach results indicated that these treatments share a number of common elements, which include: (1) psychoeducation designed to provide patients and (in the case of FFT) family members with a model of the nature and course of bipolar disorder, including risk and protective factors such as the role of sleep and lifestyle regularity, stress management, and medication adherence; (2) communication and/or problem-solving training aimed at reducing familial and external stress; and (3) a review of strategies for the early detection and intervention for mood episodes, including intensified pharmacotherapy, the activation of increased support, and more frequent treatment sessions [60, 59]. These psychosocial treatments may also be combined with cognitive restructuring, thought and activity monitoring, treatment contracting, and other interventions in individual, group, and family settings [55].

Cognitive–behavioral therapy

Cognitive–behavioral therapy is an effective and empirically supported psychosocial treatment for bipolar disorder. As an early application of CBT to bipolar disorder, it was directed successfully toward medication adherence in a brief treatment (six-session) format [57]. Since its initial success, more general applications of CBT have been adopted that focus on both relapse prevention and the treatment of bipolar depression. Some of the principles that are generally involved in this broader application of CBT are a combination of psychoeducation about bipolar disorder, cognitive restructuring, activity and lifestyle management, and active monitoring of mood states, with plans for early interventions.

Some studied have examined the direct transfer of CBT for unipolar depression to bipolar depression. For example, Lam and colleagues [61, 62] examined a brief program of individual CBT (12 to 18 sessions within the first six months and two booster sessions in the second six months of care) relative to treatment as usual. Following the promising results of a pilot study

[61], Lam *et al.* conducted a randomized controlled study of CBT in 103 bipolar patients [62]. Patients were not in an acute bipolar episode at the time of treatment; however, more than 56% had mild to moderate levels of depression when they entered the study. The results showed that patients in the CBT group had significantly reduced residual symptoms of depression at the end of treatment. Additionally, patients who received CBT had significantly fewer bipolar episodes, higher social functioning, and decreased mood symptoms. Patients in the CBT group had a relapse rate of 43.3% whereas the patients in the treatment-as-usual group had a relapse rate of 75%.

Relapse prevention was studied by Scott, Garland, and Moorhead [63]. Key elements of the CBT intervention included psychoeducation, training in medication adherence, stress management, cognitive restructuring, and regulation of activities and sleep. Patients were randomized to either CBT or a wait-list condition. Following six months of treatment, patients in the CBT group had significantly greater alleviation in depressive symptoms and higher global functioning than patients in the wait-list condition. Moreover, patients in the CBT group showed a 60% reduction in relapse rates at the 18-month follow-up point. Moreover, CBT aimed at the identification of prodromal symptoms and activation of an early intervention plan in 12 individual sessions was studied by Perry, Tarrier, Morriss, McCarthy, and Limb [64]. This intervention was compared to treatment as usual in 69 outpatients who suffered a relapse in the past year. The results indicated a significant difference in the length of time until manic relapse and improved social and employment functioning in favor of CBT over treatment as usual. However, the same results were not found for depressive relapses. Perry *et al.* hypothesized that the prodromal symptoms of mania are more distinct than those of depression, and therefore more easily identifiable to patients [64].

A recent study examined the relative benefit of seven sessions of psychoeducation (PE) vs. seven sessions of PE followed by 13 sessions of individual CBT [65]. A total of 79 adults with bipolar disorder and on stable medication regimens were studied. Patients were in full or partial remission at randomization. Following treatment, patients who received CBT in addition to PE experienced 50% fewer days of depressed mood over the course of one year. Additionally, patients who received PE alone had more antidepressant medication increases compared with those who received CBT. There were no group differences in hospitalization rates, medication adherence, psychosocial functioning, or mental health use.

Taken together, the research shows efficacy for CBT as a treatment for bipolar disorder; however, Scott *et al.* examined the impact of 22 sessions of CBT over 18 months versus treatment as usual in 253 patients with severe and recurrent bipolar disorder [66]. The overall results showed no differences between CBT and treatment as usual for time to recurrence of an episode and symptom severity ratings. However, post-hoc analyses revealed an interaction between treatment efficacy and the number of previous episodes with patients who had greater than 12 previous episodes showing no benefit from CBT, yet a benefit was evident for those with fewer than 12 previous episodes. These results emphasize the potential importance of early application of CBT in the course of bipolar disorder.

Given recent evidence for the low efficacy of, and possible increased risk of a manic episode associated with, antidepressant treatments for bipolar depression [35, 36], there is a greater emphasis on the need for psychosocial treatments for this phase of the disorder. In the large-scale National Institute of Mental Health-sponsored Systematic Treatment Enhancement Program for Bipolar Disorder (STEP-BD) protocol, psychosocial treatments for bipolar depression were examined at 15 study sites. Patients were randomized to receive intensive psychosocial treatment (up to 30 sessions of CBT, IPSRT, or FFT over nine months), or a minimal psychosocial intervention (collaborative care (CC), consisting of three sessions over six weeks) in addition to their pharmacologic treatments. Psychoeducation about bipolar disorder, relapse prevention planning, and illness management interventions were included in all four of the psychosocial interventions. Collaborative care provided a brief version of common psychosocial strategies shown to be beneficial for bipolar disorder [67, 68], while the intensive treatments were enhanced versions of CBT, IPSRT, and FFT, with additional treatment targets, including cognitive distortions and activity and skill deficits in CBT, disturbances in interpersonal relationships and social rhythms in IPSRT, and disturbances in family relationships and communication in FFT [15]. Results found all three psychotherapy approaches efficacious and indicated that these intensive psychosocial treatments are more effective than CC in alleviating bipolar depression and decreasing the risk of

relapse [15]. Rates of recovery were significantly greater (64.4% vs. 51.5%), and time to recovery was significantly shorter in the groups that received intensive psychotherapy, than among patients who received CC. Moreover, the intensive psychotherapies were efficacious in the same cohort of patients who had previously failed to respond to randomized antidepressant treatment [36]; indicating that the enhanced psychotherapies succeeded in refractory depression where the antidepressants failed.

Further analyses of the same data set, Miklowitz *et al.* [15] found that patients who received intensive psychosocial treatment had improved relationship functioning, life satisfaction and better overall functioning over the nine month study period, than patients who received CC. These results emphasize the finding that the intensive psychosocial treatments were more effective than brief psychoeducation in improving life function and satisfaction in bipolar patients.

Elements of a comprehensive CBT for bipolar disorder

One protocol of CBT for bipolar depression has been recently manualized by Otto *et al.* [69] and uses self-monitoring, role-playing, exposure, activity, and behavioral experiment assignments as core interventions. This CBT program is organized around the delivery of 30 sessions including 21 weekly and 9 biweekly sessions. The sessions are broken into four phases of treatment: (1) depression-focus phase; (2) treatment contract phase; (3) problem-list phase; and (4) well-being phase (4 sessions). In each of these phases, the target and style of interventions change. Across all phases, a patient workbook is used to aid the acquisition and independent application of therapy interventions [70].

The first phase consists of nine sessions targeted specifically at reducing symptoms of depression through interventions including psychoeducation, cognitive restructuring, and activity assignments. Initial sessions are directed at helping the patient develop a therapeutic perspective on his or her own case, and, by doing so, enlisting the patient as a "co-therapist on the case." Once the parameters of treatment and a general understanding of the CBT model are provided, cognitive restructuring techniques are emphasized. Cognitive restructuring focuses on the change of dysfunctional cognitions and core beliefs during depression and hyper-positive thinking during mania. Cognitive restructuring can be used to target several points of change such as: punitive self-talk, distortions in event interpretations, and creating more beneficial cognitive skills. In completing cognitive restructuring exercises, patients are asked to have greater awareness of their emotions in the present moment and take in both internal and external information before acting upon an emotional change. In addition to cognitive restructuring, activity assignments are used to return depressed patients to pleasant and rewarding activities and provide a routine to help with mood stability. Activity assignments evolve collaboratively, with the patient assessing current level of activity and coming up with additional activities that he/she used to enjoy or believes are important. During this phase, "behavioral experiments" can also be used to examine the accuracy of the patient's thoughts and rehearse situations relevant to the activity assignments.

Other tools that are used include mood charting, agenda setting, homework assignment and review, rehearsals, and reminder cues. A typical session is structured to include review of the patient's mood over the past week, review of the previous week's learning and homework, formulation of an agenda for the session, completion of the agenda with appropriate rehearsals, summary of session content, and, finally, assignment and troubleshooting of home practice. This format keeps the emphasis on step-by-step, goal-oriented, skill-acquisition approaches that are the basis of this treatment approach.

The second phase of treatment consists of three sessions devoted to creating the treatment contract (see Appendix 2.1 [103]), and one session devoted to hyperpositive thinking. The treatment contracting process involves several steps for the patient including: recognition of the diagnosis and its impact on functioning, identifying members of the patient's support team, specifying how to recognize if the patient is doing well (goals to be accomplished during euthymic periods), identifying early warning signs of depression and mania, and creating steps of action should the patient notice the early signs of depression or mania (steps for action might include who to call and their phone numbers, as well as taking steps to regulate sleep and maintaining a regular schedule of activities and pleasant events). Members of the patient's support team are invited to attend sessions during this phase.

The third phase of treatment consists of 13 sessions of modular design, and places emphasis on three hierarchical goals: (1) adequate acquisition of cognitive–behavioral skills emphasized to date; (2) remission of the bipolar depression; and (3) interventions for other life problems that may impact relapse, including training in problem-solving and social skills, and management strategies for anxiety, anger, and extreme emotions. The application of these modules is guided by an algorithm of treatment challenges to be assessed by the therapist.

The final phase of treatment consists of four sessions of well-being therapy [71], designed to treat residual symptoms, improve quality of life, and aid the fading of treatment sessions. In this phase, emphasis is not placed on the reduction of psychopathology, but on the identification, tracking, and enhancement of periods of well-being.

Other psychosocial treatments

In addition to CBT, several other psychosocial treatments have been applied to bipolar disorder. Interpersonal and social rhythm therapy, which is derived from interpersonal therapy for depression [72], explores the interpersonal context in which manic and depressive symptoms arise. Unlike traditional interpersonal therapy, IPSRT includes a focus on the impact of stressful life events on patients' social and circadian rhythms as well as the more traditional focus on grief over loss, interpersonal conflicts, role transitions, and interpersonal deficits. In a study conducted by Frank et al. [73], IPSRT was compared to clinical status and symptoms review treatment to determine its impact on relapse prevention [74]. Results at one-year follow-up indicated significantly greater stability of daily routines in those who received IPSRT. Frank and colleagues [75] also conducted a two-year outcome study examining varying combinations of IPSRT and clinical management (CM). While results did not reveal a significant difference between treatment modalities in time required to achieve stabilization, patients receiving IPSRT in the acute treatment phase showed a longer period of time before the development of a new affective episode indicating that this treatment promotes stability of social rhythms, which protects against future relapse.

Family-focused therapy has also been used successfully in the treatment of bipolar disorder to target the exacerbation of symptoms caused by high levels of familial expressed emotion and life events disrupting the daily routine. In a study of 101 bipolar patients conducted by Miklowitz, George, Richards, Simoneau, and Suddath [76], those assigned to FFT remained remitted or partially remitted for longer intervals than those receiving CM. Family-focused therapy also demonstrated a greater reduction in mood disorder symptoms and increased compliance with medication regimens than in the control condition. Further support for FFT was provided by Rea *et al.* [77], who compared FFT to individual treatment in a randomized clinical trial of 53 bipolar participants. Results again indicated that FFT patients were less likely to be rehospitalized during the study and showed fewer mood disorder relapses. Simoneau *et al.* also found that FFT led to more positive non-verbal interaction behavior among families one year after treatment completion than families receiving CM [78]. For patients in the FFT condition that became more non-verbally positive, greater improvements in mood were also observed. Finally, Clarkin, Carpenter, Hull *et al.* examined the effect of marital therapy and medication management finding the intervention did not effect recurrence or symptomatic status [79], but did increase global functioning and medication adherence.

Group treatment has also been used for bipolar disorder as a potentially cost-effective method to prevent recurrence. In an open treatment trial conducted by Bauer, McBride, Chase *et al.* examining the effect of the manual-based "Life Goals" program [80], patients showed increases in their knowledge about the disorder, with 70% reaching their first self-identified behaviorally based life goal. Colom *et al.* also demonstrated beneficial effects of group treatment when they compared structured group-based "psychoeducation" with a non-directive group therapy [81]. In this study, group treatment significantly reduced the number of relapsed patients and number of recurrences, in addition to fewer and less lengthy hospital stays. Increases in time to depressive, manic, hypomanic, and mixed recurrences were also noted.

Factors associated with poorer treatment outcome

High rates of comorbidity exist among patients with bipolar disorder. For comorbid anxiety disorders in epidemiologic and clinical studies, prevalence rates include ranges from 7.8 to 47.2% for social anxiety disorder, 7 to 40% for post-traumatic stress disorder, 10.6 to 62.5% for panic disorder, 7 to 32% for generalized anxiety disorder, and 3.2 to 35% for obsessive–compulsive disorder (for review, see [30]). High rates of substance use disorder comorbidity have been observed in both clinical populations [82, 83], and community samples indicating prevalence rates ranging from 21 to 45% [84, 2]. Further evidence suggests comorbidity with eating disorders [85] and attention deficit/hyperactivity disorder [86].

Psychiatric comorbidity had been linked with increased likelihood of being in a mood episode, and suicide attempts as well as reduced likelihood of recovery from a mood episode, and poorer role functioning, quality of life, and response to medications [28, 29, 42]. For bipolar patients with a comorbid substance use disorder, decreased medication compliance [83, 44], higher instances of hospitalization [82, 87], and poorer recovery are often found [88, 12]. In addition, panic disorder and/or high levels of somatic anxiety have also been identified as predictors of poorer treatment response in bipolar patients receiving IPSRT [89]. Research also indicates further predictors of poor treatment outcome include comorbidity with attention deficit/hyperactivity disorder in children and adolescents [90, 91].

In addition to Axis I comorbidity, the presence of Axis II personality disorders are also predictors of poor treatment response. Problems associated with comorbid personality disorders include poorer social and occupational functioning, increased rates of psychiatric symptoms, and decreased response to pharmacotherapy [92–94].

An early age of onset for the disorder has also been identified as a risk factor for rapid cycling, comorbidity with substance use disorders, and suicidal ideation [18, 95, 96]. Increased risk for severe course and poor treatment outcome have also been associated with early age of onset [97, 18].

Finally, suicide is of great concern as it has been found to have a particularly high association with bipolar disorder. In a study conducted by Brown, Beck, Steer *et al.* [98], results indicated that risk of suicide is four times greater in patients with bipolar disorder than average psychiatric patients and that bipolar patients also have the highest risk for completion of suicide attempts. Also, bipolar patients with a comorbid substance use disorder have a particularly elevated rate of suicide, making this a particularly at-risk population [99]. Research has shown that in some samples of bipolar patients lifetime prevalence of suicide attempts is as high as 30% [100–102].

Future directions

At the present time, the evidence for the efficacy of psychosocial interventions for bipolar disorder has never been stronger. Numerous clinical trials indicate that, on average, adding specific psychosocial interventions to an ongoing pharmacologic regimen emphasizing mood stabilizers results in both symptom reduction and enhanced protection against relapse. From this solid footing, there are a number of salient areas for expansion. The efficacy of psychosocial treatment on specific symptom areas, prominently including the role of anger and anxiety management, needs to be investigated. For example, despite the clear association between anxiety disorders and a worse course of bipolar disorder, there have not been controlled studies of the benefit of intervening with comorbid anxiety disorders for controlling the number or intensity of future mood episodes. There is also ample need for better understanding the role of sleep disruptions in bipolar disorder, and the value of adding additional psychosocial sleep interventions to the algorithm of treatment. Any of these areas of investigation offer the promise for providing additional help to patients with bipolar disorder and their families.

Appendix 2.1 Treatment contract for bipolar disorder (reprinted from Otto, MW, Reilly-Harrington NA, Knauz RO, *et al. Living with Bipolar Disorder.* New York: Oxford University Press, 2008 [103]).

Creating a Treatment Contract

Why Contract?

As part of your management of your bipolar disorder, we recommend the use of a written care plan or treatment contract. The treatment contract gives you an opportunity to decide what you want to happen when you are ill. Designing this plan when you are well allows you to specify which management strategies are preferable to cope with severe episodes. This process involves selecting and educating a support system that will participate with you on your treatment contract. Recall from Chapter 1 that your support system may include your doctors, your family members, spouse or significant other, friends, coworkers, and so on. It is important that your support system receive information about bipolar disorder. They can read this book and, most importantly, listen to you about your specific symptoms. You may also invite your support system to attend one of your meetings with your psychiatrist or therapist.

The treatment contract gives you an opportunity to decide what you want to happen when you are ill.

To involve your support system, you must specify ways in which they can be helpful to you during acute episodes. You also may wish to give permission to your support system to contact your treatment team when they detect early symptoms of mania.

We would like you to empower your support system by instructing them to anticipate problems and informing them of the types of reactions and responses you would want them to make. By planning ahead when you are feeling relatively well, you maintain maximal control. Your support team will become agents of *your plan,* not people imposing restrictions on you.

By writing a treatment contract, you and your family members will have an action plan to use in case of future episodes. The treatment contract will enable you to take part in the planning and to exercise choice and control regarding what will happen throughout the course of your bipolar mood disorder and its treatment. Once the treatment contract is signed, your clinicians and family members or support system become agents of your plan, not people controlling your decisions. This approach will allow you to plan ahead during periods of calm in anticipation of the periods of stormy weather that may lie ahead.

Format of the Contract

Your individualized treatment contract begins with a review of the purpose of the contract and an identification of your support team. Then, you specify the characteristic thoughts, feelings, behaviors, and early warning signs for your episodes of depression. Keeping in mind that the symptoms of depression can vary from person to person, you want to personalize the treatment contract to reflect your experience of depression. Next, you specify a plan for coping with depression by stating ways in which your support system can be helpful to you.

Finally, you note the thoughts, feelings, and behaviors and early warning signs of hypomania and mania. You specify a plan for coping with mania or hypomania, giving specific instructions to the members of your support system. For example, instructions might include, "Call my doctor," or "Take away my credit cards." You may also want to specify who initiates the plan for mania. It is often your family or support system who will first recognize the signs of mania. You can also include other modules that target high-risk behaviors, such as substance abuse, bulimia, gambling, and so on, if these are problematic for you.

Your Contract

The contract on the following pages is both a guide for you to use in developing your personalized treatment contract and a kind of generic contract that you may want to fill out so you can have a plan in place while you work on a more personalized plan. Use it to reach the goal of getting your first treatment contract written. As you learn more about your condition and what works or doesn't work for you, the contract can be revised.

Use the following template as a guide. As you personalize the contract to reflect your individuality, feel free to cross out any text you feel is inappropriate or add items you think will be helpful. Your contract should reflect your preferences and should incorporate as much about what you know about yourself as possible.

The most important thing about having a plan is making sure you and everyone who agrees to participate in it actually follow the plan. As you gain experience with this approach to treatment, you will see that knowing who and what you can count on can be the glue that keeps everything together.

Treatment Contract

The purpose of this contract is to organize my care for bipolar disorder, with attention to both the prevention of mood episodes and the efficient treatment of these episodes should they occur. My first step in guiding my care is the selection of my support team. The team members should include people with whom I have regular contact, who can help me identify episodes should they occur and help me put into practice some of the tools discussed in previous chapters of this book.

(Select members of your treatment team to be part of your support team; for example, you may select your psychiatrist, psychologist, social worker, or primary care physician. Other team members may be drawn from the support network identified by you in Chapter 1.)

Treatment Contract: Support Team

Role/relationship   Name   Contact information

My psychiatrist_____   Phone: _____

My therapist_____   Phone: _____

My PCP_____   Phone: _____

_____   _____   Phone: _____

_____   _____   Phone: _____

My second step in developing this contract is to identify tools I will use to help control my bipolar disorder so that I can best pursue my life goals. Many of these tools have been identified in previous chapters. My goal now is to identify some of the tools that I want to plan to use.

For every tool or strategy listed, please place a checkmark next to the ones you plan to incorporate as a part of your treatment contract.

Monitor My Mood for Early Intervention

Signs of depression and mania are listed in Chapter 2. In addition to these symptoms, I know from my own patterns that I should watch out for the following signs.

Depressed thoughts _____

_____

_____

Depressed symptoms _____

_____

_____

Depressed behavior _____

_____

_____

Hypomanic thoughts _____
_____
_____

Hypomanic symptoms _____
_____
_____

Hypomanic behaviors _____
_____
_____

Take Early Action if I Notice Signs of Depression or Mania

Contact my psychiatrist at phone no._____.
Contact my therapist at phone no._____.
Contact my support person at phone no._____.
Maintain a regular schedule of sleep and activities.
Maintain a regular schedule of pleasant events.
Evaluate my thoughts for negative or hyperpositive thinking.
Talk with my family about ways to cope.
Limit my alcohol use and avoid all non-medication drugs.
Other _____.
Other _____.
Other _____.
Other _____.

To Take Active Steps to Keep My Mood in the Desired Range

Take all medications as prescribed by my doctor.
Maintain regular appointments with my psychiatrist at _____ /month.
Maintain regular appointments with my therapist at _____ /month.
Keep a regular sleep schedule.
Maintain a schedule including at least three valued activities each day as a buffer against stress.
Avoid excessive use of alcohol.
Avoid all use of illicit drugs.
Use no alcohol for the next 30 days.
Use no recreational drugs for the next 30 days.
Keep a perspective on my thoughts and evaluate my thoughts for accuracy.
Share with my family information on communication styles that may reduce stress.
Other _____.
Other _____.
Other _____.
Other _____.

Contact the Following People Should I Ever Have Strong Suicidal Thoughts

Contact my psychiatrist at phone no. _____.
Contact my therapist at phone no. _____.
Contact my support person at phone no. _____.
Other action _____.

Keep Myself Safe Until I Can Be Seen or Go to a Local Emergency Room if I Ever Fear I May Act on Suicidal Thoughts.

If I Start to Become Depressed, I Would Like My Support Team to:

Talk to me about my symptoms (who _____)
Make plans for a pleasant event (who _____)
Discuss ways to reduce stress (who _____)

Make sure I am taking my medication (who _____)

Call my doctor if I am unable to (who _____)

Other _____

Other _____

Other _____

If I Start to Become Manic, I Would Like My Support Team to:

Talk to me about my symptoms (who _____)

Talk to me about reducing activities (who _____)

Allow me to be alone if I am irritable (who _____)

Take care of the kids/pets/other (who _____)

Take away my credit cards (who _____)

Take away my car keys (who _____)

Take me to the hospital (preferred hospital _____)

Other _____

Other _____

Other _____

I understand that this contract is designed by me so that I can take an active role in my treatment. My goal is to maximize my control by arranging for my support team to take care of me. So that any future decisions are well considered, I agree to change this contract only after giving two weeks written notice to all parties to this contract.

Signatures for Contracting Individuals

Signature	Date	Signature	Date
Signature	Date	Signature	Date

References

1. Kessler R, Chiu W, Demler O, Walters E. Prevalence, severity, and comorbidity of twelve-month DSM-IV disorders in the National Comorbidity Survey Replication (NCS-R). *Arch Gen Psychiatry* 2005; **62**: 617–27.

2. Regier D, Farmer M, Rae D, *et al.* Comorbidity of mental disorders with alcohol and other drug abuse: results from the Epidemiologic Catchment Area (ECA) study. *JAMA* 1990; **264**: 2511–18.

3. American Psychiatric Association. *Diagnostic and Statistical Manual of Mental Disorders, 4th edn., text revision.* Washington, DC: American Psychiatric Press, 2000.

4. Lish J, Dime-Meenan S, Whybrow P, Price R, Hirschfeld R.The National Depressive and Manic-depressive Association (DMDA) survey of bipolar members. *J Aff Disord* 1994; **31**: 281–94.

5. Suppes T, Leverich G, Keck P, *et al.* The Stanley Foundation Bipolar Treatment Outcome Network. II. Demographics and illness characteristics of the first 261 patients. *J Affect Disord* 2001; **67**: 45–59.

6. Colom F, Vieta E, Daban C, Pacchiarotti I, Sánchez-Moreno J. Clinical and therapeutic implications of predominant polarity in bipolar disorder. *J Affect Disord* 2006; **93**: 13–17.

7. Judd LL, Akiskal HS, Schettler PJ, *et al.* The long-term natural history of the weekly symptomatic status of bipolar I disorder. *Arch Gen Psychiatry* 2002; **59**: 530–7.

8. Judd LL, Akiskal HS, Schettler PJ, *et al.* The comparative clinical phenotype and long term longitudinal episode course of bipolar I and II: A clinical spectrum or distinct disorders? *J Affect Disord* 2003; **73**: 19–32.

9. Goldberg JF, Perlis RH, Bowden CL, *et al.* Manic symptoms during depressive episodes in 1,380 patients with bipolar disorder: findings from the STEP-BD. *Am J Psychiatry* 2009; **166**: 173–81.

10. Gitlin M, Swendsen J, Heller T, Hammen C. Relapse and impairment in bipolar disorder. *Am J Psychiatry* 1995; **152**: 1635–40.

11. O'Connell R, Mayo J, Flatlow L, Cuthbertson B, O'Brien B. Outcome of bipolar disorder on long-term treatment with lithium. *Br J Psychiatry* 1991; **159**: 123–9.

12. Tohen M, Waternaux C, Tsuang M. Outcome in mania: a 4-year prospective follow-up of 75 patients utilizing

survival analysis. *Arch Gen Psychiatry* 1990; **47**: 1106–11.

13. Yatham LN, Kauer-Sant'anna M, Bond DJ, Lam RW, Torres I. Course and outcome after the first manic episode in patients with bipolar disorder: prospective 12-month data from the systematic treatment optimization program for early mania project. *Can J Psychiatry* 2009; **54**: 105–12.

14. Keck P, McElroy S, Strakowski S, *et al.* Twelve-month outcome of patients with bipolar disorder following hospitalization for a manic or mixed episode. *Am J Psychiatry* 1998; **155**: 646–52.

15. Miklowitz D, Otto M, Frank E, *et al.* A 1-year randomized trial from the systematic treatment enhancement program. *Arch Gen Psychiatry* 2007; **64**: 419–26.

16. Kessler R, McGonagle K, Zhao S, *et al.* Lifetime and 12-month prevalence of DSM-III-R psychiatric disorders in the United States: results from the National Comorbidity Survey. *Arch Gen Psychiatry* 1994; **51**: 8–19.

17. Merikangas KR, Akiskal HS, Angst J, *et al.* Lifetime and 12-month prevalance of bipolar spectrum disorder in the National Comorbidity Survey replication. *Arch Gen Psychiatry* 2007; **65**: 543–52.

18. Perlis R, Miyahara S, Marangell L, *et al.* Long-term implications of early onset in bipolar disorder: data from the first 1000 participants in the systematic treatment enhancement program for bipolar disorder (STEP-BD). *Biol Psychiatry* 2004; **55**: 875–81.

19. Schneck C, Miklowitz D, Calabrese J, *et al.* Phenomenology of rapid-cycling bipolar disorder: data from the first 500 participants in the Systematic Treatment Enhancement Program. *Am J Psychiatry* 2004; **161**: 1902–8.

20. Suominen K, Mantere O, Valtonen H, *et al.* Early age at onset of bipolar disorder is associated with more severe clinical features but delayed treatment seeking. *Bipolar Disord* 2007; **9**: 698–705.

21. Bebbington P, Wilkins S, Jones P, *et al.* Life events and psychosis: initial results from the Camberwell Collaborative Psychosis Study. *Br J Psychiatry* 1993; **162**: 72–9.

22. Healy D, Williams J. Dysthymia, dysphoria and depression: the interaction of learned helplessness and circadian dysthymia in the pathogenesis of depression. *Psychol Bull* 1988; **103**: 163–78.

23. Healy D, Williams J. Moods, misattributions and mania: an interaction of biological and psychological factors in the pathogenesis of mania. *Psychiatr Dev* 1989; **1**: 49–70.

24. Ellicott A, Hammen C, Gitlin M, Brown G, Jameson K. Life events and the course of bipolar disorder. *Am J Psychiatry* 1990; **147**: 1194–8.

25. Johnson S, Miller I. Negative life events and time to recovery from episodes of bipolar disorder. *J Abnorm Psychol* 1997; **106**: 449–57.

26. Miklowitz D, Goldstein M, Nuechterlein K, Snyder K, Mintz J. Family factors and the course of bipolar affective disorder. *Arch Gen Psychiatry* 1988; **45**: 223–31.

27. Priebe S, Wildgrube C, Muller-Oerlinghausen B. Lithium prophylaxis and expressed emotion. *Br J Psychiatry* 1989; **154**: 396–9.

28. Henry C, Van den Bulke D, Bellivier F, *et al.* Anxiety disorders in 318 bipolar patients: prevalence and impact on illness severity and response to mood stabilizer. *J Clin Psychiatry* 2003; **64**: 331–5.

29. Otto M, Simon N, Wisniewski S, *et al.* Prospective 12-month course of bipolar disorder in outpatients with and without comorbid anxiety disorders. *Br J Psychiatry* 2006; **189**: 20–5.

30. Simon N, Otto M, Wisniewski S, *et al.* Anxiety disorder comorbidity in bipolar disorder: data from the first 500 STEP-BD participants. *Am J Psychiatry* 2004; **161**: 2222–9.

31. Calabrese J, McFadden W, McCoy R, *et al. Double-blind, placebo-controlled study of quetiapine in bipolar depression.* Abstract presented at APA 2004, NYC, USA. 2004.

32. Gao K, Gajwani P, Elhaj O, Calabrese J. Typical and atypical antipsychotics in bipolar depression. *J Clin Psychiatry* 2005; **66**: 1376–85.

33. Thase M, Macfadden W, Weisler R, *et al.* Efficacy of quetiapine monotherapy in bipolar I and II depression: a double blind, placebo-controled study (the BOLDER II study). *J Clin Psychopharmacol* 2006; **26**: 600–9.

34. Tohen M, Vieta E, Calabrese J, *et al.* Efficacy of olanzapine and olanzapine-fluoxetine combination in the treatment of bipolar I depression. *Arch Gen Psychiatry* 2003; **60**: 1079–88.

35. Nemeroff C, Evans D, Gyulai L, *et al.* Double-blind, placebo-controlled comparison of imipramine and paroxetine in the treatment of bipolar depression. *Am J Psychiatry* 2001; **158**: 906–12.

36. Sachs G, Nierenberg A, Calabrese, *et al.* Effectiveness of adjunctive antidepressant treatment for bipolar depression. *N Engl J Med* 2007; **356**: 1711–22.

37. Moller H, Grunze H. Have some guidelines for the treatment of acute bipolar depression gone too far in the restriction of antidepressants? *Eur Arch Psychiatry Clin Neurosci* 2000; **250**: 57–68.

38. Gijsman H, Gedses J, Rendell J, Nolen W, Goodwin, G. Antidepressants for bipolar depression: a systematic review of randomized, controlled trials. *Am J Psychiatry* 2004; **161**: 1537–47.

39. Leverich G, Altshuler L, Frye M, *et al.* Risk of switch in mood polarity to hypomania or mania in patients with bipolar depression during acute and continuation trials of venlafaxine, sertraline, and bupropion as adjuncts to mood stabilizers. *Am J Psychiatry* 2006; **163**: 232–9.

40. Moller H, Nasrallah H. Treatment of bipolar disorder. *J Clin Psychiatry* 2003; **64**: 9–16.

41. American Psychiatric Association. Practice guideline for the treatment of patients with bipolar disorder (revision). *Am J Psychiatry* 2002; **159**: 1–50.

42. Simon N, Otto M, Weiss R, *et al.* Pharmacotherapy for bipolar disorder and comorbid conditions: baseline data from STEP-BD. *J Clin Psychopharmacol* 2004; **24**: 512–20.

43. Johnson R, McFarland B. Lithium use and discontinuation in a health maintenance organization. *Am J Psychiatry* 1996; **153**: 993–1000.

44. Keck P, McElroy S, Strakowski S, *et al.* Factors associated with pharmacologic noncompliance in patients with mania. *J Clin Psychiatry* 1996; **57**: 292–7.

45. Allison D, Casey D. Antipsychotic-induced weight gain: a review of the literature. *J Clin Psychiatry* 2001; **62**: 22–31.

46. Gao K, Ganocy S, Gajwani P, *et al.* A review of sensitivity and tolerability of antipsychotics in patients with bipolar disorder or schizophrenia: focus on somnolence. *J Clin Psychiatry* 2008; **69**: 302–9.

47. Gao K, Kemp D, Ganocy S, *et al.* Antipsychotic-induced extrapyramidal side effects in bipolar disorder and schizophrenia: a systematic review. *J Clin Psychopharmacol* 2008 **28**, 203–9.

48. Newcomer J. Second-generation (atypical) antipsychotics and metabolic effects: a comprehensive literature review. *CNS Drugs* 2005; **19**: 1–93.

49. Bowden C, Asnis G, Ginsberg L, *et al.* Safety and tolerability of lamotrigine for bipolar disorder. *Drug Saf* 2002; **27**: 173–84.

50. Goodwin F, Jamison K. *Manic-Depressive Illness: Bipolar Disord and Recurrent Depression*, 2nd edn. New York, NY: Oxford University Press, 2007.

51. Macritchie K, Geddes J, Scott J, Haslam D, Goodwin, G. Valproic acid, valproate and divalproex in the maintenance treatment of bipolar disorder. *Cochrane Database Syst Rev* 2001; **3**: CD003196.

52. Scott J, Pope M. Nonadherence with mood stabilizers: prevalence and predictors. *J Clin Psychiatry* 2002; **65**: 384–90.

53. Perlis R, Sachs G, Lafer B, *et al.* Effect of abrupt change from standard to low serum lithium levels: a reanalysis of double-blind lithium maintenance data. *Am J Psychiatry* 2002; **159**: 1155–9.

54. Gelenberg A, Kane J, Keller M, *et al.* Comparison of standard and low serum levels of lithium for maintenance treatment of bipolar disorders. *N Engl J Med* 1989; **321**: 1489–93.

55. Otto M, Miklowitz D. The role and impact of psychotherapy in the management of bipolar disorder. *CNS Spectr* 2004; **9**: 27–32.

56. Callahan M, Bauer M. Psychosocial interventions for bipolar disorder. *Psychiatr Clin North Am* 1999; **22**: 675–88.

57. Cochran, S. Preventing medical noncompliance in the outpatient treatment of bipolar affective disorders. *J Consult Clin Psychol* 1984; **52**: 873–8.

58. Bauer, M. S. An evidence-based review of psychosocial treatments for bipolar disorder. *Psychopharmacol Bull* 2001; **35**: 109–34.

59. Otto MW, Applebaum AJ. The nature and treatment of bipolar disorder and the bipolar spectrum. In Barlow DH, ed. *Oxford Handbook of Clinical Psychology*. New York: Oxford University Press, 2010.

60. Miklowitz D, Goodwin GM, Bauer MS, Geddes JR. Common and specific elements of psychosocial treatments for bipolar disorder: a survey of clinicians participating in randomized trials. *J Psychiatr Pract* 2008; **14**: 77–85.

61. Lam D, Bright J, Jones S, *et al.* Cognitive therapy for bipolar illness: a pilot study of relapse prevention. *Cognit Ther Res* 2000; **24**: 503–20.

62. Lam D, Watkins E, Hayward P, *et al.* A randomized controlled study of cognitive therapy for relapse prevention for bipolar affective disorder: outcome of the first year. *Arch Gen Psychiatry* 2003; **60**: 145–52.

63. Scott J, Garland A, Moorhead, S. A pilot study of cognitive therapy in bipolar disorders. *Psychol Med* 2001; **31**: 459–67.

64. Perry A, Tarrier N, Morriss R, McCarthy E, Limb, K. Randomized controlled trial of efficacy of teaching patients with bipolar disorder to identify early warning signs or relapse and obtain treatment. *Br Med J* 1999; **318**: 149–53.

65. Zaretsky A, Lancee W, Miller C, Harris A, Parikh SV. Is cognitive-behavioral therapy more effective than psychoeducation in bipolar disorder? *Can J Psychiatry* 2008; **53**: 441–8.

66. Scott J, Paykey E, Morriss, *et al.* Cognitive-behavioral therapy for severe and recurrent bipolar disorders. *Br J Psychiatry* 2006; **188**: 313–20.

67. Miklowitz, D. A review of evidence-based psychosocial interventions for bipolar disorder. *J Clin Psychiatry* 2006; **67**: 28–33.

68. Miklowitz D, Otto M. New psychosocial interventions for bipolar disorder: a review of the literature and introduction of the Systematic Treatment Enhancement Program. *J Cogn Psychother* 2006; **20**: 215–30.

69. Otto MW, Reilly-Harrington NA, Kogan J, *et al. Managing Bipolar Disorder: A Cognitive-behavioral Approach (Therapist Guide)*. New York, NY: Oxford University Press, 2009.

70. Otto MW, Reilly-Harrington NA, Kogan JN, *et al. Managing Bipolar Disorder: A Cognitive-behavioral Approach (Workbook)*. New York, NY: Oxford University Press, 2009.

71. Fava GA, Ruini C. Development and characteristics of a well-being enhancing psychotherapeutic strategy: well-being therapy. *J Behav Ther Exp Psychiatry* 2003; **34**: 45–63.

72. Klerman G, Weissman M, Rounsaville B, Chevron E. *Interpersonal Psychotherapy for Depression*. New York, NY: Basic Books, 1984.

73. Frank E, Hlastala S, Ritenour A, *et al.* Inducing lifestyle regularity in recovering bipolar disorder patients: results from the maintenance therapies in bipolar disorder protocol. *Biol Psychiatry* 1997; **41**: 1165–73.

74. Frank E, Kupfer D, Perel J, *et al.* Three year outcomes for maintenance therapy in recurrent depression. *Arch Gen Psychiatry* 1990; **47**: 1093–9.

75. Frank E, Kupfer D. Thase M, *et al.* Two-year outcomes for interpersonal and social rhythm therapy in individuals with bipolar I disorder. *Arch Gen Psychiatry* 2005; **62**: 996–1004.

76. Miklowitz D, George E, Richards J, Simoneau T, Suddath, R. A randomized study of family-focused psychoeducation and pharmacotherapy in the outpatient management of bipolar disorder. *Arch Gen Psychiatry* 2003; **60**: 904–12.

77. Rea M, Tompson M, Miklowitz D, *et al.* Family-focused treatment versus individual treatment for bipolar disorder: results of a randomized clinical trial. *J Consult Clin Psychol* 2003; **71**: 482–92.

78. Simoneau T, Miklowitz D, Richards J, Saleem R, George, E. Bipolar disorder and family communication: effects of a psychoeducational treatment program. *J Abnorm Psychol* 1999; **108**: 588–97.

79. Clarkin J, Carpenter D, Hull J, Wilner P, Glick I. Effects of a psychoeducational intervention for married patients with bipolar disorder and their spouses. *Psychiatr Serv* 1998; **49**: 531–3.

80. Bauer M, McBride L, Chae C, Sachs G, Shea N. Manual-based group psychotherapy for bipolar disorder: a feasibility study. *J Clin Psychiatry* 1998; **59**: 449–55.

81. Colom F, Vieta E, Martinez-Aran A, *et al.* A randomized trial on the efficacy of group psychoeducation in the prophylaxis of recurrences in bipolar patients whose disease is in remission. *Arch Gen Psychiatry* 2003; **60**: 402–7.

82. Brady K, Castro S, Lydiard R, Malcolm R, Arana G. Substance abuse in an inpatient psychiatric sample. *Am J Drug Alcohol Abuse* 1991; **17**: 389–97.

83. Goldberg J, Garno J, Leon A, Kocsis J, Portera L. A history of substance abuse complicates remission from acute mania in bipolar disorder. *J Clin Psychiatry* 1999; **60**: 733–40.

84. Kessler R, Crum R, Warner L, *et al.* Lifetime co-occurrence of DSM-III-R alcohol abuse and dependence with other psychiatric disorders in the National Comorbidity Survey. *Arch Gen Psychiatry* 1997; **54**: 313–21.

85. McElroy S, Altshuler L, Suppes T, *et al.* Axis I psychiatric comorbidity and its relationship to historical illness variables in 288 patients with bipolar disorder. *Am J Psychiatry* 2001; **158**: 420–6.

86. Nierenberg A, Miyahara S, Spencer T, *et al.* Clinical and diagnostic implications of lifetime attention deficit/hyperactivity disorder comorbidity in adults with bipolar disorder: data from the first 1000 STEP-BD participants. *Biol Psychiatry* 2005; **57**: 1467–73.

87. Reich L, Davies R, Himmelhoch J. Excessive alcohol use in manic-depressive illness. *Am J Psychiatry* 1974; **131**: 83–6.

88. Keller M, Lavori P, Coryell W, *et al.* Differential outcome of pure manic, mixed/cycling, and pure depressive episodes in patients with bipolar illness. *JAMA* 1986; **255**: 3138–42.

89. Feske U, Frank E, Mallinger A, *et al.* Anxiety as a correlate of response to the acute treatment of bipolar I disorder. *Am J Psychiatry* 2000; **157**: 956–62.

90. Masi G, Perugi G, Toni C, *et al.* Predictors of treatment nonresponse in bipolar children and adolescents with manic or mixed episodes. *J Child Adolesc Psychopharmacol* 2004; **14**: 395–404.

91. Strober M, DeAntonio M, Schmidt-Lackner S, *et al.* Early childhood attention deficit hyperactivity disorder predicts poorer response to acute lithium therapy in adolescent mania. *J Affect Disord* 1998; **51**: 145–51.

92. Carpenter D, Clarkin J, Glick I, Wilner P. Personality pathology among married adults with bipolar disorder. *J Affect Disord* 1995; **34**: 269–74.

93. Dunayevich E, Sax K, Keck P, *et al.* Twelve-month outcome in bipolar patients with and without personality disorders. *J Clin Psychiatry* 2000; **61**: 134–9.

94. Kutcher S, Maton P, Korenblum, M. Adolescent bipolar illness and personality disorder. *J Am Acad Child Adolesc Psychiatry* 1990; **29**: 355–8.

95. Tohen M, Greenfield S, Weiss R, Zarate C, Vagge L. The effect of comorbid substance use disorders on the course of bipolar disorder: a review. *Harv Rev Psychiatry* 1998; **6**: 133–41.

96. Tsai S, Chen C, Kuo C, *et al.* 15-year outcome of treated bipolar disorder. *J Affect Disord* 2001; **63**: 215–20.

97. Carter T, Mundo E, Parikh S, Kennedy J. Early age at onset as a risk factor for poor outcome of bipolar disorder. *J Psychiatr Res* 2003; **37**: 297–303.

98. Brown G, Beck A, Steer R, Grisham J. Risk factors for suicide in psychiatric outpatients: a 20-year prospective study. *J Consult Clin Psychol* 2000; **68**: 371–7.

99. Dalton J, Cate-Carter T, Mundo E, Parikh S, Kennedy J. Suicide risk in bipolar patients: the role of comorbid substance use disorders. *Bipolar Disord* 2003; **5**: 58–61.

100. Chen Y, Dilsaver, S. Lifetime rates of suicide attempts among subjects with bipolar and unipolar disorders relative to subjects with other Axis I disorders. *Biol Psychiatry* 1996; **39**: 896–9.

101. Oquendo M, Waternaux C, Brodsky B, *et al.* Suicidal behavior in bipolar mood disorder: clinical characteristics of attempters and nonattempters. *J Affect Disord* 2000; **59**: 107–17.

102. Oquendo M, Mann J. Identifying and managing suicide risk in bipolar patients. *J Clin Psychiatry* 2001; **62**: 31–4.

103. Otto MW, Reilly-Harrington NA, Knauz RO, *et al. Living with Bipolar Disorder.* New York: Oxford University Press, 2008.

Generalized anxiety disorder

Adrian Wells and Peter Fisher

The diagnosis of generalized anxiety disorder (GAD) has become more reliable and the features better defined since the change of this disorder from a residual category in the third edition of the *Diagnostic and Statistical Manual of Mental Disorders* (DSM-III; [1]). Consequently GAD is now recognized as a prevalent disorder associated with significant disability, impaired quality of life, and health costs [2].

In this chapter we review the nature of GAD, describe the most common treatments, and evaluate their efficacy. The chapter focuses on the metacognitive model of GAD and describes the structure, choice, and implementation of treatment strategies in metacognitive therapy (MCT).

Diagnostic features

The central diagnostic feature of DSM-IV GAD is the occurrence of excessive anxiety and worry about a number of events occurring more days than not [3], for at least six months. The worry usually concerns a number of different domains such as work, health, family, and finances. Individuals must report difficulty controlling worry and there must be at least three other symptoms from among the following: (1) restlessness; (2) easily fatigued; (3) difficulty concentrating or mind going blank; (4) irritability; (5) muscle tension; (6) sleep disturbance.

The focus of worry and anxiety in GAD must not be confined to the features of another Axis I disorder. For example, worry should not be about having a panic attack, as is the case in panic disorder, or of being embarrassed in public, as in social anxiety disorder. The anxiety, worry, or symptoms should cause significant distress or impairment in social or occupational functioning, and must not be due to a medical condition or use of substances. In DSM-IV a hierarchical exclusion is maintained in which GAD is not diagnosed if it occurs exclusively during a mood disorder, a psychotic disorder, or developmental disorder.

Prevalence, course, and comorbidity

The 12-month prevalence of DSM-III-R and DSM-IV GAD ranges from 1.1% to 3.6% [4,5], but rates defined by less stringent ICD-10 criteria are higher at around 5% [6]. Commensurate with an effect of this disorder on healthcare utilization, the prevalence is much higher in patients in primary care than in the general community. Data from studies in several countries show that GAD is one of the most frequently identified mental disorders in primary care with a current prevalence rate of 3.7 to 8% [7,8], and a 12-month prevalence of 10.3% [9].

Studies of the course of GAD show that the disorder is chronic and unremitting. Yonkers *et al.* reported that only 40% of individuals with GAD were in full remission after two years [10], with a full remission rate of only 38% after five years [11].

High rates of comorbidity are found in DSM-III-R GAD in clinical samples but the rates in community samples are similar to the rates observed among individuals with other anxiety and mood disorders [6]. Wittchen explained this discrepancy by showing that comorbidity was a predictor of help-seeking among people with the disorder [6]. The most prevalent comorbidity is major depressive disorder, followed by social phobia, specific phobia, and panic disorder. In people with comorbid GAD and depression, GAD typically develops first [12]. The age of onset for GAD is typically between the late teenage years and late twenties.

The nature of worry

Difficult to control worry is the central feature of GAD. Worry is a predominantly verbal conceptual process involving chains of negative thoughts. An early definition of worry was provided by Borkovec, Robinson, Pruzinsky, and DePree [13: p. 10]:

> Worry is a chain of thoughts and images, negatively affect-laden and relatively uncontrollable; it represents an attempt to engage in mental problem-solving on an issue whose outcome is uncertain but contains the possibility of one or more negative outcomes; consequently worry relates closely to the fear process.

More recent definitions have included extended reference to the goals and function of worrying:

> Worry is a chain of catastrophising thoughts that are predominantly verbal. It consists of the contemplation of potentially dangerous situations and of personal coping strategies. It is intrusive and controllable although it is often experienced as uncontrollable. Worrying is associated with a motivation to prevent or avoid potential danger. Worry may itself be viewed as a coping strategy but can become the focus of an individual's concern.
>
> (Wells [14: p. 87])

The definition above recognizes that worry can be turned on itself, a phenomenon that has been labeled as meta-worry, or worry about worry [15]. This is a concept central in the metacognitive model of GAD.

Several studies have compared worry with other types of intrusive and repetitive thinking. In particular, normal worry and obsessions appear to differ [16], with worry being of longer duration than an obsessional thought and being more verbal. Diagnostically a useful distinction between obsessional thoughts and worry can be made. Obsessions are defined as ego-dystonic, meaning that they are experienced as senseless, repugnant, or out of character (DSM-IV, [3]). In contrast, worrying is often seen as a more useful process that is characteristic of the self. Individuals with GAD often report that they have been worriers for a significant portion of their lives and they see it as part of their personality.

Worry has been viewed as a dimensional construct, with normal and pathological worry occupying opposite ends of a continuum. However, it may not be the case that GAD simply represents the high-end of a normal worry continuum, after all not all high-frequency worriers have GAD. Drawing on Wells' metacognitive model [15], Ruscio and Borkovec explored the characteristics of worry and appraisal of worry among high worriers with and without GAD [17]. Comparison of these groups revealed that the experience of worry and consequences of worry were similar. However, more substantial differences emerged in beliefs about worry. Individuals with GAD endorsed greater beliefs about the uncontrollability and danger of worrying. Thus, differences in actual worry severity do not distinguish GAD from high worriers without GAD, but negative beliefs about worry appear to be distinctive of GAD. These results suggest that worry in GAD may differ in some important respects from non-GAD high worry levels because it is associated with specific negative appraisals and beliefs (i.e., worry about worry).

Psychological treatments for GAD

The majority of psychotherapy outcome research conducted on GAD has focused on interventions that fall under the rubric of cognitive–behavioral therapy (CBT). Clinical trials have predominantly tried to answer the question of whether behavioral therapy (typically, applied relaxation), cognitive therapy, or a combination of these two approaches (cognitive–behavioral therapy), is most effective. In addition to these generic treatments, a number of disorder-specific models or theories and associated interventions have been developed over the past decade. Among the most promising approaches is the meta-cognitive model and treatment of GAD [15, 14], presented in detail later in this chapter. A second innovative approach is a form of cognitive therapy that specifies a central role for intolerance of uncertainty (IOU) [18]. This intervention is briefly described below with the earlier cognitive and behavioral approaches.

Applied relaxation

This approach is derived from the work of Jacobson who developed progressive muscle relaxation (PMR) to target the physiological effects of anxiety [19], in the case of GAD this predominately focuses on the somatic symptom of muscle tension. Jacobson also advocated that PMR would help people to have a more relaxed attitude to life and that deep states of muscle relaxation are incompatible with anxiety and stress. Abridged versions of PMR are used in the two most frequently used relaxation therapies, namely applied relaxation (AR; [20]) and self-control desensitization (SCD; [21]).

Applied relaxation begins by providing the patient with a cogent rationale for the use of relaxation in treating GAD, followed by self-monitoring to help the patient recognize early physiological signs of anxiety and worries. Patients are initially trained in PMR, followed by a variety of relaxation methods including differential relaxation and rapid relaxation over the course of therapy. The goal is to enable patients to rapidly induce (in 20 to 30 seconds) a relaxed state in response to anxiety cues. Application training is the final step in which patients practice inducing relaxation in real-life situations. The other main form of relaxation training evaluated in GAD is SCD, which has been used as a component of the relaxation treatment package in clinical trials conducted by Borkovec and colleagues [22]. Importantly, Borkovec's relaxation treatment includes all aspects of AR but as it incorporates SCD [20], it differs in a number of ways. First, a wider array of relaxation methods are utilized including meditational and imaginal relaxation. Second, the main aim of AR is to enable the patient to cope with anxiety, and not to extinguish anxiety responses. In SCD, the central premise is extinction as well as developing new coping skills. Third, AR does not use imaginal exposure to worry cues, whereas considerable time is spent on imaginal rehearsal to anxious thoughts in SCD. In the GAD outcome literature, AR and SCD are treated as essentially the same intervention as their similarities substantially outweigh their differences.

Cognitive therapy

Cognitive therapy (CT) for GAD is based on a generic schema model of anxiety and corresponding treatment protocol [23]. This theory asserts than individuals with high levels of anxiety have core beliefs/schemas that overestimate the dangerousness of the world, with a corresponding underestimate of their ability to cope. Core beliefs give rise to negative automatic thoughts in the form of worries relating to threat: "What if I fail?" "What if people don't like me?" These negative thoughts are perceived as accurate reflections of reality and the person therefore feels compelled to respond to the thoughts by further worrying or by engaging in coping strategies such as extensive reassurance seeking. The final element of this model is cognitive distortions such as selective abstraction or dichotomous thinking. These biases are typically congruent with the danger-related schema and tend to both elevate levels of anxiety and contribute to the individual developing an unrealistic appraisal of the level of threat.

Cognitive therapy aims to modify each of these three aspects of negative thinking and begins by providing a formulation based on the cognitive model. Self-monitoring is also used in CT, but the focus is on identifying danger-related thoughts about the future, the self, and the world. The therapist works with the patient to modify anxiety-related cognitions through verbal reattribution methods. Negative thoughts are subjected to logical disputation including strategies such as evaluating evidence for and against the thought, labeling the cognitive distortion contained within the thought, and generating alternative views to the negative appraisal. Changes in negative beliefs need to be consolidated through behavioral experiments in real-life settings. Typically, this involves identifying and empirically testing the patient's negative predictions. Generalized anxiety disorder patients often engage in behaviors such as avoidance or reassurance seeking, which maintain the sense of threat and prevent discovery of information that can disconfirm their worrying thoughts.

Cognitive–behavioral therapy

Cognitive–behavioral therapy for GAD comprises a package of treatment involving both behavior (relaxation strategies) and cognitive approaches. It is predicated on the assumption that there is a need for specific treatment strategies tailored to the main cognitive, behavioral, and physiological features of GAD. As described above, treating the physiological component involves a variety of relaxation strategies, the behavioral component focuses on modifying problematic coping strategies such as reassurance seeking, avoidance, and procrastination using in vivo exposure methods. As GAD patients often avoid situations, there is a reduced opportunity for engaging in pleasurable activities; therefore activity scheduling can be used to counteract low mood as well as providing opportunities to modify anxiogenic cognitions. Strategies for modifying the cognitive component are as described in the cognitive therapy section above, and involve reality-testing negative thoughts about the dangerousness of the world and the individual's inability to cope.

Intolerance of uncertainty (IOU)

This model gives a central role to a specific schema regarding being intolerant of uncertainty, rather than the broader generic schema regarding an overestimation of the dangerousness of the world. Intolerance of uncertainty is defined as the tendency to respond negatively in uncertain situations [18]. More specifically, GAD patients use worry in ambiguous situations to try and eliminate uncertainty by attempting to think through all possible permutations and outcomes. Of course, life is uncertain and therefore it is impossible to remove uncertainty, therefore the GAD patient is repeatedly exposed to cues that trigger bouts of worry. The main aim of treatment is to enable the patient to become more tolerant of uncertainty.

Treatment based on the IOU model consists of four main elements. First patients are introduced to the concept of intolerance and uncertainty and socialized to the model, which includes highlighting the negative consequences of worrying, followed by worry awareness training to help patients recognize the worry process. Second, positive beliefs about the usefulness of worry as a method of coping with uncertainty are challenged and modified. Third, patients tend to avoid uncertain or difficult situations and view problem-solving negatively, therefore they are helped to develop both problem-solving skills and confidence in their ability to solve problems. Finally, the IOU model distinguishes between worries that can be effectively solved and worries that cannot be resolved or that may never happen. Accordingly, worries that can be solved are subjected to problem-solving, whereas imaginal exposure is used to treat the irresolvable worries by facilitating emotional processing.

Meta-analytic reviews

A considerable number of meta-analytic reviews and over 30 clinical trials have resulted in clinical guidelines recommending CBT as a first line treatment for GAD [24]. Early meta-analytic reviews concluded that CBT was superior to a range of control conditions including non-directive therapy, wait-list controls, and pill placebo [25, 26]. The Gould *et al.* meta-analysis calculated effect sizes across 13 studies that compared cognitive–behavioral approaches with a control condition and 22 studies that compared various forms of pharmacotherapy with pill placebo [26]. At post-treatment, CBT and pharmacologic approaches were equivalently efficacious and both were more effective than the control conditions. An updated review of the Gould study obtained very similar results and concluded that treatments that fall under the banner of cognitive and behavioral approaches are at least as effective as pharmacotherapy for GAD [27].

Borkovec and Ruscio conducted the first meta-analytic review that explored whether there were differential efficacy rates between treatments that are typically grouped together as CBT [28]. Four aggregate comparison groups were developed: (1) CBT; (2) cognitive therapy or behavior therapy; (3) non-specific treatments, which included non-directive therapy and pill placebo conditions, as well as any other form of therapy; and (4) wait-list/no treatment. Cognitive–behavioral therapy produced the largest within-group effect sizes at post-treatment and at follow-up, on measures of both anxiety and depression. Between-group comparisons also demonstrated that CBT was more effective than the single components of behavior therapy or cognitive therapy. Interestingly, the wait-list condition demonstrated almost no change, with a mean within-group effect size at post-treatment of 0.01. This lack of change concurs with the estimated 5% recovery rate in wait-list conditions derived by Fisher and Durham [29], highlighting the chronicity of GAD and the very low probability of remission without treatment.

A Cochrane systematic review concluded that psychological therapies using a CBT approach are more effective than treatment as usual/wait-list control [30]. Estimates of clinical response suggested 46% of patients in receipt of CBT made a clinical response at post-treatment compared with 14% in wait-list control/treatment-as-usual control conditions. However, the eight studies that contributed to the clinical response data did not use a standardized operational definition of response, making interpretation of the results problematic.

Most recently, Covin *et al.* conducted a meta-analysis of CBT for pathological worry [31], indexed by the Penn State Worry Questionnaire (PSWQ; [32]) in order to determine the extent to which treatments modified the cardinal component of GAD. Overall, CBT was effective in reducing levels of worry, with the treatment targeting IOU being the most effective. The study is noteworthy for including clinical studies of CBT for both working age and older adults, with the younger client group achieving higher pre- to post-treatment effect sizes. This meta-analysis focused on CBT, rather than cognitive therapy or behavior therapy alone. However, the IOU treatment is labeled as CBT, it does not contain any form of relaxation training and it achieved the largest within-group effect sizes. This meta-analysis leaves an important question unanswered: does applied relaxation produce changes in levels of worry?

Results from the above meta-analytic reviews highlight that a range of psychological treatments within the CBT class produce greater pre- to post-treatment change than placebo, wait-list control, or therapies designed to control for non-specific effects. Furthermore, individual CBT appears to be a very acceptable form of treatment with very low attrition rates of approximately 9% [33]. Hunot *et al.* also reported reasonably low attrition rates [30], 15% across psychological treatment studies, but highlighted that individual approaches have lower drop-out rates than group interventions. However, some of the findings obtained require further exploration. Norton and Price in a meta-analytic review of CBT for anxiety disorders [34], obtained weighted pre- to post-effect sizes for GAD that were larger than those obtained for panic disorder, social phobia, and obsessive–compulsive disorder. This finding runs contrary the result of another meta-analysis of randomized placebo-controlled trials and the general impression held by clinicians that CBT for GAD is not as effective as CBT for panic disorder and social phobia [35]. Westen and Morrison also obtained much larger pre- to post-treatment effect sizes for GAD relative to panic disorder [36], but the reverse was true in terms of improvement rates. Specifically, the pre- to post-treatment effect sizes were 1.5 for panic disorder and 2.1 for GAD, whereas the improvement rates were 63% and 52%, respectively. Many reasons could account for this finding, including (1) treatment response and decreases in the severity of symptoms is not uniform across anxiety disorders, or (2) disorder-specific outcome measures differ in their sensitivity to treatment effects [34]. Regardless of the reason(s) for the discrepancy, reliance on effect-size estimates to indicate relative treatment efficacy is unwise. Effect sizes are also limited in their ability to convey an estimate of the absolute efficacy of a treatment, and alternative methods are needed to determine the clinical significance of treatments. In the next section, we consider the extent to which

psychological treatments produce clinically significant change.

Do psychological therapies produce clinically significant change?

Fisher and Durham conducted a clinical significance review of six clinical trials conducted between 1990 and 1998 [29]. All studies used the trait version of State-Trait Anxiety Inventory (STAI-T; [37]) permitting standardized outcome criteria to be established using clinical significance methodology proposed by Jacobson and colleagues (e.g., [38]. In summary, the two most effective psychological treatments for GAD were individual AR and CBT. A limitation of the Fisher and Durham analysis was that it relied solely on the STAI-T to index clinically significant change [29].

Fisher addressed this limitation [39], in an updated clinical significance review by including and developing standardized clinical significance criteria for the PSWQ as well as the STAI-T [32]. Raw data were pooled across 11 randomized controlled trials for GAD conducted between 1990 and 2006 (see [39] for full details of the review). The final data set comprised only treatment completers, and clinical studies had to use the STAI-T and/or the PSWQ to be eligible for inclusion. For the STAI-T, ten controlled studies are included ($n = 495$) and the reanalysis on the PSWQ is based on five studies ($n = 223$). The development of standardized clinical significance criteria provides a benchmark figure against which to judge the efficacy of emerging therapies. Accordingly, the first comparative controlled trial of MCT and group cognitive therapy based on the IOU model were included [40, 41]. A summary of the recovery rates as indexed by the STAI-T and the PSWQ for the three most widely evaluated psychological treatments (CBT, CT, and AR) aggregated across clinical trials, together with MCT and group IOU therapy can be seen in Table 3.1. Although, evaluation of CT based on the IOU model and MCT are in their infancy, both treatments appear to hold promise for improving the efficacy of psychological treatments for GAD. Both approaches focus on modifying excessive and uncontrollable worry, but target different underlying psychological mechanisms. Group IOU CT was equivalent to CBT at post-treatment, with both treatment approaches achieving a 48% recovery rate on the PSWQ. However, at

Table 3.1 Aggregated recovery rates by treatment type

Treatment	STAI-T				PSWQ			
	n	Post-treatment	n	One-year follow-up	n	Post-treatment	n	One-year follow-up
Applied relaxation	95	34%	57	46%	65	37%	56	38%
Cognitive therapy	109	36%	74	37%	41	37%	39	33%
Cognitive–behavioral therapy	97	46%	40	63%	42	48%	40	53%
Group IOU therapy	–	–	–	–	23	48%	22	64%
Metacognitive therapy	10	80%	10	60%	10	80%	10	80%

(Adapted from Fisher [39])

12-month follow-up, the recovery rates for IOU substantially increased to 64%, which outperforms the aggregated recovery rates for AR, CT, and CBT.

How well does MCT for GAD perform? Metacognitive therapy achieved recovery rates of 80% at post-treatment on both the STAI-T and the PSWQ, with the gains largely maintained through to one-year follow-up. Metacognitive therapy achieved the highest recovery rates at post-treatment by any treatment condition across all studies on both the STAI-T and the PSWQ. In addition MCT was relatively brief with a range of eight to twelve sessions delivered suggesting that it could prove to be a time efficient, as well as a very effective, intervention. However, the small sample precludes drawing firm conclusions and clearly larger scale comparative trials and independent replication are required to further establish the efficacy of MCT for GAD.

The two versions of the analysis of clinical significance lead to quite different conclusions in terms of the relative efficacy of psychological treatments for GAD. Aggregated recovery rates from the earlier review suggested that AR and CBT were the most effective treatments, with a slight advantage for AR. The inclusion of a further four studies evaluating the main forms of CBT significantly revises the hierarchy of treatment efficacy. In Fisher [39], the recovery rates on both the STAI-T and PSWQ suggests that CBT is more effective than either AR or CT alone.

This concurs with the meta-analytic results obtained by Borkovec and Ruscio [28]. However, the disorder-specific treatments, especially MCT are both more effective than the older treatments. This suggests that identifying and modifying the psychological mechanisms responsible for pathological worry could result in a significantly greater number of GAD patients making clinically significant change.

The metacognitive model

Wells advanced a metacognitive model and treatment of GAD with the aim of improving therapeutic outcomes (see Figure 3.1) [15]. The model provides an explanation of the development and persistence of excessive and difficult-to-control worry in people with the disorder. At the center of the model are metacognitive beliefs, metacognitive appraisals, and patterns of unhelpful regulation of thinking. The person with GAD experiences disabling anxiety and worry because s/he holds particular negative metacognitive beliefs.

On experiencing a negative thought, the person with GAD activates extended negative thinking in the form of worry. This process is termed Type I worry and consists of thinking about a range of potential threats and ways of dealing with them or avoiding them. For example, while reading a newspaper an individual may see an item about crime and has the

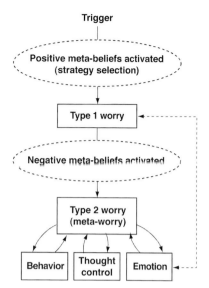

Figure 3.1 The metacognitive model of generalized anxiety disorder. From Wells A. *Cognitive Therapy of Anxiety Disorders: A Practice Manual and Conceptual Guide*. Chichester, UK: Wiley. 1997, p. 204 [45]. ©1997 John Wiley & Sons Limited. Reprinted with permission.

triggering thought: "What if that happened to me?" This is followed by extended worry about crime and how to avoid it and prevent oneself and one's family becoming a victim. This worry process persists because the individual holds positive beliefs about the usefulness of worrying. Positive metacognitive beliefs include the following:

"If I think of everything that can go wrong I can avoid it."
"Worrying about the future means I'll be prepared."
"If I worry I will be more thorough."
"Worrying stops me from missing something important."
"Worrying helps me cope."

Positive beliefs like this are not specific to GAD, and according to the model most people hold them to some degree. Holding such beliefs simply means the person is prone to engage in extended worry in response to negative ideas. This extended negative conceptual activity or Type I worry can increase anxiety and influence mood but these feelings are alleviated when the person appraises that their worrying is having the desired effect of meeting their goals. However, the person prone to GAD may be less flexible in their control of thinking styles, which

manifests as a tendency to overuse worrying at the expense of alternative means of dealing with negative thoughts and potential threats.

As a result of social learning and the consequences of repeated worrying, negative beliefs about worrying develop. Events that can lead to negative belief formation include negative interpretation of anxiety symptoms caused by Type I worry, exposure to negative information about stress and mental health, and the effect that worry can have on adaptive processes such as emotional processing. For example, a patient with GAD described how she had been a worrier from an early age, and later in life her mother suffered a "nervous breakdown" after which she reasoned that this fate also awaited her if she could not stop worrying. Negative beliefs about worrying and heightened distress developed from this time.

Two broad domains of negative beliefs are important: (1) beliefs about the uncontrollability or worry; and (2) beliefs about the meaning and harmful effects of worrying. Once negative beliefs develop these become activated in worry episodes and lead to an increased sense of threat. The activation of these beliefs gives rise to Type II worry (meta-worry) in which the person with GAD negatively interprets their process of worrying and associated symptoms. Examples of negative beliefs are:

"My worrying is uncontrollable."
"I cannot stop myself from worrying."
"Worrying can damage my body."
"Worrying could make me mentally ill."
"My worrying is a sign that I'm crazy."
"Worrying will damage my heart."

Type II worry increases the sense of immediate threat and as a consequence anxiety is heightened. When threat is seen as impending (e.g., "I'm having a nervous breakdown"), sudden increases in anxiety in the form of panic attacks may occur. As a result of Type II worry and intensified anxiety the individual finds it harder to achieve the internal subjective criteria that they use to signal that it is safe to stop worrying. Furthermore, greater anxiety can lead to lowered perceptions of the self as able to cope.

Two other sets of factors contribute to problem maintenance because they interfere with self-regulation strategies that could challenge erroneous negative metacognitive beliefs. These factors are: *behaviors* and *thought control* strategies.

Behaviors can vary, but include strategies such as seeking reassurance, avoiding triggers for worry such as news items, and adhering to familiar routines. Behaviors are a problem when they prevent the person discovering that worry is harmless and can be controlled. For example, if a person seeks reassurance when they are worried they are effectively transferring the control of their worry to another person. This interferes with the individual discovering that they can control worry themselves and erroneous beliefs about uncontrollability persist. When behaviors are successful in terminating worry this is also a problem because it can prevent the person discovering that worry does not lead to catastrophic outcomes such as mental breakdown as portrayed by their negative beliefs.

Thought-control strategies are also used that set up unhelpful patterns of self-regulation. In particular, the person with GAD often tries to suppress negative thoughts that trigger worrying, such as thoughts about illness, work situations, or accidents. The problem is that suppression is not entirely effective and its failure can reinforce negative beliefs about loss of control. However, the person with GAD rarely tries to interrupt the sustained worry process when activated and is motivated to continue with worry in order to be able to cope, further depriving themselves of consistent experiences of successful worry-control. When worry is interrupted this can have the unhelpful effect of preventing the person discovering that worry is harmless.

It is clear from this account that the model posits a range of problematic maintenance cycles. They involve negative metacognitive appraisals and beliefs about worry, and unhelpful patterns of metacognitive control in the distressing experience of worry in people with GAD.

Metacognitive therapy

Metacognitive therapy aims to modify negative beliefs about the uncontrollability and danger of worrying [15], and provide the patient with alternative non-conceptually based strategies for reacting to negative thoughts.

Treatment commences with developing an idiosyncratic case formulation based on the metacognitive model. This can be facilitated by using a case formulation interview schedule and a measure of metacognitions, behavior, and distress called the Generalized Anxiety Disorder Scale – Revised (GADS-R: [42]).

In generating a case formulation, first the therapist identifies a recent "distressing" worry episode and seeks to determine the "trigger" for the episode. The trigger is represented by the first negative thought that starts off the worry sequence. Once this is identified the therapist asks for a brief description of the content of the Type I worry and the resulting emotion. From emotion, the next stages in tracing out the formulation focus on the negative and positive metacognitions. Type II worry is elicited by asking: "When you felt anxious and experienced symptoms, did you think anything bad could happen as a result of worrying and being anxious?" Follow-up questions are also used such as: "What's the worst that could happen if you continue to worry?"

The identification of Type II worry is used as the pathway to exploring negative and positive metacognitive beliefs. Direct questions such as: "How much do you believe worry is uncontrollable?" and "What are the dangers of worrying?" can be used to elicit negative beliefs. Questions such as: "What are the advantages of worrying?" and "Is worrying helpful in some way?" are used to access positive beliefs. The therapist then goes on to determine the nature of behaviors used to cope with anxiety by asking: "Do you do anything to stop yourself worrying?" and direct questions are used that seek to determine the presence of avoidance, reassurance seeking, and using familiar routines, etc. Finally, questioning turns to elucidating the nature of "thought control" by asking: "Do you ever try not to think certain things in case it activates worry?" and "Have you ever just decided not to continue with worry when you have a negative thought?" These latter questions aim to identify the presence of thought suppression and failure to disengage the worry process.

Following on from case formulation the therapist socializes the patient by introducing the idea that the central problem is not worry (since most people worry), but beliefs about worry and the use of unhelpful responses to negative thoughts. In sharing the case formulation with the patient the initial aim is to help the patient understand how metacognitive beliefs are a problem. The therapist asks questions in order to facilitate this such as: "If you believed you could control worry how much of a problem would worry be?" and "If you believed that worry made you a better person, how distressing would worry be for you?"

The next step in socialization involves showing how the self-regulatory strategies used by the patient contribute to the problem and reinforce negative beliefs about worrying. The therapist uses a *thought suppression experiment* to show how trying not to have thoughts that might trigger worrying is not helpful in the long term. For example, the therapist suggests that an experiment is attempted in which the patient tries not to think about a "purple elephant" for the next two minutes. After this period the patient is asked what happened to their thoughts. Usually, the patient describes how the target thought occurred and this is the basis of discussion concerning how suppression of thoughts that might trigger worrying is unhelpful. If the patient was able to suppress the thought then the therapist questions why the patient cannot consistently apply this strategy to worry triggers and a discussion follows concerning the inconsistent effectiveness of this strategy.

The therapist then introduces the idea that it is beneficial to discover the truth about worrying and first of all to discover that it is not uncontrollable. Uncontrollability beliefs are modified first in MCT because these beliefs are always present in GAD, and because weakening these beliefs also weakens beliefs about the danger of worry and increases compliance with subsequent behavioral experiments aimed at testing the danger of worrying. As a prelude to an experimental test of uncontrollability an experiential technique is introduced in which the therapist suggests that instead of suppressing or worrying in response to a thought the patient tries "detached mindfulness." Detached mindfulness (DM) refers to being aware of a thought and disengaging any coping or further appraisal process from it [43]. Several exercises have been developed to facilitate this experience [14]. In order to facilitate this experience the therapist can suggest that first suppression is tried, and then the target thought is allowed to remain in consciousness and the patient watches it in a detached way without influencing the thought or analyzing it. This technique is helpful in enabling the patient to discriminate between an initial thought (trigger) and sustained responses to that thought. It also enables patients to exercise appropriate control over thinking processes rather than inappropriate suppression of content.

In addition to introduction of DM, the therapist also introduces the worry-postponement experiment. It is suggested that the next time the patient notices a worry trigger, that s/he applies DM and postpones any reactive worrying until a specified 15-minute worry period at the end of the day. All worry triggers during the day should be treated in this way. This is set as a homework task. The therapist is explicit in giving a rationale for this experiment as a "means of testing your belief that worrying is uncontrollable." In introducing this experiment the therapist takes the utmost care to be sure that the patient understands the difference between "suppression" and worry postponement. In postponement the patient is not asked to remove the content of a negative thought from consciousness, but to simply suspend any sustained worry response normally made to that content.

Further verbal and behavioral reattribution strategies are undertaken over the next few sessions to fully challenge belief in uncontrollability. For example, the patient can be encouraged to worry more and try to lose control of worry in the session, and for homework to provide more evidence that worrying cannot become uncontrollable.

Throughout these and the other strategies of MCT the therapist monitors the patient's belief level using verbal ratings and the GADS-R. Once beliefs concerning uncontrollability are at zero percent, the therapist decides to focus on modifying beliefs about the danger of worrying. It is important to deal with these beliefs because the patient should not simply be allowed to think that they now have control over worrying and therefore can avert any danger associated with it.

Verbal methods such as questioning the evidence for the dangerous effects of worry, challenging the purported mechanism of such effects, and examining counter-evidence is undertaken. Behavioral experiments are run in which dangerous outcomes are tested. For example, a patient believed that worrying would damage her heart because it elevated her heart rate. The therapist ran an experiment with her in which the effects of worrying on heart rate were compared with the effects of physical exercise. The patient learned that exercise increased her heart rate more than worry did, and the therapist was able to question whether this meant that exercise was more dangerous than worry, and thereby weaken the patient's belief.

The therapist moves onto the next stage of treatment consisting of challenging positive beliefs about worry once beliefs about danger have been effectively challenged (i.e., they are all at zero percent). Why challenge positive beliefs when these are not the direct cause of GAD in the model? The answer to this is that the model predicts that use of worrying as a predominant mode of dealing with negative thoughts and stress can generate its own problems, such as failed emotional processing, that increase vulnerability to psychological disorder. Thus, dealing with positive beliefs is a means of further increasing metacognitive flexibility and reducing general vulnerability.

Positive beliefs are modified using standard verbal reattribution techniques of questioning the evidence and generating counter-evidence, and through specially designed behavioral experiments such as the *worry modulation experiment*. The therapist asks the patient to deliberately increase worry on a particular occasion and then abandon worry to test whether increasing the activity increases positive outcomes. For instance, a patient who believed that worrying made him more thorough at work was asked to worry more on one work day and to abandon worry on the next to see if it influenced how many mistakes he made. After conducting the experiment the patient found that he was thorough in his job, irrespective of his level of worry.

After positive beliefs have been challenged, the final stage of treatment is consolidating the range of new ways of relating to negative thoughts that are an alternative to the old worry routine. The therapist and patient work together to compile and write out a therapy blueprint containing the case formulation evidence against negative and positive beliefs, and a plan of how to respond to negative thoughts and worries in the future. Any work on residual metacognitive beliefs as indicated on the GADS-R is undertaken, and the patient is discharged to follow-up when this is complete.

Conclusion

This chapter presented an overview of the nature and prevalence of GAD and the cognitive–behavioral approaches used to treat this disorder. Empirical analysis of the efficacy of treatments shows that cognitive–behavioral interventions, especially those involving cognitive restructuring, are effective. However, only approximately 50% of patients can be classified as recovered using formal criteria when the outcomes are aggregated. These figures reveal scope for significant improvements to be made in the efficacy of treatments.

One way to improve outcome is to base treatment on a model that explains the mechanisms giving rise to difficult to control and distressing worry, the most central feature of GAD. Earlier treatments have tended to be based more on techniques (e.g., relaxation) and general models of anxiety rather than a specific model of worry, with a few exceptions [41, 15].

One of those exceptions – the metacognitive model and treatment – was described in this chapter with consideration of the stages of treatment and the decision criteria for sequencing and moving between the stages. It is beyond the scope of this chapter to review evidence for the metacognitive model, but support is accumulating and the interested reader can find reviews in other sources [44, 42].

Preliminary indications suggest that MCT is an effective treatment for GAD and it can be delivered in a small number of sessions, typically ten to twelve. Recovery rates appear to be high with 70 to 80% of patients meeting criteria for recovery as indexed by trait-anxiety in the two trials conducted to date. However, one of these studies is uncontrolled, and both of them use relatively small samples meaning that caution should be exercised in extrapolating from these data. A comparison between the effects of MCT and other treatments must await larger well controlled comparative evaluations before firm conclusions can be drawn.

References

1. American Psychiatric Association. *Diagnostic and Statistical Manual of Mental Disorders, 3rd edn.* Washington DC: APA, 1980.

2. Kessler RC, Dupont RL, Berglund P, Wittchen HU. Impairments in pure and comorbid generalized anxiety disorder and major depression at 12 months in two national surveys. *Am J Psychiatry* 1999; **156**, 1915–23.

3. American Psychiatric Association. *Diagnostic and Statistical Manual of Mental Disorders, 4th edn.* Washington DC: APA, 1994.

4. Offord DR, Boyle MH, Campbell D, *et al.* One year prevalence of psychiatric disorder in Ontarians 15 to 64 years of age. *Can J Psychiatry* 1996; **41**: 559–63.

5. Hunt C, Issakidis C, Andrews G. DSM-IV generalized anxiety disorder in the Australian National Survey of Mental Health and Well-being. *Psychol Med* 2002; **32**: 649–59.

6. Wittchen HU, Zhaos S, Kessler R, Eaton W. DSM-III-R generalized anxiety disorder in the National Comorbidity Survey. *Arch Gen Psychiatry* 1994; **51**: 355–64.

7. Maier W, Gansicke M, Freyberger HJ, *et al.* Generalized anxiety disorder (ICD-10) in primary care from a cross-

cultural perspective: a valid diagnostic entry? *Acta Psychiatrica Scandinavica* 2000; **101**: 29–36.

8. Olfson M, Fireman B, Weissman MM, *et al.* Mental disorders and disability among patients in a primary care group practice. *Am J Psychiatry* 1997; **154**: 1734–40.

9. Ansseau M, Dierick M, Buntinkx F, *et al.* High prevalence of mental disorders in primary care. *J Affect Disord* 2004; **78**: 49–55.

10. Yonkers K, Massion A, Warshaw M, Keller M. Phenomenology and course of generalised anxiety disorder. *Br J Psychiatry* 1996; **168**: 308–13.

11. Yonkers K, Dyck I, Warshaw M, Keller M. Factors predicting the clinical course of generalised anxiety disorder. *Br J Psychiatry* 2000; **176**: 544–9.

12. Kessler RC, Nelson CB, McGonagle KA, *et al.* Comorbidity of DSM-III-R major depressive disorder in general population: results from the US National Comorbidity Survey. *Br J Psychiatry* 1996; **168**: 17–30.

13. Borkovec TD, Robinson E, Pruzinsky T, DePree JA. Preliminary exploration of worry: some characteristics and processes. *Behav Res Ther* 1983; **21**: 9–16.

14. Wells A. A metacognitive model and therapy for generalised anxiety disorder. *Clin Psychol Psychother* 1999; **6**: 86–96.

15. Wells A. Meta-cognition and worry: a cognitive model of generalised anxiety disorder. *Behav Cogn Psychother* 1995; **23**: 301–20.

16. Wells A, Morrison T. Qualitative dimensions of normal worry and normal obsessions: a comparative study. *Behav Res Ther* 1994; **32**: 867–70.

17. Ruscio AM, Borkovec TD. Experience and appraisal of worry among high worriers with and without generalized anxiety disorder. *Behav Res Ther* 2004; **42**: 1469–82.

18. Dugas MJ, Gagnon F, Ladouceur R, Freeston MH. Generalized anxiety disorder: a preliminary test of a conceptual model. *Behav Res Ther* 1998; **36**(2): 215–26.

19. Jacobson E. *Progressive Relaxation*. Chicago, IL: University of Chicago Press, 1938.

20. Ost L. Applied relaxation: description of a coping technique and review of controlled studies. *Behav Res Ther* 1987; **25**: 397–409.

21. Goldfried MR. Systematic desensitization as training in self control. *J Consult Clin Psychol* 197; **137**: 228–34.

22. Borkovec TD, Newman M, Pincus A, Lytle R. A component analysis of cognitive behavioral therapy for generalized anxiety disorder and the role of interpersonal problems. *J Consult Clin Psychol* 2002; **70**(2): 288–98.

23. Beck AT, Emery G, Greenberg R. *Anxiety Disorder and Phobias: A Cognitive Perspective*. New York: Basic Books, 1985.

24. National Institute for Health and Clinical Excellence. Anxiety (amended): management of anxiety (panic disorder, with or without agoraphobia, and generalized anxiety disorder) in adults in primary, secondary or community care. NICE Clinical Guideline 22 (amended). London: NICE, 2007.

25. Chambless DL, Gillis MM. Cognitive therapy of anxiety disorders. *J Consult Clin Psychol* 1993; **61**(2): 248–60.

26. Gould R, Otto M, Pollack M, Yap L. Cognitive behavioural and pharmacological treatment of generalized anxiety disorder: a preliminary meta-analysis. *Behav Ther* 1997; **28**: 285–305.

27. Mitte K. Meta-analysis of cognitive-behavioral treatments for generalized anxiety disorder: a comparison with pharmacotherapy. *Psychol Bull* 2005; **131**(5): 785–95.

28. Borkovec TD, Ruscio A. Psychotherapy for generalized anxiety disorder. *J Clin Psychiatry* 2001; **62** (suppl 11): 37–42.

29. Fisher PL, Durham RC. Recovery rates in generalised anxiety disorder following psychological therapy: an analysis of clinically significant change in STAI-T across outcome studies since 1990. *Psychol Med* 1999; **29**: 1425–34.

30. Hunot V, Churchill R, Teixeira V, Silva De Lima M. Psychological therapies for generalised anxiety disorder. *Cochrane Database Syst Rev* 2007; **1**: CD001848.

31. Covin R, Ouimet AJ, Seeds PM, Dozois DJA. A meta-analysis of CBT for pathological worry among clients with GAD. *J Anxiety Disord* 2008; **22**(1): 108–16.

32. Meyer TJ, Miller ML, Metzger RL, Borkovec TD. Development and validation of the Penn State Worry Questionnaire. *Behav Res Ther* 1990; **28**: 487–95.

33. Borkovec TD, Newman MG, Castonguay LG. Cognitive-behavioral therapy for generalized anxiety disorder with integrations from interpersonal and experiental therapies. *CNS Spectr* 2003; **8**(5): 382–9.

34. Norton PJ, Price EC. A meta-analytic review of adult cognitive-behavioral treatment outcome across the anxiety disorders. *J Nerv Ment Dis* 2007; **195**(6): 521–31.

35. Hofmann SG, Smits JAJ. Cognitive-Behavioral Therapy for adult anxiety disorders: a meta-analysis of randomized placebo-controlled trials. *J Clin Psychiatry* 2008; **69**: 621–32.

36. Westen D, Morrison, K. A multi-dimensional meta-analysis of treatments for depression, panic and

generalized anxiety disorder: an empirical examination of the status of empirically supported therapies. *J Consult Clin Psychol* 2001; **69**: 875–99.

37. Spielberger CD, Gorsuch RL, Lushene R, Vagg PR, Jacobs GA. *Manual for the State-Trait Anxiety Inventory (Form Y Self-evaluation Questionnaire)*. Palo Alto, CA: Consulting Psychologists Press, 1983.

38. Jacobson NS, Truax P. Clinical significance: a statistical approach to defining meaningful change in psychotherapy research. *J Consult Clin Psychol* 1991; **59**(1): 12–19.

39. Fisher PL. The effectiveness of psychological treatments for Generalized Anxiety Disorder. In Davey G, Wells A, eds. *Worry and Psychological Disorders: Assessment and Treatment*. Chichester: John Wiley & Sons Ltd, 2006.

40. Wells A, Welford M, King P, *et al.* A pilot randomized trial of metacognitive therapy vs applied relaxation in the treatment of adults with generalized anxiety

disorder. *Behav Res Ther* 2010; doi:10.1016/j.brat.2009.11.013.

41. Dugas MJ, Ladoucer R, Leger E, *et al.* Group cognitive-behavioural therapy for generalized anxiety disorder: treatment outcome and long-term follow-up. *J Consult Clin Psychol* 2003; **71**(4): 821–5.

42. Wells A. *Metacognitive Therapy for Anxiety and Depression*. New York: Guilford Press, 2008.

43. Wells A, Matthews, G. *Attention and Emotion: A Clinical Perspective*. Hove UK: Erlbaum, 1994.

44. Wells A. The metacognitive model of worry and generalized anxiety disorder. In Davey GCL, Wells A, eds. *Worry and its Psychological Disorders: Theory, Assessment and Treatment*. Chichester, UK: Wiley. 2006, pp. 179–99.

45. Wells A. *Cognitive Therapy of Anxiety Disorders: A Practice Manual and Conceptual Guide*. Chichester, UK: Wiley, 1997.

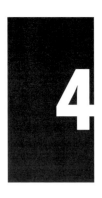

Social anxiety disorder

Tejal A. Jakatdar and Richard G. Heimberg

The nature of social anxiety disorder

Social anxiety disorder (also known as social phobia) is defined as "a marked or persistent fear of one or more social or performance situations" by the *Diagnostic and Statistical Manual of Mental Disorders*, 4th edition, text revision [1]. Individuals with social anxiety disorder may experience anxiety and/or avoidance of a variety of social situations, including parties, public speaking, dating situations, and expressing onself assertively, among others. Most socially anxious individuals are afraid of being judged negatively and/or doing something that would be perceived as humiliating or embarrassing. Common somatic symptoms include palpitations, dizziness, numbness or tingling sensations, abdominal distress, dry mouth, sweating, and blushing. These symptoms may be the same as those experienced in other anxiety disorders; however, in socially anxious individuals, they are situationally bound, that is, cued by anxiety-provoking social situations or thoughts in anticipation of them. To meet criteria for social anxiety disorder, individuals must realize that the fear they experience in these situations is excessive or unreasonable.

In the current diagnostic system, socially anxious individuals fall into one of two subcategories depending on the pervasiveness of their fears. Individuals who fear most social situations (typically involving social interaction, public speaking, or performance of other activities in front of others) meet the criteria for the generalized subtype of social anxiety disorder. Individuals whose fear is related to a specific social situation or a limited number of situations are said to have non-generalized social anxiety disorder [1]. A number of authors have questioned the utility of this subtyping scheme, as it appears to have simply dichotomized the continuum of number of feared social situations [2, 3]. However, generalized social anxiety disorder is more likely to aggregate in families [4] and is associated with greater comorbidity and impairment [5] than non-generalized social anxiety disorder.

Socially anxious individuals typically experience significant impairment in their social, educational, and occupational functioning [6]. More individuals with social anxiety seek public assistance, and they are more likely to work at jobs that are below their capacity and believe that their supervisors think poorly of them than their non-socially anxious counterparts [7]. A significant number of individuals with social anxiety disorder experience a lack of friendships/social support, fewer dating partners, and hence, a lower quality of life [6, 8]. In one study, a larger percentage of the individuals with social anxiety disorder had never married compared to individuals with panic disorder and agoraphobia [9].

Social anxiety disorder is a common psychiatric disorder. According to Kessler and colleagues, the 12-month prevalence rate is 6.8% and the lifetime prevalence rate is 12.1% [10, 11]. Social anxiety disorder often begins during early childhood or adolescence, and the disorder may follow a chronic course [12]. However, individuals with the generalized subtype may have an earlier onset than individuals with the non-generalized subtype [13]. The average elapsed time between development of social anxiety disorder and the time at which individuals seek treatment is about 20 years, and treatment is most often sought when the person has developed a comorbid disorder or other complications of social anxiety disorder [12]. Epidemiological studies suggest gender differences, in that women are more likely to suffer from the disorder than men [10]. Although Rapee and

Cognitive–behavioral Therapy with Adults: A Guide to Empirically Informed Assessment and Intervention, ed. Stefan G. Hofmann and Mark A. Reinecke. © Cambridge University Press 2010.

colleagues suggest that men and women seek treatment at about equal rates [14], others suggest that the ratio in both treatment and epidemiological samples is closer to 3:2, favoring women in the community samples and men in treatment samples [15, 16].

More than 80% of individuals suffering from social anxiety disorder meet criteria for at least one additional Axis I diagnosis, and the onset of social anxiety disorder most commonly precedes the onset of the comorbid condition [17]. Most common comorbid Axis I diagnoses include specific phobia, agoraphobia, major depression, and alcohol abuse and dependence [17]. Social anxiety disorder, which has an early onset, may be a marker for other comorbid conditions developing later in life, including other anxiety disorders, mood disorders, and substance use disorders [13]. Comorbidity of psychiatric conditions complicates treatment and may lead to a poorer prognosis in general. Moreover, individuals with social anxiety and comorbid depression or substance abuse may have a greater number of suicide attempts and are more likely to report a poorer quality of life and greater use of medications to control their symptoms [17]. Studies by Katzelnick and colleagues [5] and Stein and colleagues [18] also suggest a higher rate of suicide attempts among individuals with generalized social anxiety disorder and comorbid depression than individuals without generalized social anxiety disorder without comorbid depression.

Family studies suggest that social anxiety disorder may be at least partially inherited; there may be a threefold increase in the rate of social anxiety disorder in the relatives of patients [19]. Furthermore, twin studies suggest that the heritability of social anxiety disorder is 30 to 50% [20]. The comorbidity between social anxiety and depression may also be genetically mediated [20]. Environmental factors such as parental anxiety and parental attitudes about child rearing may influence the development and maintenance of social anxiety [21]. Children may learn from parents that the world is a dangerous place and that they have little control over the outcomes of social situations. Furthermore, negative peer and social experiences or embarrassing social incidents may contribute to the development and maintenance of social anxiety disorder [17].

Cognitive models of social anxiety disorder

The core cognitive feature of social anxiety disorder is *fear of negative evaluation* [22, 23]. In the model proposed by Rapee and Heimberg [23, 24], the cycle of social anxiety is initiated with the perception of an *audience*, that is, someone who may potentially evaluate the person, whether this potential evaluation is real or imagined (see Figure 4.1 for a schematic presentation of Rapee and Heimberg's model). In the presence of the perceived audience, the individual forms a *mental representation of the self as seen by the audience*, that is, he or she forms an image of how he or she appears to the other person [23]. The mental representation is informed by distorted negative images based to varying degrees on real or perceived negative feedback from others, biased attention for threat in past social situations, and the biased memory for the outcome of these events that may have been created in part by attention to threat at the time of these events, as well as current fears of negative evaluation.

Socially anxious individuals may compare this mental representation of the self as seen by the audience to their perception of the audience's standards for their performance. On the one hand, we have a self-image that is negatively distorted and, on the other hand, we have perceived expectations that are likely to be distorted in the opposite direction. This comparison leads to a significant discrepancy between what the individual believes himself or herself to be able to do and what the individual believes is expected of him or her by the other person(s); thus, the socially anxious individual believes that he or she will almost always fall short of expectations and be negatively evaluated by the audience. The perception of negative evaluation gives rise to physical (heart pounding, sweating, dry mouth, etc.), cognitive (negative thoughts about oneself and one's performance – e.g., "I will make a fool of myself," "I will fail," etc.), and behavioral (avoidance of social situations, stuttering, fidgeting, etc.) symptoms of anxiety, in rough proportion to the degree of discrepancy between the mental representation of the self as seen by the audience and the perception of the audience's standards. These symptoms in turn lead the individual to believe that he or she has, "in fact," been perceived negatively by others. This judgment may be further "supported" by internal physiological sensations. Importantly, external indicators provide further information (e.g., somebody looking at their watch may give the indication that they are bored) that feeds into the mental representation of the self as seen by the audience, ratcheting it toward the negative, and the cycle begins

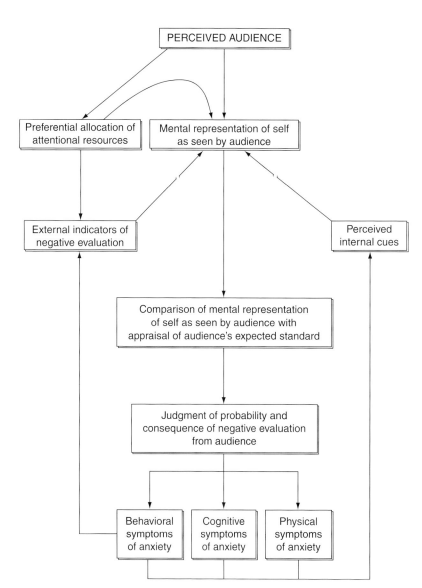

Figure 4.1 A model of the generation and maintenance of anxiety in social/evaluative situations. Reprinted from Rapee RM, Heimberg RG. A cognitive-behavioral model of anxiety in social phobia. *Behav Res Ther* 1997; **35**(8): 743 [23]. ©1997, with kind permission from Elsevier.

anew. Unfortunately for socially anxious persons, it is this perception of the situation that is likely to be encoded into memory, setting them off on bad footing for the next social situation. Furthermore, it is quite likely that the person's focus of attention on these mental representations interferes with the quality of his or her actual behavioral performance, which can only exacerbate the cycle described above.

Clark and Wells [22] have discussed the role of *safety behaviors* in the maintenance of social anxiety disorder. A safety behavior is a behavior that the individual will perform in order to feel less anxious or to avoid the feared outcome in a social situation.

For example, a person who fears that she will have nothing to say during social conversations may rehearse what she will say next rather than allow herself to participate in the conversation and participate spontaneously; similarly, a person fearful of public speaking may prepare for hours on end, far beyond that required by the nature of the upcoming speaking engagement. As socially anxious individuals may not engage in social situations without using safety behaviors, they may attribute social successes to these behaviors and discount information that might otherwise serve to disconfirm their negative beliefs about themselves in social situations. In addition Clark and

Wells have also discussed post-event processing, that is, the tendency of persons with social anxiety to ruminate about the outcomes of social situations. Usually the processing is negative and leads to more negative cognitions and emotions, thereby helping maintain social anxiety (see [25] for a review of the construct).

Hofmann [26] has recently proposed a model of the maintenance of social anxiety disorder. According to this model, a socially anxious individual enters a situation with high perceived social standards and poorly defined social goals. These factors lead to social apprehension – the expectation that things will not work out well – which, in turn, leads to heightened self-focused attention. A number of other cognitive processes are also called into play – negative self-perception, high estimated social costs, low perceived emotional control, and perceived poor social skills. These processes further increase the person's belief that the situation will turn out badly, which, in turn, leads to avoiding the situation and/or using safety behaviors in the situation to avoid the anxiety or the feared consequences. Most individuals will engage in post-event rumination (same as post-event processing described above) of the actual or perceived specific negative aspects of the situation or their behaviors, cognitions, and physiological symptoms. The rumination will feed back into the social apprehension. This chain will help maintain the high perceived social standards and the tendency to set unachievable social goals.

The models by Rapee and Heimberg [23] and by Clark and Wells [22] have great similarities in that they both emphasize the importance of internal representations in socially anxious individuals in social situations. The major difference between the models appears to be on the relative emphasis placed on the role of external threat [24]. Clark and Wells focus only on internal representations, placing great emphasis on the notion that the person turns inward to gather further information once a social threat has been detected in the environment. In contrast, Rapee and Heimberg have described both internal and external cues and how they may influence formation or (re)calibration of the mental representation of the self as seen by the audience as a social situation unfolds. Changes in audience behavior can impact individuals' responses. Hofmann's [26] promising new model emphasizes different elements in the cognitive–behavioral cycle of the maintenance of social anxiety but requires further evaluation.

Empirical support for efficacy and effectiveness of treatment

Although there have been a multitude of studies of the efficacy of cognitive–behavioral therapies and pharmacotherapies for social anxiety disorder (and a smaller number of studies of dynamically oriented and interpersonal psychotherapies), this review will focus on the combination of exposure and cognitive techniques (a broader qualitative review of the cognitive–behavioral treatment outcome literature is provided by [27], and a recent meta-analysis of placebo-controlled studies of cognitive–behavioral therapy, CBT, is provided by [28]; a review of pharmacotherapy for social anxiety disorder is provided by [29]).

A substantial literature demonstrates that the combination of exposure and cognitive techniques leads to strong treatment gains. These treatments are superior to wait-list control groups [30, 31, 32], educational-supportive control therapy [33, 34], and pill placebo [34, 35]. Furthermore, gains are maintained over follow-up periods of up to five years [36, 37]. Cognitive–behavioral therapies have been demonstrated to produce response rates equivalent to the monoamine oxidase inhibitor phenelzine [34] and equal to [38] or superior to the selective serotonin reuptake inhibitor fluoxetine [35]. However, gains following CBT are more resistant to relapse following the discontinuation of medication [39]. Recent research indicates that the administration of D-cycloserine, the partial agonist of N-methyl-D-aspartate, may potentiate the effects of cognitive–behavioral treatment [40].

It is of great import to demonstrate that treatments tested under highly controlled conditions can be successfully administered in clinical settings, and three studies of this nature have been conducted for the cognitive–behavioral treatment of social anxiety disorder. Gaston and colleagues [41] compared the effectiveness of group CBT for social anxiety disorder developed and evaluated in a research unit to that of the same cognitive–behavioral treatment administered in a private practice setting. Treatment was equally effective for both groups, and gains were maintained at a three-month follow-up. Additional studies by Lincoln and colleagues [42] and McEvoy [43] examined the effectiveness of individual or group CBT in community settings and demonstrated effects comparable to those reported in randomized controlled trials.

Introduction to a clinical case

Monica was a 25-year-old woman who presented with significant anxiety in social situations. She had finished college with a degree in psychology three years prior to evaluation and was unemployed despite significant financial need. Monica described herself as having always been shy and inhibited in social situations. As a child, it was difficult for her to make friends. In school, Monica was severely and repeatedly teased for stuttering. She had seen a speech therapist for several years when she was in school. Although she rarely stuttered in the present day, it sometimes did occur when she was very anxious in social situations.

At intake, Monica lived alone. She avoided taking on a roommate even though she could have benefited from the financial support that a roommate would provide. She had a few friends, and she socialized with them only occasionally. Monica had been on a handful of dates, but she had not enjoyed the experience and decided that she did not want to put herself through the anxiety of dating any longer. She had attended a few parties in college, but she was always quite anxious doing so, and she rarely attended parties after graduation. When she did go to parties, she drank alcohol to feel more comfortable and did not believe that she could cope with the anxiety she experienced without drinking. She would only interact with people she knew well and would avoid making new acquaintances.

Monica also reported trouble with public speaking and with stating her opinion. In college, she avoided taking courses that would require her to speak up in class, answer questions, or make presentations. Monica was very interested in pursuing a doctoral degree in psychology but had shied away from doing so because of the heavy emphasis on presentation and participation in class discussion. Furthermore, she was terrified at the prospect of presenting her academic work at professional conferences and answering questions about her work. Monica was also very interested in the clinical aspect of the field, but she was very anxious about developing rapport with clients and conducting psychotherapy with them. At the time of the evaluation, Monica reported being depressed and unhappy about the many opportunities she felt she had lost, not only socially but also professionally. She described herself as feeling very isolated.

In addition to a diagnosis of generalized social anxiety disorder, Monica was assigned a diagnosis of depressive disorder not otherwise specified. Monica had some depressive symptoms but did not meet criteria for a diagnosis of major depressive disorder. She had, at times in the past, met criteria for alcohol abuse, but this was not currently the case, as she was more likely to avoid problematic situations than drink in them.

Overview of the treatment protocol

General structure of sessions

The treatment protocol summarized in this chapter was developed by Hope, Heimberg, Juster, and Turk [44, 45]. It is a manualized protocol that incorporates cognitive restructuring and exposure to feared social situations. Clients learn cognitive restructuring skills that they can utilize during exposures conducted both in session and as part of between-session homework assignments. As with any manualized treatment, therapists must flexibly implement the protocol in a manner that suits the needs of the individual client [46]. In Monica's case, special attention was paid to her fears of stuttering and her anxious thoughts related to it.

The *Managing Social Anxiety* client workbook [44] consists of 14 chapters that guide treatment over the course of 16 to 20 weekly sessions. Treatment may vary, depending on the nature of the social anxiety, treatment compliance, therapeutic alliance, comorbid conditions, and extra-therapeutic events such as holidays, vacations, and illnesses. Clients are assigned readings and other homework tasks at the end of every session, which are then reviewed at the beginning of the subsequent session. The treatment is broken down into five segments that are presented below. Monica's treatment lasted 19 sessions that included all of these segments.

The therapeutic relationship

In this protocol, the therapeutic relationship is collaborative in nature. In the first segment of treatment (see below), the therapist takes an active role in educating the client about social anxiety disorder and developing a mutual understanding of the client's specific concerns. The therapist involves the client as much as possible to draw parallels between concepts raised in the workbook and the client's experiences, but respects the reticence that is often present at the beginning of treatment of socially anxious persons. The client is very much involved in the development of his or her fear and avoidance hierarchy and during the cognitive restructuring and exposure phases of the treatment. The therapist and client work collaboratively to develop the content of in-session and in vivo exposures.

Although this is a manualized treatment protocol, empathy, mutual respect, and trust are emphasized and considered an integral part of therapy adherence [46]. Therapists are rated on different dimensions such as active listening, responding to verbal and non-verbal cues, communicating support and investment in the client, and facilitating the client's investment in the treatment. A recent study by our group [47] demonstrated that the therapeutic relationship was, in fact, related to successful outcome. Client ratings of therapeutic alliance were positively related to session helpfulness.

When Monica first started treatment, she was shy, spoke little, and made very little eye contact. The therapist respected her anxiety and carried much of the interaction in the first few sessions, allowing Monica to habituate to the therapeutic context. Over time, she became more willing to speak and risk the evaluation of the therapist, who maintained a positive stance toward her at all times. Monica developed a warm relationship with the therapist, and as she became more trusting, she was more willing and able to share the details of her fears. She became an active participant in treatment and took well to the interactive nature of training in cognitive restructuring skills and in-session exposures (see below). Exposures to feared situations began slowly, given her anxiety and the therapist's desire to involve her as a collaborative partner. However, this strategy paid dividends later in therapy when Monica was hesitant to begin work on more difficult situations. The trust that had been built up in the earlier sessions allowed the therapist to ask her to push herself a bit more than she might otherwise have done and thereby facilitated the outcome of her treatment. Monica and her therapist negotiated a series of exposures to situations that she had previously avoided, and (although it is not possible to be definitive in the description of an individual client) it appears that these exposures propelled her toward a successful termination.

Strategies and techniques

Segment one: psychoeducation

The client workbook contains much of the material and strategies that drive the treatment. The first segment of treatment utilizes material from chapters 1 to 4 in the client workbook [44], which focus primarily on psychoeducation about social anxiety disorder. During this segment, much attention is paid to the therapeutic relationship (as noted above), and the therapist helps the client to gain a broader perspective on social anxiety and how it is affecting their life. This segment, especially the first three sessions, is more didactic than later sessions. The therapist attempts to engage the client as much as possible, taking into consideration the client's anxiety in session and fears of being evaluated by the therapist for sharing his or her social fears. In Monica's case, the therapist allowed her to participate as much or as little as she desired in the earlier sessions, gently encouraging her to talk about her experience of social anxiety as she became more comfortable.

Typically, one chapter a week is assigned for reading in advance of sessions, especially in the first two segments of treatment. The client is also asked to complete forms included in the assigned chapter and which are intended to teach specific concepts of relevance to social anxiety disorder. Examples of completed forms are provided. The therapist explains the homework to the client when it is assigned. At the beginning of subsequent sessions, the therapist reviews the homework with the client and asks the client to express questions, concerns, thoughts, and emotions about the homework experience. If the client has not completed the assigned homework, the therapist and client will troubleshoot the obstacles that interfered with homework completion and re-emphasize the importance of attempting these assignments.

Certain topics are reviewed in each chapter. The first session and chapter 1 focus on understanding the meaning of social anxiety from the client's perspective. The therapist presents a series of case vignettes that help the client understand that social anxiety falls on a continuum. It is strongly emphasized that social anxiety is a normal part of life. Although social anxiety may be debilitating at clinical levels, it is unrealistic to strive toward a state of perpetual freedom from it. The first session also includes a brief explanation of what the treatment program will encompass and what the client needs to do to take the most from it.

Chapter 2 focuses on describing and helping the client understand the three components of anxiety: (1) the physiological component, consisting of bodily reactions such as pounding heart; (2) the cognitive component, consisting of thoughts that the person may have in anxiety-evoking social situations such as "I will have nothing to say", and (3) the behavioral component, consisting of what the person does (behaviors that either express anxiety or are intended to control it) or does not do (avoidance) in that situation. The therapist helps the client identify each of the components that he or she experiences in anxiety-evoking situations. Finally, the therapist describes how the three components interact to create a "downward spiral" of anxiety and negative affect. Like many clients, Monica spontaneously reported a number of physiological symptoms but only came to recognize the contributions of her thoughts and behaviors as a result of this discussion and the accompanying homework assignments. She acknowledged that, in a typical social situation, she first becomes aware of irregularities in her heart rate and breathing, which lead her to think about how poorly she will be/is performing in the social situation, which lead her to break eye contact and reduce her verbal output. Self-observation of her social withdrawal leads to negative self-evaluation and fear of the same from others, which is followed by another burst of physiological arousal.

The third chapter gives the client a chance to reflect on how his or her social anxiety may have originated and been maintained. The roles of genetics, family interactions, and important life events are discussed. The client is given the opportunity to discuss how these factors may have played a role in the development of his or her social anxiety. Monica related to all three aspects – she mentioned that her mother was socially withdrawn and always paid a great deal of attention to the evaluation of others. Furthermore, Monica also related several instances of severe teasing about her stuttering and problems with obesity that she experienced as a child that helped to shape and maintain her social anxiety. The therapist empathized with Monica's history and pointed out that social anxiety is primarily learned and can be changed through new learning and experiences. After some further discussion of dysfunctional thinking and how

it may relate to physiological and behavioral symptoms of anxiety, the therapist laid the groundwork for the combination of cognitive restructuring and exposures to come.

The fourth session is an important one in which the client and therapist collaboratively discuss the client's feared social situations and work together to develop a fear and avoidance hierarchy, a graduated list of feared social situations that will provide both a roadmap to the development of exposure exercises and one method of evaluating progress in treatment. The therapist also helps the client examine subtle nuances and variations on the situations that may bring about more or less anxiety. For Monica, feared situations ranged from interactions with sales people to dating situations. Monica was eager to find a job, look for a roommate, and finally start dating. The subjective units of distress scale (SUDS) [48] is described and used to rate anxiety in each situation, and a similar rating of avoidance is completed. In addition, two relevant social situations are selected for self-monitoring during the week and the client also rates daily average anxiety and depression. Self-monitoring is continued throughout treatment and provides another means for evaluating clients' progress.

Segment two: training in cognitive restructuring skills

About two to three sessions are devoted to the development of cognitive restructuring skills. In session 5 and chapter 5, the training begins with the basic principle that it is not the situation itself but how we interpret it that determines our emotional and behavioral reactions. Ellis [49] referred to this idea as the ABCs – "A" is the activating event, i.e., the event that starts the process. "B" is the person's thoughts and beliefs about the situation, and "C" is the consequence or outcome of the situation (the emotional and behavioral reactions of the person, the response of others, etc.). Monica described an incident in which she approached a female classmate to study together. However, the woman gave a rather abrupt and rude response and declined to make plans with her (A, the activating event). Monica reported several thoughts in response, including "She does not see me as a good enough study partner" and "She doesn't like me because I'm so quiet" (B, her beliefs about the situation). Monica immediately withdrew from the situation, felt embarrassed and sad, and did not try to find another study partner during the remainder of her college career (C, the consequence).

It is possible that if Monica had pursued another study partner, she would have been successful. However, this would have happened only if Monica could have found alternative explanations for why the woman responded as she did when Monica approached her. A different interpretation of the situation (e.g., attribution to the classmate's issues rather than her own) may have facilitated further approach attempts. This brings us to the next concept of "automatic thoughts."

Automatic thoughts (ATs) are thoughts that pop into our heads during or in anticipation of specific situations. Among clients with anxiety or mood disorders, these thoughts are typically negative, distorted, and associated with unpleasant emotions, but they are accepted as valid without conscious examination [50]. Several exercises in the workbook facilitate the understanding of this concept and provide practice identifying ATs in different anxiety-evoking situations. Exercises for the identification of ATs are conducted both in session and as homework assignments.

The next step is identifying "thinking errors" [51]. Thinking errors are negative and irrational ways of thinking about oneself, the world, and the future that are common in ATs. Clients are trained to identify various thinking errors such as mind reading, overgeneralization, emotional reasoning, etc. The process of identifying ATs and thinking errors that occur within them forms the basis of cognitive restructuring. Some of Monica's common ATs and the thinking errors she identified with them include (1) "I will stutter and people will laugh at me" – fortune telling (predicting negative outcomes), mind reading (presuming to know what others are thinking in the absence of evidence); (2) "I will have nothing interesting to say" – fortune telling, all-or-nothing thinking (polarized thinking); and (3) "I have nothing to offer anybody" – all-or-nothing thinking, overgeneralization (making all-encompassing sweeping statements). Clients are also taught to identify emotions that are stimulated by their ATs.

The therapist next focuses on the idea that we typically do not challenge our ATs but take them as fact. Furthermore, we do not examine any evidence that may be contrary to what we believe to be true and accurate. At this stage, the client is instructed on different ways of questioning or challenging his or her ATs. The client verbalizes the dialogue between the "anxious self" (ATs) and the "coping self" (questions to dispute the evidence on which the ATs are based) to come to a rational and realistic understanding and belief about the AT (see an example of an "anxious self/coping self dialogue" in the next section). The therapist then encourages the client to generate a "rational response," which is a brief phrase that summarizes the evidence derived from this dialogue. Whenever the anxiety-provoking ATs occur during or in anticipation of the target situation, the client is instructed to use the rational response to combat them. Clients practice the cognitive restructuring steps outlined above before using them in exposures. Chapter 6 worksheets instruct them to pick anxiety-provoking situations and proceed step-by-step through the process. When they become familiar with the process, they are ready to start using cognitive restructuring during in-session exposures.

Segment three: exposures

In-session exposures begin in session 7 or 8. The first exposure session lasts 90 minutes (all other sessions are 60 minutes in duration). The therapist and client select a situation with a moderate SUDS rating (~50) from the fear and avoidance hierarchy to serve as the basis for the exposure. The therapist must be reasonably certain that the client will be able to successfully negotiate the situation to be role-played, as the nature of this in-session exposure experience will influence the client's willingness to engage in later exposures both in session and as homework assignments. In our research studies, a minimum of four in-session exposures must be completed over the course of therapy, but more is better. Every exposure session follows the format described in Table 4.1 and as described for the client in chapter 7 of the workbook. The session begins with homework review, and the client and therapist then move on to formulate the details of the exposure. A situation is selected, and the client identifies the ATs that are elicited as he or she imagines the situation. Thinking errors are identified, and disputing questions are used to help the client generate an anxious self/coping self dialogue and rational response. Finally, the client is asked to set non-perfectionistic behavioral goals for the exposure. A good behavioral goal is one that is objective, under the control of the client, can be quantified, and can be observed by others. Conversely, a poor goal is one that is based on management of the situation without anxiety or with an excessively high standard for performance.

Monica's first in-session exposure was to have a casual conversation with a neighbor. Her ATs were as

Table 4.1 Outline of exposure sessions

1. Review homework from previous week
2. Complete in-session exposure
   a. Exposure pre-processing
      (1) Briefly negotiate details of exposure
      (2) Elicit automatic thoughts
      (3) Client labels thinking errors in automatic thoughts
      (4) Client disputes one or two automatic thoughts
      (5) Client develops a rational response
      (6) Client sets non-perfectionistic, behavioral goals
   b. Conduct role-play for approximately ten minutes
      (1) Request SUDS and the rational response every minute
      (2) Track client's progress on behavioral goals
   c. Exposure post-processing
      (1) Review whether goals were attained
      (2) Discuss how well the rational response worked
      (3) Discuss any unexpected or new automatic thoughts
      (4) Client, therapist, and role-players react to client's performance
      (5) Graph and interpret SUDS ratings pattern
      (6) Client states what was learned from the exposure
3. Assignment of homework
   a. Related in vivo exposures with associated cognitive restructuring
   b. Continued self-monitoring of depression, general anxiety, and social anxiety
   c. Other assignments as appropriate

follows: "I will have nothing interesting to say"; "I will stutter"; "I will make a fool of myself"; and "I will make a very bad impression." After Monica identified the thinking errors in each of the ATs, the therapist helped her pick ATs that would be most productive to challenge. What follows is a portion of the anxious self/coping self dialogue that was conducted in preparation for the in-session exposure:

ANXIOUS SELF – I will have nothing interesting to say.

COPING SELF – Am I a 100% certain that I will have nothing interesting to say?

ANXIOUS SELF – No, but in the past I didn't have anything interesting to say.

COPING SELF – How did I decide that what I said wasn't interesting?

ANXIOUS SELF – I just feel its not interesting, but I know that's just emotional reasoning.

COPING SELF – Right, "feeling" something doesn't make it a fact. What do other people talk about, and how interesting is that anyway?

ANXIOUS SELF – They talk about lots of silly stuff – the weather, what they did for the weekend, you know, stuff like that.

COPING SELF – And what do you talk about?

ANXIOUS SELF – Same stuff. I guess that's OK, huh?

COPING SELF – Yes, it is. That's how we get to know each other. It's just a conversation and not the end of the world. It's important to say something and leave it at that.

Monica came to the rational response – "It's just a conversation." This simple statement captured for her many of the subtleties of the above dialogue – that she believes that she has little to say, but that is based on feeling rather than fact, that people talk about mundane things, that she can do that as well, and that it is most important to just get in there and participate. Monica's behavioral goals were to continue the conversation for five minutes and to say three things about herself. For the first session, the therapist typically serves as the role-player; role-play assistants are often utilized in later sessions.

The therapist records the client's SUDS ratings, before the exposure, at one-minute intervals during the exposure, and at the end of the exposure. Every time a SUDS rating is requested, the therapist also asks the client to repeat the rational response aloud. The purpose of this intervention is to help the client develop the habit of using the rational response during anxiety-provoking situations in the future. The exposure usually lasts approximately ten minutes (it may be more or less depending on the client's level of anxiety and the nature of the situation) and may continue until the SUDS have dropped and a plateau has been reached. The therapist may provide encouragement as needed so that the client will attempt the behavioral goals and will refrain from using safety behaviors.

Next is the debriefing of the in-session exposure. The therapist and client review whether the client attained the agreed-upon behavioral goals, if the client had the expected ATs, if the rational response was a useful tool for combatting these ATs, and the relative weight of the evidence from the exposure in favor of the AT versus the rational response. It is also typical to inquire whether other, unexpected ATs occurred that might require attention at that moment or in a future exposure. The therapist often graphs the SUDS ratings collected during the exposure, and the pattern of these SUDS ratings is examined. These ratings sometimes demonstrate that the anxiety decreased as the client stayed in the situation over an extended period of time. At other times, the message may be different – anxiety may not decrease by much, but the client was able to accomplish the behavioral goals despite his or her anxiety, or anxiety may have moved up and down over the course of the exposure, depending on whether the client adopted a coping stance or not. However, most all of these are positive outcomes, as they represent new learning for the client and a new perspective on his or her anxiety. As a final step in the debriefing, the therapist asks the client to verbalize what has been learned from the exposure experience and how it may be applied to real-life situations. The debriefing helps the client process the exposure in a productive way and minimizes focusing on self-perceived failure because the client was anxious during the exposure. Most often, clients obtain evidence that disconfirms their negatively biased beliefs about their performance or about how they are perceived by others.

At the end of the session, the therapist and client collaboratively pick a situation for an in vivo exposure for the client to complete as homework before the next session. The client uses a worksheet that takes him or her step by step through the cognitive restructuring process in advance of the exposure assignment. The worksheet also includes questions that are used for debriefing after the exposure has been completed. In future in-session exposures, the therapist and the client tackle more difficult variations on the same situation or progress toward other situations higher on the fear and avoidance hierarchy, and these are followed by related homework assignments. Additional reading assignments from the client workbook include an overview of issues related to ongoing exposures (chapter 8), as well as optional chapters that focus on specific topics that may be more or less central to the concerns of a specific client: chapter 9: Observational fears; chapter 10: Interaction fears; chapter 11: Public speaking fears. Monica and the therapist worked on each of the different topics mentioned above as her fears spanned the entire range. They conducted in-session and in vivo exposures to combat her fears of public speaking, doing things while being observed, and interacting with groups of varying sizes.

Segment four: advanced cognitive restructuring

Chapter 12 of the client workbook introduces the concept of "core beliefs" – the beliefs that underlie and provide the power behind ATs. After a few in-session exposures, the therapist and client may begin to notice common themes in the client's most frequent ATs. This segment focuses on understanding these themes and moving beyond situation-specific ATs. There is a helpful worksheet called "Peeling the onion" in this chapter which assists the client in peeling layers and going deeper to understand the core beliefs. Core beliefs such as "I'm worthless," "I'm unlovable," or "I'm a fraud" commonly underlie ATs such as "I won't be able to think of anything to say" or "They'll think I'm boring," which are commonly reported by socially anxious clients. These beliefs can be challenged in the same way as ATs, and this work can be conducted in-session and in vivo exposures.

Monica's core belief was that she was worthless. The therapist worked with her to restructure this core belief and also helped her realize that it was quite inaccurate. By this point, Monica had engaged in several exposures, both in and out of session. Her confidence had grown and she had started thinking differently about her abilities. Monica completed an anxious self/coping self dialogue and came to the realization that not only did her core belief rest on a number of thinking errors, but she did have something to offer to the world and she was far from worthless. This was a powerful realization that had been building throughout the treatment and that she was able to flesh out and really make her own.

Segment five: termination

Chapter 13 of the client workbook is devoted to termination. Termination may take place around session 16 for most clients. However, depending on individual client needs, the termination session may be delayed. In this session, the therapist and client review the fear and avoidance hierarchy and re-rate each item. The new ratings are compared to the ratings made earlier in treatment. With successful treatment, the fear and avoidance ratings are usually substantially reduced. This is a good place to acknowledge the progress made in treatment and to discuss future goals and relapse prevention (see below). Monica acknowledged that she had made progress in every area that she worked on and was on her way to achieving the goals she had set for herself.

Relapse prevention

In the final session, the therapist and the client address the important issue of relapse prevention. First, the therapist and client come to a mutual agreement that regularly scheduled treatment sessions have come to an end. Next, they discuss the areas that may require additional work on the part of the client in order to consolidate or build upon gains made in treatment. Collaboratively, they generate a list of goals and potential exposures to help the client move toward these goals in the upcoming months. Planning of this nature will help the client continue to use his or her newly acquired cognitive restructuring and behavioral approach skills in future social situations and reduce the chances that he or she will fall back into old avoidant habits. The therapist and Monica developed goals for her to work on and set timelines. Some of her goals included going to meetings of the local chapter of Toastmasters International and continuing her public speaking exposures, continuing to talk to people who may become potential roommates, working on finding a job and continuing to go on interviews, and continuing to go on dates.

The therapist acknowledges that there may be certain situations and life events that may set the client off course to a certain extent. Progress in the treatment of social anxiety may expose the client to situations never previously confronted (e.g., the client who has never dated has yet to experience the ups and downs of relationship conflicts). The therapist may offer two to three booster sessions to help the client troubleshoot and stay on track. Oftentimes, this offer of future assistance is helpful for clients and will make it easier for both client and therapist to terminate on a positive note.

Difficulties encountered during treatment

Expectations for treatment outcome

When clients are excited about the therapy and motivated to make changes, it bodes well for therapeutic progress. However, our clients may sometimes have unrealistic expectations about the time frame in which they will start to see progress or the amount of progress they may ultimately achieve. It is easy to see how a client may become disillusioned with the process of therapy or even discontinue therapy prematurely as a result. Several aspects of the psychoeducation sessions are devoted to this important topic – social anxiety is a normal part of life and it is unrealistic to expect that treatment will make it all go away. Self-monitoring is also instituted in the psychoeducation segment so that clients will be able to see small changes before bigger ones have a chance to occur. Throughout treatment, however, it is important for the therapist to be responsive to verbal and non-verbal cues of disappointment, frustration, and disillusionment.

In contrast to unrealistic expectations is the problem of negative expectations. In two studies, patients who found treatment to be credible and expected treatment gains did better than those who held more negative expectations regarding treatment [52, 53]. Our protocol contains assessment of expectancies for treatment outcome, which can then be discussed with the therapist. In addition, one of the exercises in the current protocol used to educate clients about the nature of ATs elicits negative thoughts about starting treatment for social anxiety disorder.

Treatment compliance issues

Although the protocol described in this chapter is flexible enough to fit individual client needs, therapists may encounter circumstances in which clients are not "on board" with various aspects of the treatment. Some clients may be resistant to engaging in in-session exposures. There are a number of possible reasons for this, and it is important for the client and therapist to discuss the client's reactions. One obvious and common cause is the clients' beliefs that they will achieve little benefit from putting themselves in a potentially anxiety-evoking situation. After all, an in-session exposure involves being observed by others doing something that you are admittedly anxious about, and this should raise the anxiety of any client with social anxiety disorder. It may be necessary to select a less anxiety-evoking situation at the start; however, there must be a careful balance here, as the client is likely to discount the meaningfulness of success if the situation can be discounted as "too easy." Another cause is the client's belief that because the exposure takes place in session, it is not real and therefore not worthwhile. In fact, being turned down for a date or a raise, or expressing an opinion to a boss who may hold a grudge, does have fewer potentially negative consequences in the session than in the world outside. Nevertheless, this is typically an avoidance strategy, and on questioning, most clients will admit to this. It is important to discuss with these clients the need to suspend disbelief and to let the situation unfold. Even if the worst of negative consequences will not occur, there remains much to be learned and practice to be gotten once the client agrees to participate. Typically, this concern will abate after a single in-session exposure yields results that the client sees as useful.

Homework compliance may be an issue for certain clients, and it is very important as homework is the bridge between in-session activity and change of emotions and behavior in the world beyond. A study by Edelman and Chambless [54] showed that clients who were compliant with homework made more treatment gains than their counterparts both immediately and at a six-month follow-up. However, another study by Woody and Adessky [55] did not find the significant differences between those who were and were not compliant with homework.

The study by Woody and Adessky [55] notwithstanding, non-completion of homework assignments should be addressed early in treatment. Homework assignments other than readings or exercises from the client workbook are designed collaboratively, and the client should be instructed that he or she should suggest an alternative task if the one being discussed is unlikely to be completed. It should also be kept in mind that failure to complete homework is not always about unwillingness. It may take the form of avoidance as well. For instance, a client may put off doing the homework until the end of the week as a way to avoid thinking about it and then find out that the person he or she wanted to talk to was not available in the little time remaining before the next session. Alternatively, homework may not be completed because a planned event did not actually occur. A homework assignment to attend a picnic and make conversation with acquaintances or strangers can be foiled by the weather! It is important in these situations that the client thinks about the homework early in the week, thinks about alternatives if the initial idea does not work out, and generally comes to think of the time that he or she is in treatment as a time to experiment with new behaviors, every day if possible.

Comorbid disorders

Depression and substance use disorders are among the more common disorders comorbid with social anxiety disorder. Here we focus on depression. In a study by Erwin and colleagues, clients with social anxiety disorder and comorbid depressive disorders demonstrated greater pre-treatment severity of social anxiety than clients with either no comorbidity or social anxiety disorder comorbid with another anxiety disorder. Although these clients demonstrated greater post-treatment severity as well, the rate of change in treatment was equivalent across groups [56]. In a study by Ledley and colleagues [57], individuals with higher levels of depressive symptoms also reported higher levels of social anxiety and less change in the symptoms of social anxiety during treatment. This was the case regardless of the type of treatment (CBT, pharmacotherapy, combined treatment), but both studies suggest that additional treatment *might have* benefited the clients with comorbid depression. Regardless of the outcomes of these studies, therapists need to make decisions about the best ways to deal with comorbid clients. Generally, one may focus on the disorder that is the most pertinent for the client and then potentially proceed to treat the other condition(s). However, if the therapist determines that there is a functional relationship between the comorbid conditions, they should be treated in the order that the functional analysis suggests. For example, unless a client with social anxiety and comorbid depression is highly lethargic or presents a risk of imminent self-harm, a functional analysis that social anxiety has led to social isolation, and social isolation has resulted in depression suggests that social anxiety disorder be the first disorder treated. In support of this position, one study (58) determined that changes in social anxiety mediated changes in depression among socially anxious clients, whereas changes in depression did not have the same impact on changes in social anxiety. To the extent possible, our experience suggests that a sequential approach is often best, but many of the techniques described herein have substantial applicability to depression as well.

Clinical decision making: integrating science and practice

Clinical practice is the integration of empirical science, data available in support of various techniques and strategies, the skill of the clinician in putting them into practice, and the goals and values of the client. In the treatment protocol described in this chapter, there are several points at which the therapist has to make decisions about the specific strategies to be employed. Below, several decision points of relevance for therapists using this protocol are described.

When developing a fear and avoidance hierarchy, the therapist and client work together to determine what items should be included. The items should represent situations that are important to the client and reflect goals that he or she wishes to accomplish in treatment. Clients may present situations that do not represent the full range of anxiety experience, providing only a list of highly anxiety-evoking situations. At such times, the therapist can discuss and come up with alternative situations that are suitable for exposures and that also capture the client's feared situations. Here, the therapist can facilitate the process of hierarchy formation by discussing with the client the factors that make one situation more difficult than another and examining variations on a situation that may be more or less anxiety evoking. The most useful hierarchy is one that spans the range of moderate to more severe anxiety, with relatively equal SUDS rating differences between items, and which includes a relatively small number of discrete situations (but with multiple variations on each). This set of characteristics is likely to increase the chances that successful completion of one item will leave the client in a state of readiness to address the next one. It is also important to note that all hierarchy items should have relevance to the client's personal values and goals; that is, does completing a hierarchy task move the client closer to accomplishing something that is important to him or her?

Before each in-session exposure, the therapist and client examine the client's ATs about the situation. Clinical judgment is very important when deciding what ATs should be targeted for attention. Early in treatment, the therapist is likely setting the stage for failure if he or she decides to challenge a thought that is an expression of a core belief (e.g., "I am a failure"). This thought is central to the client's psychological schema, and it is supported by numerous other negatively biased thoughts. One can think of a three-dimensional lattice work – the closer to the center, the less movement will be evident at any intersection or node. Using the same logic, however, if the therapist starts with the thought that is more related to the specifics of the particular situation (e.g.,

"I will have nothing to say" in a conversation at a party at a friend's house), it becomes easier to challenge the thought, and it is more likely that the client may consider the evidence in support of the rational response as well. This thought is less central to the client's schema, and therefore it should be more open to modification. Core beliefs can be challenged later in treatment when doing so will lead to better outcomes.

Both the therapist and the client should agree on what exposures to work on and the pace of movement up the hierarchy. Exposures should be based not only on the hierarchy but also on a discussion between the client and therapist about the level of comfort with the exposures. If the client is asked to move too far too soon, either in session or for homework, little good can result. The client may comply but feel overwhelmed, may not be able to absorb the positive aspects of this learning experience, and may feel betrayed (or at least unsupported) by the therapist. Oftentimes, the hierarchy is modified or intermediate items are created based on the progress made during exposures in and out of session. Duration of the role-play, number, gender, and age of role-players, the specific nature of the situation, and the behavior required of the client, etc., are important considerations when setting up in-session exposures.

Clients often feel quite anxious during in-session exposures, and the therapist will often feel the urge to rescue the client from that anxiety. However, that decision should always be made thoughtfully rather than impulsively. For instance, if a client is afraid that he cannot fill silences, a pause of just a few seconds can jump-start the therapist's empathy and lead him or her to cut the exposure short or cue a role-player to pick up the conversation. Clearly, if a client is really struggling, such a move may be called for. However, one of the goals of exposures is to have the client experience success and experience an increased sense of self-efficacy. Jumping in quickly to save the client from distress may defeat this purpose. In order to help the client maximize progress, it may be important to let clients see that they truly can "make the save." It is the therapist's responsibility to determine what is too much for the client to carry off and what is just right.

Research by Hayes and colleagues [47] demonstrates that the nature of the working alliance is important in the conduct of in-session exposures.

These researchers demonstrated that the relationship of the working alliance between the therapist and the client and the client's SUDS ratings during in-session exposures is curvilinear – less anxiety reduction was reported when the client rated the working alliance as poor and when the client rated the alliance as very good. Greater anxiety reduction was reported during exposures when the alliance was rated as moderate. It is probable that a weak alliance is not helpful in any way. A strong alliance may actually interfere with therapeutic progress because the level of comfort between the therapist and the client may suppress anxiety and limit the opportunity for the experience of anxiety reduction. A moderate alliance in this case, appeared to be most beneficial. Further research is needed in this area, but these findings suggest that it is possible to inhibit client progress by being too warm and supportive!

Conclusion

The main goal of this chapter was to provide a combination of empirical evidence along with an emphasis on clinical skills and techniques for the treatment of social anxiety disorder. Social anxiety disorder is a debilitating disorder that follows a chronic course. We have outlined the nature and the diagnostic criteria of the disorder. We have reviewed different cognitive, behavioral, affective, and social factors implicated in the etiology and/or maintenance of the condition that serve as the focus of treatment. We have provided a bit of empirical data on the efficacy and effectiveness of treatment. Inclusion of a clinical case gives the readers a flavor for the types of clients with social anxiety disorder we treat in our clinic, although these clients cover a wide spectrum of severity and impairment. We have described in detail the treatment protocol that we use to treat the disorder. However, the clinical application of this protocol also requires a great deal of flexibility, knowledge of cognitive–behavioral models of social anxiety disorder, and attention to the conceptualization of each individual client.

We have discussed some common problems that we encounter when treating social anxiety disorder and provided troubleshooting advice for clinicians. Every therapist struggles when making moment-to-moment clinical decisions. We have highlighted certain key areas in our treatment protocol in which the therapist makes such decisions based on empirical evidence and to a great extent on their clinical skills and experience. We hope that this brief chapter will provide readers with a good understanding of the different topics mentioned above, and that the resources and suggested readings will fill in any gaps.

Suggested readings

Bandelow B, Stein DJ (eds). *Social Anxiety Disorder*. New York: Marcel Dekker, 2004.

Crozier WR, Alden LE (eds). *The Essential Handbook of Social Anxiety for Clinicians*. Chichester, United Kingdom: John Wiley & Sons, Ltd, 2005.

Heimberg RG, Becker RE. *Cognitive-Behavioral Group Therapy for Social Phobia: Basic Mechanisms and Clinical Strategies*. New York: Guilford Press, 2002.

Hope DA, Heimberg RG, Juster H, Turk CL. *Managing Social Anxiety: A Cognitive-Behavioral Therapy Approach (Client Workbook*, 2nd edn*)*. New York: Oxford University Press, 2010.

Hope DA, Heimberg RG, Turk CL. *Managing Social Anxiety: A Cognitive-Behavioral Therapy Approach (Therapist Guide*, 2nd edn*)*. New York: Oxford University Press, 2010.

Ledley DR, Heimberg RG. Social anxiety disorder. In Antony MM, Ledley DR, Heimberg RG, eds. *Improving Outcomes and Preventing Relapse in Cognitive Behavioral Therapy*. New York: Guilford Press. 2005, pp. 38–76.

Turk CL, Heimberg RG, Magee L. Social anxiety disorder. In Barlow DH, ed. *Clinical Handbook of Psychological Disorders*, 4th edn. New York: Guilford Press. 2008, 123–63.

Online resources

www.academyofct.org (Academy of Cognitive Therapy)

www.temple.edu/phobia (Adult Anxiety Clinic of Temple University)

www.adaa.org/GettingHelp/AnxietyDisorders/SocialPhobia.asp (Anxiety Disorders Association of America)

www.abct.org (Association for Behavioral and Cognitive Therapies)

www.nimh.nih.gov/HealthInformation/socialphobiamenu.cfm (National Institute of Mental Health)

www.nmha.org/go/information/get-info/anxiety-disorders/social-phobias (National Mental Health Association)

www.socialphobia.org (Social Anxiety/Social Phobia Association)

www.paruresis.com (International Paruresis Association)

References

1. American Psychiatric Association. *Diagnostic and Statistical Manual of Mental Disorders*, 4th edn., text revision. Washington, DC: APA. 2000, p. 456.

2. Vriends N, Becker E, Meyer A, *et al.* Recovery from social phobia in the community and its predictors: data from a longitudinal epidemiological study. *J Anx Dis* 2007; **21**: 320–37.

3. Hook JN, Valentiner DP. Are specific and generalized social phobias qualitatively distinct? *Clin Psy Sci Prac* 2002; **9**: 379–95.

4. Stein MB, Chartier MJ, Hazen AL, *et al.* A direct-interview family study of generalized social phobia. *Am J Psychiatry* 1998; **155**: 90–7.

5. Katzelnick DJ, Kobak KA, DeLeire T, *et al.* Impact of generalized social anxiety disorder in managed care. *Am J Psychiatry* 2001; **158**: 1999–2007.

6. Schneier FR, Heckelman LR, Garfinkel R, *et al.* Functional impairment in social phobia. *J Clin Psychiatry* 1994; **55**: 322–31.

7. MA Bruch, Fallon M, Heimberg RG. Social phobia and difficulties in occupational functioning. *J Counseling Psychol* 2003; **50**: 109–17.

8. Safren SA, Heimberg RG, Brown EJ, Holle C. Quality of life in social phobia. *Depress Anxiety* 1997; **4**: 126–33.

9. Sanderson WC, DiNardo PA, Rapee RM, Barlow DH. Syndrome comorbidity in patients diagnosed with a DSM-III-R anxiety disorder. *J Abnormal Psychol* 1990; **99**: 308–12.

10. Kessler RC, Chiu WT, Demler O, Merikangas K, Walters EE. Prevalence, severity, and comorbidity of 12-month DSM-IV disorders in the National Comorbidity Survey Replication. *Arch Gen Psychiatry* 2005; **62**: 617–27.

11. Kessler RC, Berglund P, Demler O, *et al.* Lifetime prevalence and age-of-onset distributions of DSM-IV disorders in the National Comorbidity Survey Replication. *Arch Gen Psychiatry* 2005; **62**: 593–602.

12. FR Schneier, Johnson J, Hornig CD, Liebowitz MR, Weissman MM. Social phobia: comorbidity and morbidity in an epidemiologic sample. *Arch Gen Psychiatry* 1992; **49**: 282–8.

13. Ruscio AM, Brown TA, Chiu WT, *et al.* Social fears and social phobia in the USA: results from the National Comorbidity Survey Replication. *Psychol Med* 2008; **38**: 15–28.

14. Rapee RM, Sanderson WC, Barlow DH. Social phobia features across the DSM-III-R anxiety disorders. *J Psychopathology Behav Assess* 1998; **10**: 287–99.

15. Heimberg RG. Cognitive and behavioral treatments for social phobia: a critical analysis. *Clin Psychol Rev* 1989; **9**: 187–228.

16. Chapman TF, Mannuzza S, Fyer AJ. Epidemiology and family studies of social phobia. In: Heimberg RG, Liebowitz MR, Hope DA, Schneier FR, eds. *Social Phobia: Diagnosis, Assessment and Treatment.* New York, Guilford Press. 1995, 21–40.

17. Magee WJ, Eaton WW, Wittchen H-U, McGonagle KA, Kessler RC. Agoraphobia, simple phobia, and social phobia in the National Comorbidity Survey. *Arch Gen Psychiatry* 1996; **53**: 159–68.

18. Stein MB, Fuetsch M, Muller N, *et al.* Social anxiety disorder and the risk of depression: a prospective community study of adolescents and young adults. *Arch Gen Psychiatry* 2001; **158**: 251–6.

19. Merikangas KR, Angst J. Comorbidity and social phobia: evidence from clinical, epidemiologic, and genetic studies. *Eur Arch Psychiatry Clin Neurosci* 1995; **244**: 297–303.

20. Kendler KS, Karkowski LM, Prescott CA. Causal relationship between stressful life events and the onset of major depression. *Am J Psychiatry* 1999; **156**: 837–41.

21. Rapee RM, Melville LF. Recall of family factors in social phobia and panic disorder: comparison of mother and offspring reports. *Depress Anxiety* 1997; **5**: 7–11.

22. Clark DM, Wells A. A cognitive model of social phobia. In: Heimberg RG, Liebowitz MR, Hope DA, Schneier FR, eds. *Social Phobia: Diagnosis, Assessment and Treatment.* New York, Guilford Press. 1995, pp. 69–93.

23. Rapee RM, Heimberg RG. A cognitive-behavioral model of anxiety in social phobia. *Behav Res Ther* 1997; **35**: 741–56.

24. Schultz LT, Heimberg RG. Attentional focus in social anxiety disorder: potential for interactive processes. *Clin Psychol Rev* 2008; **28**(7): 1206–21.

25. Brozovich F, Heimberg RG. An analysis of post-event processing in social anxiety disorder. *Clin Psychol Rev* 2008; **28**: 891–903.

26. Hofmann SG. Cognitive factors that maintain social anxiety disorder: a comprehensive model and its treatment implications. *Cogn Behav Ther* 2007; **36**: 193–209.

27. Rodebaugh TL, Holaway RM, Heimberg RG. The treatment of social anxiety disorder. *Clin Psychol Rev* 2004; **24**: 883–908.

28. Hofmann SG, Smits JAJ. Cognitive-behavioral therapy for adult anxiety disorders: a meta-analysis of randomized placebo-controlled trials. *J Clin Psychiatry* 2008; **69**(4): 621–32.

29. Schneier FR, Erwin BA, Heimberg RG, *et al.* Social anxiety disorder and specific phobias. In: Gabbard GO, ed. *Gabbard's Treatments of Psychiatric Disorders*, 4th edn. Washington, DC: American Psychiatric Press, Inc. 2007, 495–506.

30. Butler G, Cullington A, Munby M, Amies P, Gelder M. Exposure and anxiety management in the treatment

of social phobia. *J Consult Clin Psychol* 1984; **52**: 642–50.

31. Clark DM, Ehlers A, Hackmann A, *et al*. Cognitive therapy versus exposure and applied relaxation in social phobia: a randomized controlled trial. *J Consult Clin Psychol* 2006; **74**: 568–78.

32. Hope DA, Heimberg RG, Bruch MA. Dismantling cognitive-behavioral group therapy for social phobia. *Behav Res Ther* 1995; **33**: 637–50.

33. Heimberg RG, Dodge CS, Hope DA, *et al*. Cognitive-behavioral group treatment of social phobia: comparison to a credible placebo control. *Cognit Ther Res* 1990; **14**: 1–23.

34. Heimberg RG., Liebowitz MR, Hope DA, *et al*. Cognitive-behavioral group therapy versus phenelzine in social phobia: 12-week outcome. *Arch Gen Psychiatry* 1998; **55**: 1133–41.

35. Clark DM, Ehlers A, McManus F, *et al*. Cognitive therapy versus fluoxetine in generalized social phobia: a randomized placebo-controlled trial. *J Consult Clin Psychol* 2003; **71**: 1058–67.

36. Heimberg RG, Salzman DG, Holt CS, *et al*. Cognitive-behavioral group treatment for social phobia: effectiveness at five-year follow-up. *Cognit Ther Res* 1993; **17**: 325–39.

37. Taylor S. Meta-analysis of cognitive-behavioral treatments for social phobia. *J Behav Ther Exp Psychiatry* 1996; **27**: 1–9.

38. Davidson JRT, Foa EB, Huppert J, *et al*. Fluoxetine, comprehensive cognitive behavioral therapy, and placebo in generalized social phobia. *Arch Gen Psychiatry* 2004; **61**: 1005–13.

39. Liebowitz MR, Heimberg RG, Schneier FR, *et al*. Cognitive-behavioral group therapy versus phenelzine in social phobia: long-term outcome. *Depress Anxiety* 1999; **10**: 89–98.

40. Hofmann SG, Suvak M. Treatment attrition during group therapy for social phobia. *J Anxiety Disorders* 2006; **20**: 961–72.

41. Gaston JE, Abbott NJ, Rapee RM, Neary SA. Do empirically supported treatments generalize to private practice? A benchmark study of a cognitive-behavioural group treatment programme for social phobia. *Br J Clin Psychol* 2006; **45**: 33–48.

42. Lincoln TM, Rief W, Hahlweg K, *et al*. Effectivenness of an empirically supported treatment for social phobia in the field. *Behav Res Ther* 2003; **41**: 1251–69.

43. McEvoy PM. Effectiveness of cognitive behavioural group therapy for social phobia in a community clinic: a benchmarking study. *Behav Res Ther* 2007; **45**: 3030–40.

44. Hope DA, Heimberg RG, Juster, H, Turk CL. *Managing Social Anxiety: A Cognitive-Behavioral Therapy Approach (Client Workbook)*. San Antonio, TX: The Psychological Corporation, 2000.

45. Hope DA, Heimberg RG, Turk CL. *Managing Social Anxiety: A Cognitive-behavioral Therapy Approach (Therapist Guide)*. New York: Oxford University Press, 2006.

46. Hope DA, Van Dyke M, Heimberg RG, Turk CL, Fresco DM. *Cognitive-behavioral therapy for social anxiety disorder: Therapist adherence scale*. Unpublished manuscript, Available from Heimberg RG, Temple University, 2002.

47. Hayes SA, Hope DA, VanDyke M, Heimberg RG. Working alliance for clients with social anxiety disorder: relationship with session helpfulness and within-session habituation. *Cognitive Behav Ther* 2007; **36**: 34–42.

48. Wolpe J, Lazarus A. *Behavior Therapy Techniques*. New York: Pergamon Press, 1966.

49. Ellis A, Grieger R. *Handbook of Rational-Emotive Therapy*. New York: Springer, 1977.

50. Beck AT, Rush AJ, Shaw BF, Emery G. *Cognitive Therapy of Depression*. New York: Guilford Press, 1979.

51. Beck JS. *Cognitive Therapy: Basics and Beyond*. New York: Guilford Press, 1995.

52. Chambless DL, Tran GQ, Glass CR. Predictors of response to cognitive-behavioral group therapy for social phobia. *J Anx Dis* 1997; **11**: 221–40.

53. Safren SA, Heimberg RG, Juster HR. Client expectancies and their relationship to pretreatment symtomatology and outcome of cognitive-behavioral group treatment for social phobia. *J Consult Clin Psychol* 1997; **65**: 694–8.

54. Edelmann RE, Chambless DL. Adherence during session and homework in cognitive-behavioral group treatment of social phobia. *Behav Res Ther* 1995; **33**: 537–77.

55. Woody SR, Adessky RS. Therapeutic alliance, group cohesion, and homework compliance during cognitive-behavioral group treatment of social phobia. *Behav Ther* 2002; **35**: 5–27.

56. Erwin BA, Heimberg RG, Juster HR, Mindlin M. Comorbid anxiety and mood disorders among persons with social phobia. *Behav Res Ther* 2002; **40**: 19–35.

57. Ledley DR, Huppert JD, Foa EB, *et al*. Impact of depressive symptoms on the treatment of generalized social anxiety disorder. *Depress Anxiety* 2005; **22**: 161–7.

58. Moscovitch DA, Hofmann SG, Suvak M, In-Albon T. Mediation of changes in anxiety and depression during treatment for social phobia. *J Consult Clin Psychol* 2005; **75**: 945–52.

Specific phobia

Naomi Koerner, Jenny Rogojanski, and Martin M. Antony

Descriptive psychopathology and diagnostic considerations

As outlined in the 4th edition of the *Diagnostic and Statistical Manual of Mental Disorders* (DSM-IV-TR) [1], specific phobia is characterized by clinically significant anxiety that is experienced in response to particular feared objects or situations. Exposure to the feared stimulus results in an immediate anxiety response that the individual recognizes as being in excess of what is reasonable. Fear of the object or situation leads to anxiety when an encounter is anticipated, often causing the individual to avoid exposure to the feared object or situation. Lastly, the specific phobia is associated with significant distress or interference with the individual's functioning and is not better accounted for by another mental disorder.

The DSM-IV-TR describes five types of specific phobia, including *animal type* (e.g., fears of dogs, spiders, snakes), *natural environment type* (e.g., fears of heights, storms, being near water), *blood-injection-injury type* (e.g., fears of receiving an injection, seeing blood, undergoing surgery), *situational type* (e.g., fears of flying, closed spaces, driving), and *other type* (e.g., vomiting, costumed characters such as clowns).

Regardless of type, in most cases, the focus of the individual's concern is that some aspect of the feared object or situation will cause harm to the self. It should be noted that recent research indicates that strong feelings of *disgust* may also motivate individuals to avoid particular objects or situations [2]. Individuals may also report being concerned about panicking, experiencing anxious arousal, losing control, or fainting during an encounter with the feared object or situation. It is not uncommon for individuals to experience a panic attack upon confronting the feared stimulus, and fainting is common among people with phobias of blood or injections. Anxiety is typically felt immediately upon exposure to the feared object or situation, and the level of anxiety experienced typically varies as a function of the proximity to the object and the degree to which escape from the feared encounter is possible. Panic attacks may also occur prior to or following exposure to a feared stimulus [3, 4].

Course

It is common for initial symptoms of a specific phobia to emerge in childhood or early adolescence, with the mean age of onset varying according to type. However, the fear of an object or situation must be sufficiently distressing or impairing before it can be considered a fully fledged specific phobia, and one study found an average lapse of nine years between the onset of fear and the point at which the fear was impairing enough to warrant the label phobia [5]. Without intervention, specific phobias typically persist over time.

Epidemiology

Specific phobia is one of the most common psychiatric disorders in the general population, with documented lifetime prevalence estimates ranging between 9.4% [6] and 12.5% [7]. It has also been found that the prevalence rates of specific fears vary according to type, with animal and height phobias being the most commonly reported [6]. Furthermore, subclinical fears that do not meet diagnostic criteria for specific phobia are even more prevalent [8]. In a study of 267 patients with a principal diagnosis of an anxiety disorder [9], 28% reported subclinical specific fears that did not meet the diagnostic threshold for distress or functional impairment.

There are also sex and ethnic differences associated with the diagnosis of specific phobia. Certain

Cognitive–behavioral Therapy with Adults: A Guide to Empirically Informed Assessment and Intervention,
ed. Stefan G. Hofmann and Mark A. Reinecke. © Cambridge University Press 2010.

specific phobias (e.g., animals, lightning, enclosed spaces) are more commonly reported by women than by men. Men may underreport their levels of fear [10], which may partially explain these sex differences. Additionally, in Western cultures women tend to present for treatment more readily than do men, which may contribute to larger sex differences found in studies of individuals presenting for treatment in clinical settings versus those in epidemiological studies [11]. Sex differences are minimal for fear of heights, flying, and blood-injection injury [6, 8, 12, 13]. Recent epidemiological data indicate that specific phobias are less common among Asian and Hispanic adults than among Caucasian adults [6], the reasons for which have not yet been determined.

Comorbidity

When specific phobia is the principal diagnosis, rates of comorbidity with other Axis I disorders tend to be lower than those associated with principal diagnoses of other mood and anxiety disorders [14]. However, it has been found that having a specific phobia of one type makes an individual more likely to have another specific phobia, particularly of the same type [15]. For example, Öst [16] found that approximately 70% of individuals with blood phobia also reported having a clinically-significant fear of injections. A more recent study of 1,127 outpatients showed that 15% of individuals diagnosed with a specific phobia reported symptoms that met criteria for an additional specific phobia [14].

Specific phobias also frequently co-occur with other DSM-IV disorders as an additional diagnosis, particularly when the predominant diagnosis is an anxiety disorder or a mood disorder [6, 14]. Among the anxiety and mood disorders, comorbidity is highest with panic disorder with agoraphobia and bipolar II disorder, respectively [6]. Specific phobias tend to co-occur less frequently with major depressive disorder [6, 17], bulimia nervosa [18], and alcohol use disorders [19].

Psychological models of specific phobia

There continues to be considerable debate over which factors are implicated in the etiology and maintenance of specific phobias. Behavioral treatments for specific phobias are rooted in Mowrer's [20] classic two-stage theory of fear development. The model proposes that specific phobias develop when a neutral stimulus becomes associated with an aversive stimulus through the process of classical conditioning. This newly formed association is then maintained through negative reinforcement, as avoidance of the feared stimulus allows the individual to minimize his or her fear reaction.

Although the parsimony of Mowrer's theory is compelling, a number of limitations associated with conditioning as an explanation for the acquisition and maintenance of phobias have been noted [for reviews, see 21, 22]. In several seminal papers, Rachman [23–25] described a number of phenomena that he proposed could not be fully accounted for by conditioning theories, including Mowrer's model. He argued that classical conditioning is not a sufficient explanation for phobia development because many individuals with phobias cannot recall a specific conditioning event that led to the onset of their fear, and conversely, many individuals who have had traumatic experiences do not develop a phobia. Furthermore, Rachman hypothesized that fear can be acquired through two additional pathways that operate via "social learning" and do not require direct contact with the feared stimulus: (1) *informational transmission* – learning from information transmitted by others (e.g., via television, newspapers, a parental figure) that an object or situation is dangerous; and (2) *vicarious acquisition* – observing someone else's overtly fearful reactions to an object or situation.

There is empirical support for both of these pathways. Field, Lawson, and Banerjee [26] examined the influence of verbal threat information about animals on fear cognitions and immediate avoidance behavior in children. Participants were shown pictures of rare animals with which they were not familiar (a cuscus, a quoll, and a quokka) and were provided with either no information, positive information, or threat information for each of the animals. Participants then completed measures of explicit and implicit fear cognitions as well as a behavioral approach test (BAT). In the BAT, children were presented with three closed boxes that they were led to believe contained the animals and were asked whether they wanted to pet the animals (this required inserting their hand inside each of the three boxes). Participants took longer to approach the box that supposedly contained the animal about which they received threat information. Furthermore, the experimental manipulation led to changes in explicit and implicit fear beliefs that varied as a function of the type of information that was received about the animals, which persisted for up to six months post-intervention.

Although the vicarious acquisition hypothesis has been based to a large extent on retrospective research using self-report measures [for a review, 27], existing findings from experimental research designs provide some support for the role of social observation as a mechanism of fear acquisition. Animal work by Cook, Mineka, and colleagues [28] has provided, to our knowledge, what is probably the best direct evidence for this mechanism. In their classic study, baby rhesus monkeys that observed an adult rhesus monkey display a fearful reaction to a snake on video, acquired a fear of snakes that persisted for three months. Fear acquisition has also been examined in human infants and toddlers with the use of *social referencing* paradigms. Social referencing refers to infants' use of adults' expressions of emotion to inform their own responses in novel or ambiguous situations [29]. The ability to engage in social referencing is considered to be adaptive in that it allows infants to learn about and avoid situations that are potentially dangerous. It has been suggested that enhanced attentional processing of adults' negative vocal and facial expressions of emotion may be one mechanism by which infants learn to associate novel situations and stimuli with possible negative outcomes [29]. Social observation as a mechanism for fear acquisition in humans has been investigated in a small number of studies. Studies by Dubi and colleagues [30], and Egliston and Rapee [31] have shown that toddlers display more pronounced fear and avoidant reactions in response to a toy snake or spider when their mothers react negatively to the objects, as compared to when they react positively to them. Observing positive maternal reactions to fear-relevant stimuli may even "inoculate" young children from acquiring fears of such stimuli. In a recent study by Egliston and Rapee [31], toddlers observed their mothers display either positive or neutral reactions to a plastic snake or spider. Following the observation, toddlers were exposed to an experimenter who expressed fear and disgust in response to the same stimulus toys. In the last phase of the experiment, the toddlers were presented with the toys. Toddlers who initially observed positive maternal reactions to the stimulus toys displayed more positive affect when presented with the toys and approached the toys more closely compared with toddlers who initially observed neutral maternal reactions.

In a classic paper, Seligman [32] discussed the notion of "biologically prepared" fears – phobias that appear to be selective, persistent in course, and easily acquired. To account for biologically prepared fears, Menzies and colleagues [33–35] proposed the addition of a *non-associative* pathway to Rachman's three pathways to fear acquisition. This fourth pathway is conceptualized as innate and attempts to account for fears that develop without any overt evidence of prior learning. Menzies and colleagues proposed that many biologically prepared fears fall into this category. The non-associative pathway hypothesis suggests that so-called biologically relevant fears, such as fear of heights and fear of being near water, may have evolved through natural selection to promote avoidance, and by extension, an increased likelihood of survival. It is further hypothesized that biologically-relevant fears extinguish for most individuals, but can persist for certain individuals or become re-activated during a stressful period. Most individuals adjust to these stimuli through normal developmental processes, and those who do not seem to have a higher likelihood of developing clinically significant phobias in adulthood. While there is some support for the proposal of a non-associative fear pathway [34], concerns about the hypothesis have been raised as well. For example, Mineka and Öhman [36] suggested that the non-associative pathway hypothesis does not consider the important role of interoceptive cues in conditioning events. Further, it has been argued that the non-associative pathway hypothesis is essentially unfalsifiable because support for the hypothesis relies on the *absence* of a detectable or identifiable associative history [37, 38]. Davey [37] remarked that the non-associative pathway hypothesis also relies too heavily on explanations that are based in evolution, that by necessity are constructed post hoc.

In conclusion, a number of conceptual models have been advanced to explain the processes by which fears are acquired. Mowrer's model emphasized basic conditioning processes, while Rachman's theory highlighted "non-conditioning" routes to fear acquisition such as information transmission and observation. Menzies and colleagues suggested that "non-associative pathways" may account for the acquisition of some fears. In a recent review, Hofmann [39] points out that none of these theories provide an explicit explanation of the role of *cognitive processes* in fear acquisition, even though changes in cognition have been shown to mediate changes in fear following exposure-based treatment. Hofmann proposes that two "higher order" cognitive processes may be particularly important in fear acquisition: *harm expectancy* and *perceptions of predictability and controllability*. He suggests that these cognitive processes likely have a role in all forms of fear learning, even basic Pavlovian conditioning. It remains to be determined whether harm expectancy and beliefs about predictability and controllability are *causal* factors in phobias.

Constitutional factors in specific phobia

The contributions of *biology and genetics* to specific phobia have been examined. As noted earlier, Seligman [32, 40] posited that humans are predisposed to acquire fears of stimuli that are relevant to their survival more readily than other kinds of fears. In an observational learning experiment, Cook and Mineka [28] demonstrated that rhesus monkeys developed a fear of biologically-relevant stimuli (a toy snake) but not of biologically-irrelevant stimuli (flowers) after watching spliced video footage of monkeys appearing to respond fearfully to both kinds of stimuli. While these data appear to provide some support for Seligman's hypothesis, there are other data to suggest that the biological relevance of stimuli may not have as profound an influence on the ease with which a fear is acquired as was initially hypothesized. For example, in a study by Dubi and colleagues [30], toddlers were exposed to a rubber snake or spider (presumed to be biologically relevant) and a rubber flower or mushroom (presumed to be biologically irrelevant) after they observed their mothers express negative or positive affect in response to these stimuli. The toddlers expressed more fear and engaged in greater avoidance of objects that had been paired with negative expressions of emotion, irrespective of the biological relevance of the stimulus.

Genetic vulnerability to specific phobia has been examined using family and twin studies (for a review, see [41]). There is some evidence that specific phobias run in families [42]. The findings regarding the heritability of specific phobias have been mixed. For example, Kendler and colleagues report heritability estimates of 25 to 67% depending on subtype [43, 44]. In a twin study conducted by Skre, Onstad, Torgersen, Lygren, and Kringlen [45], fear of small animals had moderate heritability; on the other hand, there was no evidence of a genetic influence in natural environment fears and situational fears.

Behavioral inhibition is a temperamental trait that promotes sensitivity to, and avoidance of, novel situations. Behavioral inhibition is characterized by heightened reactivity to aversive events and is considered to be a putative risk factor for various forms of psychopathology, including anxiety disorders [46, 47]. In one study, behavioral inhibition at 21 months of age was shown to be a significant predictor of the onset of multiple specific phobias at age eight [48]. Goodwin, Fergusson, and Horwood [49] followed a cohort of over 1,000 children longitudinally and found that anxious/withdrawn behavior at age eight was significantly related to increased risk of specific phobia at ages 16 to 21, even after controlling for potentially confounding factors such as stressful life events, parental internalizing disorders, and child abuse.

Cognitive factors in specific phobia

The role of *cognitive factors* in specific phobia has also been examined. It has been suggested that individuals with certain forms of specific phobia (e.g., situational phobias) may be concerned not only about encounters with their feared object or situation, but also their own anxiety-related physical sensations in an encounter with the object or situation. In other words, individuals with certain types of specific phobia may be high in *anxiety sensitivity*. Anxiety sensitivity is a dispositional characteristic that reflects individual differences in fear of anxiety-related physical sensations that arise from the belief that the experience of anxious arousal is harmful [50]. Individuals with situational phobias have been shown to respond strongly to panic induction challenges [51] and engage in more avoidance behaviors in claustrophobic situations [52], which provides some basis for the hypothesis. It is noted, however, that some studies have not found significant differences between phobia subtypes in levels of anxiety sensitivity (e.g., Antony, Brown, & Barlow, [53]).

Researchers have also examined the role of *attentional bias* in specific phobia. Öhman and colleagues [54] suggest that the capacity for selective attention evolved, in part, to enable individuals to rapidly detect threats to survival. They further proposed that stimuli such as snakes and spiders are especially likely to elicit automatic attentional capture because of their evolutionary relevance. A number of studies have examined attentional processing in individuals with a specific phobia of spiders. Some studies have produced evidence of enhanced attentional bias in individuals with a fear of spiders; however, other findings suggest that spider-fearful individuals *avoid* attending to spider-relevant stimuli (for a review, see [55]). Yet another set of findings suggests that spider-fearful individuals selectively attend to *safety cues* when presented with spider-relevant stimuli [56]. Differences across studies in the tasks that are used to assess attentional bias likely account for the mixed findings in the literature.

In a recent paper, Teachman and colleagues [57] proposed that *perceptual bias* may play an important role in some forms of specific phobia. In earlier studies by Rachman and Cuk [58] and Riskind and colleagues [59], individuals with a fear of spiders reported greater perceptions of spider movement when presented with spider-related stimuli than did individuals without a fear of spiders. In a study by Teachman [57], individuals with a fear of heights were asked to stand on a 26-feet high balcony, look over the ledge, and estimate the vertical distance to the ground. All participants over-estimated the height of the balcony and individuals with a fear of heights provided significantly higher estimates than did individuals who were low on fear of heights. Furthermore, differences in height perception could not be fully accounted for by cognitive biases, suggesting that perceptual biases may be a separate mechanism by which fear of heights is maintained.

Mental imagery in specific phobia

Recent research suggests that *visual and somatic mental imagery* may also play a role in the maintenance of specific phobia [60]. Distressing mental imagery plays a role in many forms of anxiety, including specific phobia [61, 62]. Studies suggest that the presence of recurring or persistent distressing mental images interferes with cognitive processing, contributes to the maintenance of fear and avoidance, and may prolong the course of anxiety disorders [60]. In a study by Hunt and colleagues [60] of 92 participants, 78% reported experiencing vivid and horrifying visual and somatic images related to their feared object or situation. In two experimental investigations, Hunt and colleagues [60, 63] examined the impact of directly modifying fear imagery on fear of snakes and found that the modification of these images via cognitive strategies led to a significant reduction in behavioral avoidance of snakes.

Taken together, it appears that a number of different factors may play a role in the maintenance and

possibly the etiology of specific phobia. However, to our knowledge, there are no integrative models of risk for specific phobia that take into account the interaction between biology, genetics, temperament, and cognitive/perceptual processes.

Efficacy and effectiveness of treatment

Much of the evidence converges on in vivo exposure being the most efficacious treatment for most specific phobias compared with wait-list and placebo interventions [see 64 and 65 for reviews]. The Task Force on the Promotion and Dissemination of Psychological Procedures (Society of Clinical Psychology, Division 12, American Psychological Association) published a set of guidelines for the definition of empirically supported treatments [66] and according to those guidelines, in vivo exposure has been identified as a *well supported* treatment for specific phobia. Canadian clinical practice guidelines published recently by the Canadian Psychiatric Association also recommend exposure for the treatment of specific phobia [67]. In in vivo exposure, clients confront their feared object or situation in a controlled and systematic fashion. The vast majority of individuals are able to perform the terminal task in the BAT after completing a course of in vivo exposure [e.g., 68, 69]. Furthermore, a recent analysis suggests that treatment gains are maintained for at least one year, particularly when treatment completers continue exposure practices after treatment has ended [64].

In the case of blood and needle phobias, the treatment of choice is applied tension. Applied tension involves tensing the muscles of one's body during exposure to feared situations, which triggers a temporary increase in blood pressure and prevents fainting. A study comparing applied tension to exposure without the tension exercises found that applied tension led to better outcomes for the treatment of blood phobia [70].

Studies have examined predictors of treatment outcome in specific phobia. Öst and colleagues [71] examined whether treatment outcome for claustrophobia varied as a function of individuals' response style in encounters with their feared object or situation. They compared *behavioral responders* (individuals whose primary response was avoidance) and *physiological responders* (individuals whose primary response was anxious arousal) and found that exposure led to greater improvement in symptoms in behavioral responders than did applied relaxation. On the other hand, physiological responders made greater gains with applied relaxation than with exposure.

Hellström and Öst [72] conducted a study to identify predictors of outcome associated with in vivo exposure for spider phobia and injection phobia, and in vivo exposure and applied tension for blood phobia. Proposed predictors included demographic variables (age and family history), clinical variables (e.g., age of onset of phobia, duration of phobia, pathway by which fear was acquired, severity of anxious and depressive symptoms) and cardiovascular reactivity during a behavioral approach test. The proposed predictors were not found to be associated with treatment outcome for any of the specific phobias under study.

There has been an increase in research on the use of technology in the treatment of specific phobia. In virtual reality treatments, a computer program is used to generate a three-dimensional digitized version of the feared object or situation, and clients carry out exposure practices in the simulated environment [73]. The advantages of virtual reality treatments include that they are cost and time effective and enable individuals to expose themselves to objects and situations that would otherwise be difficult or impractical to access (e.g., airplanes, in the case of flying phobia). Furthermore, virtual reality exposure may be a viable alternative for individuals who refuse in vivo exposure. There are limited data to suggest that virtual reality exposure may be as efficacious as therapist-guided in vivo exposure for flying phobia [74] and height phobia [75], though more research is needed to establish the relative effectiveness of these approaches. There are data on the long-term maintenance of gains following virtual reality treatment for these phobias; however, these should be interpreted conservatively as they are based on self-report measures of fear, and not behavioral measures [64].

The consensus has been that psychotropic medication, either in isolation or in combination with psychological treatment, does not lead to appreciable improvement in specific phobias [64]. The data indicate by and large that psychotropic medications are not incrementally beneficial to treatment [for a review, see 76]. However, recent evidence suggests that the use of D-cycloserine (DCS), an established antibiotic medication for the extended treatment of tuberculosis, may enhance fear extinction in exposure treatment [77, 78]. The efficacy of DCS for reducing fear has

been demonstrated in animal studies [79, 80], and recent research has provided preliminary support for the use of acute doses of DCS as an adjunct to exposure in the treatment of specific phobia [77, 78]. However, considerable research is needed to determine whether DCS is in fact a reliable pharmacologic enhancer for exposure-based treatments for specific phobia. In addition, questions remain about the mechanisms by which DCS facilitates new learning in exposure and about the long-term consequences, if any, of DCS use [81].

Assessment of specific phobias

Before starting treatment, it is important to conduct a comprehensive evaluation of clients' symptoms. Semistructured diagnostic interviews such as the Structured Clinical Interview for DSM-IV Axis I Disorders (SCID-I/P; [82]) and the Anxiety Disorders Interview Schedule for DSM-IV (ADIS-IV; [83]) can be used to establish the diagnosis of specific phobia.

Clinicians should obtain information about the physiological reactions (e.g., racing heart, sweating, rapid breathing, fainting) that their clients experience in the presence, or in anticipation of their feared object or situation. Clinicians should also ask about behavioral responses to feared objects and situations, including overt (i.e., observable) and covert (i.e., unobservable) strategies that are used to avoid them. Attention should be paid to safety-seeking strategies that may contribute to the maintenance of fears and therefore have the potential to undermine the effectiveness of exposure treatment. Clinicians may also find it useful to ask their clients about the anxiety-provoking thoughts that they have when they encounter their feared object or situation (e.g., "the dog will know that I am scared and will want to jump on me"). In preparation for exposure, clinicians should collect information on the factors that influence level of fear (e.g., size of an airplane, proximity of a spider) and on clients' access to individuals who can provide instrumental support with exposure practices (e.g., individuals who can control an animal during exposure practices). Finally, it is important to obtain information about clients' treatment history to identify potential obstacles in treatment (e.g., a prior history of terminating treatment prematurely).

There are a number of validated self-report scales for the assessment of phobic fears that can be used to measure changes in symptoms over the course of

Table 5.1 Self-report measures for the assessment of specific phobia

Acrophobia Questionnaire (AQ; [107])

Claustrophobia Questionnaire (CLQ; [108])

Dental Anxiety Inventory (DAI; [109])

Fear of Flying Scale (FFS; [110])

Fear Questionnaire (FQ; [111])

Fear of Spiders Questionnaire (FSQ; [112])

Fear Survey Schedule (FSS; [113–116])

Medical Fear Survey (MFS; [117])

Phobic Stimuli Response Scales (PSRS; [118])

Snake Questionnaire (SNAQ; [119])

Adapted from: McCabe RE and Antony MM. Anxiety disorders: social and specific phobias. In *Psychiatry*, 3rd edn. Tasman A, Kay A, Lieberman JA, First MB, Maj M (eds). Chichester, UK: John Wiley & Sons, Ltd. 2008 [106].

treatment (refer to Table 5.1; for a review of these measures, including their psychometric properties, see [84, 85]). Scales should be given out before treatment begins, periodically over the course of treatment, and again after treatment has ended.

Behavioral assessment

The BAT is a controlled assessment of behavioral reactions to feared stimuli. Behavioral approach tests are conducted before, during, and after treatment to assess changes in fear over the course of therapy. The BAT provides clinicians with an opportunity to observe how clients react in the presence of their feared object or situation and to obtain clinically relevant information that clients may have difficulty reporting in the interview, or may not be fully aware of (e.g., subtle avoidance behaviors). In a typical BAT, clients are asked to carry out a series of approach tasks (e.g., five to ten), starting with easier steps and progressing to more difficult ones. For example, in the case of an animal phobia, the first step of a BAT might involve looking at a photograph of the feared animal, and the final task might involve touching the feared animal (e.g., holding a spider, stroking a cat's face). Before and after every task in the BAT, clients are asked to indicate the intensity of their fear using a 100-point scale. Severity of the client's fear is indicated by his or her fear ratings as well as the number of steps

taken during the BAT. As treatment progresses, clients are typically able to complete more steps in the BAT, and with less fear. In some BAT procedures, the clinician models each task before the client attempts it [e.g., 63]. To our knowledge, there are no data to suggest that this is a necessary component of the BAT; however, modeling might help to facilitate engagement in the assessment if clients are highly fearful. Clinicians may also find it useful to obtain information about clients' anxiety-provoking cognitions during the BAT to determine whether maladaptive thoughts and mental images are contributing to the maintenance of fear.

Treating specific phobias

Structure of sessions

A considerable amount of research has been carried out to establish guidelines for the structuring of sessions. Findings regarding the optimal timing of exposure sessions have been inconsistent (for a review, see [86]). However, it is generally recommended that clients practice exposure at least several times during the course of the week, in light of findings from other anxiety disorders demonstrating that daily exposures (i.e., massed exposure practices) are more effective than exposures conducted once per week (i.e., spaced exposure) [87]. In addition, longer exposures tend to be more effective than briefer exposures [see 86]; practices should generally last one to two hours, or until the individual learns that his or her feared consequences do not occur.

A small number of studies have compared the efficacy of individual versus group treatment for specific phobia. A study by Öst [88] suggests that both formats are equally effective. However, given the effectiveness of single-session exposure-based treatments for specific phobia, clinicians may find it more practical and efficient to deliver treatment on an individual basis [11].

Strategies and techniques

Psychoeducation

A question that clients are likely to ask, particularly ones who cannot trace the origin of their fear to a traumatic event (e.g., a bite, an accident), is "Why did I get this fear?" Clinicians can address this question by engaging clients in a discussion of the pathways to fear discussed earlier.

In preparation for exposure, it is also important to engage clients in a discussion of the short-term and long-term effects of avoidance. Avoidance reduces fear in the short term, but prevents recovery from fear in the long term because fear-driven predictions and assumptions are never disconfirmed. Clinicians can also provide information about the nature of anxiety more generally (i.e., its function and its adaptive aspects). This may be particularly important for clients who are concerned about losing control over their anxious reactions when encountering their feared object or situation.

It is not uncommon for clients to state that exposing themselves to their feared object or situation has not worked for them in the past. Clinicians can address this by explaining the difference between therapeutic exposure and the "sporadic" exposure that clients have likely experienced previously. Specifically, therapeutic exposure should be prolonged, frequent, and systematic, and proceed at a pace that is directed by the client [89]. On the other hand, impromptu encounters with a feared object or situation are often infrequent, brief, unpredictable, and outside of the client's control, all of which prevent such encounters from being helpful.

Development of the exposure hierarchy

In preparation for exposure, clients (in collaboration with the therapist) should develop a hierarchy of situations that they fear or avoid. Clients' exposure hierarchies should consist of 10 to 15 items, ranging from very difficult (e.g., 90 to 100, on a 0- to 100-point scale) at the top of the hierarchy to mildly difficult (e.g., about 30 out of 100) at the bottom of the hierarchy. The hierarchy should include items that are specific, concrete, and take into consideration the factors that influence the client's fear. For example, the task of "looking at a spider" can be broken up into several items and arranged in order of difficulty based on *realness* and *movement* (if these factors influence the client's fear): looking at a picture of an animated spider; looking at a photograph of a real spider; watching a video clip of a still spider; watching a video clip of a spider moving quickly toward the camera; looking at a live spider in a glass container. An example of an exposure hierarchy is provided in Table 5.2.

Exposure

In preparation for exposure, clients will have to take into consideration how they are going to obtain the materials they will need to carry out the tasks in their

Table 5.2 Exposure hierarchy for Anna's fear of dogs

Item	Description	Fear rating (0 to 100)
1	Touch the face of a large dog	100
2	Touch the back of a large dog	95
3	Walk by an unleashed large dog without crossing the street	90
4	Stand one foot from a large dog on a leash	80
5	Sit on a bench in a dog park and watch dogs	75
6	Hold a puppy or small dog	75
7	Touch the face of a puppy or small dog	70
8	Stand one foot away from a puppy or small dog	65
9	Stand four feet from a large dog on a leash	65
10	Stand eight feet from a large dog on a leash	55
11	Stand four feet away from a puppy or small dog	50
12	Go to the animal shelter or pet store and look at dogs behind a cage or glass	50
13	Stand eight feet away from a puppy or small dog (e.g., boyfriend's pug)	40
14	Watch video clips with close-up shots of dogs	30

hierarchy (e.g., photographs, film clips, access to specific objects or locations; see [90] for suggestions). Some clients may need access to an individual who can provide instrumental support with specific aspects of the exposure homework practices. The helper should be a trusted and supportive individual (e.g., a family member, a friend) who knows about the client's fear, who is not afraid of the client's feared object or situation, and perhaps most importantly, will not be critical toward or demanding of the client during exposure practices. The role of the helper is to provide support and encouragement, model non-fearful behavior, and assist with the practical aspects of exposure (e.g., provide access to and be present during exposure involving animals). Clients can provide their helpers with readings on the treatment of phobias, so the helper understands the rationale and exposure procedures. If possible, helpers can also sit in on an exposure session conducted by the therapist.

Clients should begin exposure with a task on their hierarchy that is associated with a moderate level of fear (typically in the range of 40 to 60). It is also fine for clients to start with easier items or more difficult items if they prefer. The initial task should be challenging, but one that the client will likely be able to complete successfully. The pace at which clients progress through their exposure hierarchy is, to a large extent, self-directed. Clients can use their fear ratings to gauge their readiness to proceed to the next step. Generally, clients should stay with a task until their fear has decreased to a level at which they are willing to try the next task on the hierarchy. The quicker clients progress through their hierarchy steps, the quicker they will experience a reduction in fear. However, clients who prefer to take steps more gradually will generally still experience a reduction in fear over time. Clients are encouraged to conduct regular "checks" on their progress by re-attempting earlier tasks to ensure that they have in fact mastered the easier steps in their hierarchy. Clients should be encouraged to stay in the situation until they feel more comfortable. If they must leave the situation, they should be encouraged to return to the situation as soon as possible after leaving. It is not necessarily a problem if a client's fear does not decrease within an exposure session. In such cases, clients typically still experience a reduction in fear across sessions [91].

To benefit maximally from exposure, practices should be frequent and planned in advance. Clients should set aside one to two hours for their exposure practices, as longer exposures are generally more effective than shorter exposures. Clients should also work toward reducing the use of safety behaviors. Safety behaviors are overt or subtle behaviors that individuals engage in to reduce fear or prevent a feared outcome (e.g., getting hurt) in encounters with their feared object or situation. Over the long term, use of these behaviors may undermine treatment outcome by preventing clients from learning that the feared situation is in fact not dangerous. However, early in treatment, continued use of safety behaviors may help to facilitate engagement in exposure practices (see [92] for a detailed discussion of the role of safety behaviors in exposure therapy).

Other strategies

Systematic desensitization [93] is similar to in vivo exposure in that clients expose themselves to their feared object or situation in a graduated fashion. However, in systematic desensitization, clients receive training in progressive muscle relaxation (PMR) as a first step in treatment and engage in PMR during the exposure [94]. Another distinction is that clients expose themselves to *mental images* of their feared stimulus. The use of relaxation is based in reciprocal inhibition [93], the notion that fear associations can be weakened via the repeated pairing of mental images of anxiety-provoking stimuli with a response that is incompatible (i.e., relaxation). Although studies have been conducted to examine the efficacy of systematic desensitization for specific phobia (for a review, see [64]), for a number of reasons, it is seldom recommended in current practice. First, there has been little empirical support for the notion that anxiety can be counter-conditioned using systematic desensitization [95]. Furthermore, the effectiveness of systematic desensitization is dependent upon the client's ability to generate vivid and concrete mental images of their feared object or situation [94], and not everyone has this ability.

As mentioned earlier, *applied tension* involves tensing the muscles of the body while engaging in exposure practices. This strategy is used in the treatment of blood and needle phobias that are associated with a history of fainting. Two controlled investigations of the efficacy of applied muscle tension for blood phobia suggest that it is more efficacious than in vivo exposure [64]. A more detailed description of this procedure is provided elsewhere [96].

Only a small number of studies have examined the use of *cognitive strategies* (i.e., examining the evidence for negative beliefs about feared situations) in the treatment of specific phobia. For example, there are a few studies supporting the use of cognitive strategies for the treatment of dental phobia. In addition, cognitive therapy may help in some cases of claustrophobia, though the gains obtained tend not to be as great as those obtained during exposure (for a review, see [76]).

Difficulties encountered during treatment

There are a number of challenges that clinicians and clients may encounter during exposure treatment for

Table 5.3 Troubleshooting in exposure-based treatments for specific phobia

Problem	Strategies
The client is having difficulty scheduling regular exposure practices	Encourage the client to schedule practices in a diary or planner. Remind the client that regular exposure practices will lead to a better treatment outcome.
The exposure object or situation is difficult to control	Minimize the unpredictability and uncontrollability of the exposure as much as possible, particularly in the beginning stages of treatment. For example, use cages and leashes if the exposure object is an animal
The client's fear does not decrease during the exposure session or across sessions	Assess whether the client is engaging in subtle or covert (i.e., non-observable) safety behavior. Encourage client to minimize engagement in these behaviors and to phase them out at later stages of treatment. Assess whether the exposure exercise is too difficult for the client; if so, return to a less difficult exercise.
The client is unwilling to engage in an exposure practice	Assess whether the exposure exercise is too difficult for the client and modify the exercise as appropriate.
The exposure situation is brief in duration (e.g., taking an elevator)	Repeat the exercise a number of times to ensure prolonged practice.
The client experiences an unanticipated or unpredictable negative event during an exposure practice (e.g., client gets scratched by a cat)	Remind the client that return of fear is expected after the experience of an unanticipated negative event. Encourage the client to continue with exposure practices. The client may have to return to tasks that are less difficult before moving forward in their exposure hierarchy. Assess the client's fear cognitions to determine whether the client is engaging in unhelpful thinking that may prevent continuation with exposure exercises (e.g., "cats *always* seem to want to attack me"). Use cognitive restructuring to re-evaluate such beliefs.

Adapted from: Antony MM, Swinson RP. *Phobic Disorders and Panic in Adults: A Guide to Assessment and Treatment.* Washington, American Psychological Association, 2000 [89].

specific phobia. For a list of these challenges, refer to Table 5.3. Due to space limitations, we discuss just two of these here: difficulty scheduling time to practice and unpredictable events occurring during practices. For a more detailed discussion of obstacles that often arise during exposure therapy, see Antony and Swinson [89].

Scheduling time to practice

Exposure is most effective when clients practice between treatment sessions; however, clients commonly report difficulty finding time to practice exposure between sessions. Clients should be encouraged to plan practices in advance, and to schedule practices in a planner or calendar, just as they would any appointment. Clients may be more likely to schedule practices in advance if exposure exercises involve making a commitment to another individual (e.g., an individual who will be helping the client with the practice). For some clients, it may be easiest to conduct practices more

intensively. For example, rather than finding an hour or two to practice driving each day over the course of several weeks, it may be easiest to take a week off work and to practice driving for six or eight hours each day during the week. Some practices can also be conducted during the course of a client's day (e.g., driving to work instead of taking the bus, for a client who fears driving), in which case practices need not take up much extra time. It is often helpful to remind clients that repeated practice between sessions will accelerate treatment progress.

Minimizing unpredictability during exposures

It is important to minimize unpredictability as much as possible during exposure treatment. Planning and scheduling exposures in advance increases the predictability of exposure. Careful selection of the target for exposure can also minimize unpredictability. This is particularly important at the beginning of treatment as setbacks in the early stages of exposure may undermine the confidence of clients. When working with animals, it is important to choose animals that are familiar (e.g., a dog that is unlikely to growl or bite) and that can easily be restrained (e.g., with a leash). As exposure progresses and the client begins to make measurable gains, it may be useful for the client to have contact with stimuli that are less predictable (e.g., unleashed dogs in a dog park).

In rare cases, clients may experience an unpredictable negative event involving their feared object or situation (e.g., getting scratched by a cat, getting stuck in an elevator, experiencing a car accident). Typically, such events can lead to an increase in fear. It is important for both clinicians and clients to be realistic about the possibility (albeit remote) of a traumatic event occurring. Clinicians should underscore the importance of continuing exposure practices following such an event to prevent entrenchment of the fear.

Preventing recurrence of fear

Although in vivo exposure is considered to be the "gold standard" treatment for specific phobia (as well as other forms of anxiety that are characterized by situational avoidance), *return of fear* is a common phenomenon that clinicians and clients must contend with. Return of fear [97] refers to the renewed experience of fear that occurs with the passage of time after it has diminished spontaneously or via repeated and systematic exposure. Rachman proposed that return of fear (1) may occur between sessions of in vivo exposure or long after the fear has been treated; and (2) is not synonymous with relapse. Given that return of fear is not uncommon, it is important for clinicians to inform their clients that they may experience a recurrence of fear after successful treatment, but that this does not indicate that a relapse has occurred or that treatment was not effective. The factors that give rise to renewed fear after a period of partial or complete extinction have been studied extensively [e.g., 98, 99]. Although it was initially thought that the fear reduction observed with *in vivo* exposure was the result of the "undoing" of fear associations, it is now understood that fear associations are not eradicated with repeated exposure to fear stimuli; but instead are *replaced with non-fearful associations*. As such, newly formed associations are likely to be fragile and vulnerable to disintegration, paving the way for return of

fear. In an effort to optimize long-term treatment outcomes, strategies for the prevention of return of fear have been developed and empirically tested. Most of the research on return of fear extends from basic research on the factors that affect the acquisition and retention of new learning and has shown that treatment outcomes may be optimized with careful consideration of factors that influence learning. One factor that has garnered attention in the experimental and clinical literature is the effect of context during exposure (discussed below). In addition, continued engagement in exposure practices after the completion of treatment can contribute to the maintenance of gains [64].

Varying the exposure context

Animal research by Bouton and colleagues [100, 101] has had a significant influence on our understanding of the role of *context effects* in fear renewal. Bouton and colleagues have shown that when fear is extinguished in a context that differs from the context in which it was initially acquired and an animal is then returned to the fear acquisition context, fear renewal is observed. Return of fear is also observed when an animal is exposed to a context that differs from the ones in which fear was acquired and extinguished, respectively. A number of studies with humans similarly indicate that return of fear is more pronounced when individuals' fear is assessed in a context that is entirely different from the treatment context [102]. External context effects may explain, for example, why a client can successfully encounter his or her feared object in the therapist's office after several exposure practices, only to experience increased difficulty when the feared object is encountered at home or in a completely different environment. Research suggests that it may be important for clients to conduct exposure in multiple external contexts (i.e., physical locations), to ensure generalization of new, non-fearful learning.

The importance of varying the *internal* context has also been discussed extensively in the phobia literature. Principles of state-dependent learning suggest that when new information is learned in a particular state, it may be difficult to retrieve new learning if there is a mismatch between the state that the individual was in at the time the information was learned and the state that the individual is in when he or she is trying to retrieve it. Regarding phobia, Mystkowski and colleagues [103] showed that when participants ingested caffeine before a one-session exposure treatment for spider phobia, return of fear was more pronounced at follow-up in participants who did not ingest caffeine before the follow-up session compared with those who *did* ingest caffeine. If internal contexts are as powerful as research suggests, this implies that clients who are taking antidepressant or anxiolytic medications during exposure treatment may be more likely to notice a return of fear when they stop taking the medications at post-treatment, due in part to neurochemical changes [104]. More research is needed to test this hypothesis.

Clinical case example: specific phobia of dogs

Anna was a 29-year-old graduate student who was afraid of dogs most of her life. She traced the origin of her fear to an event that occurred when she was eight years old. Anna was playing with her friend's German shepherd when the dog suddenly took hold of her hand with its mouth. Anna avoided dogs ever since this incident and would go to great lengths to reduce the possibility of coming into contact with them. When she walked outside, she scanned the sidewalks to ensure that she would not encounter a dog. If she caught a glimpse of a dog from a distance, she crossed the street or took a different route, even if the alternate route was inconvenient. She avoided going for walks in her neighborhood, because many of her neighbors frequently walked their dogs. She preferred not to visit the homes of friends with pet dogs. Although she did not like looking at large dogs in photographs or on television, her anxiety was only mild in these situations.

Anna managed to keep her fear of dogs under control until one year prior to treatment, when she started dating her boyfriend, Michael. Michael was a self-proclaimed "dog person" and had a small pug named Toby. When they first started dating, Anna was concerned about what Michael might think if he found out about her fear of dogs. At first, she told Michael that she did not like dogs and "preferred" cats. She also made sure that she and Michael never spent time together at his apartment. Michael's apartment was located a fair distance outside the city center, so he never questioned it. Given that their relationship was going well, Michael suggested that they move in together. The situation became complicated for Anna

when Michael indicated that he wanted the two of them, along with Toby, to find a new apartment close to a dog park. At first, Anna thought about how she might avoid living with Michael. However, Anna realized that she needed to address her fear of dogs head on if she wanted her relationship with Michael to progress to the next level. Anna told Michael about her fear of dogs and after doing research on the Internet, they discovered that in vivo exposure might help Anna overcome her fear of dogs.

Anna's initial session consisted of a thorough clinical interview. Her fear of dogs was assessed using the ADIS-IV and the interview confirmed that her symptoms were consistent with a diagnosis of specific phobia, as defined in DSM-IV. She did not endorse fear of other animals or objects, nor symptoms of any other anxiety disorder or depression. In the clinical interview, Anna reported that her heart raced and that she became short of breath in the presence of dogs. Thoughts that crossed her mind when she saw dogs included, "The dog will jump on me and I won't be able to get away" and "Dogs can sense that I'm afraid and that makes them want to bite me." During the BAT, Anna was able to comfortably look at and touch photographs of dogs, but experienced mild anxiety when watching video clips with close-up shots of large dogs. She pushed her chair back a few inches when the dogs in the videos jumped. Although Anna was able to stand in the same room as a Labrador retriever on a leash, her fear was very high, and she was unable to get any closer than ten feet from the dog. After the BAT, Anna provided a list of strategies she typically used to avoid contact with dogs. Next, Anna received two 120-minute sessions of therapist-assisted exposure, spaced three days apart. Although there are a number of ways to organize treatment sessions (single-session, multiple consecutive sessions, once-weekly sessions), the decision was made to schedule the second session three days after the first session for two main reasons. First, exposure is most effective when practices are spaced close together. Second, the three days between sessions provided Anna with sufficient time to carry out exposure practices on her own.

Treatment session 1

First, Anna was provided with psychoeducation on animal phobia and was introduced to the cognitive–behavioral model of specific phobia. Then, the rationale and procedure for exposure was explained to Anna and she spent the majority of the session developing an exposure hierarchy (see Table 5.2). Anna was also assigned readings from the book, *Overcoming Animal and Insect Phobias* [105].

Next, Anna practiced being in the same room as Michael's pug Toby, with Michael present at the session. Prior to introducing Toby into the session, Michael was provided with information on exposure. Anna and her therapist explained to Michael the rationale for exposure and they explained his role as a helper in the exposure. As mentioned earlier, when the client enlists the assistance of a helper, it is important for that individual to have a good understanding of what treatment will involve for the client to ensure that the client and the helper have a shared understanding of the process.

To start, Anna stood about eight feet away from the dog, while Michael held Toby by the leash. Her initial fear level was a 40, so she quickly moved closer (to about three feet away), until her fear was at a level of 80. After about 15 minutes, her fear decreased to a level of 55, and she decided she could get a bit closer. As mentioned earlier, clients can proceed to the next task in their hierarchy if they feel prepared to attempt it, even if they are continuing to experience a moderate level of fear. If a client attempts the next task and the task turns out to be much more challenging than the client estimated it would be, the therapist and client can work together to modify the task so it becomes more feasible. The client may also decide to return to less difficult tasks in the hierarchy to ensure that these have been mastered. Anna moved to about a foot away from Toby, and her fear increased to a level of about 75. Her fear remained at a level of about 75 for the next 10 or 15 minutes, though it temporarily increased to a level of 100 each time Toby moved quickly. Over the next 30 minutes her fear began to decrease considerably, and she was ready to try touching Toby. Michael held Toby on the leash, facing away from Anna. Anna quickly touched Toby's back. Over the next 15 minutes, she continued to practice touching Toby's back until her fear decreased to a level of about 50. At the end of the session, Anna agreed to try several practices over the next few days. Anna and her therapist discussed ideas for exposure practices that she could engage in between sessions. She agreed to visit an animal shelter and look at dogs through their cages. In addition, she agreed to continue to practice touching Toby for at least an hour per day. The therapist asked Anna whether she could think of any factors that might make it less likely that she would engage in practices between sessions and she could not think of any. This is an important question to ask clients when deciding on between-session exercises, as this provides clients with an opportunity to troubleshoot in session, which in turn increases the likelihood that between-session exposure practices will be completed, or at least attempted.

Treatment session 2

Anna reported successfully completing her homework. She was able to visit the animal shelter with minimal anxiety (at first about a 40 out of 100). Although touching Toby's back was initially more difficult at Michael's apartment than it was in the therapist's office, her fear quickly decreased. After watching Michael pat Toby's head for about five minutes, Anna agreed to touch Toby's head. Her fear was initially at a level of 80, but it decreased to about a 30 after approximately 20 minutes. Over the next two days, Anna continued to practice touching Toby's back and head. By the time she returned to her second therapy session, she was able to play with Toby off leash, with only minimal anxiety.

Given her success with Toby, Anna and her therapist decided to try exposure to larger dogs at a nearby dog park. On the way there, Anna was able to refrain from crossing the street when she saw dogs and she allowed them to sniff her. At the dog park, Anna sat on a bench and watched leashed and unleashed dogs for one hour. Anna rated her initial level of fear at a 75. After 20 minutes, it decreased to a 40 and she stood up and started walking toward the dogs on leashes. In the first session, the therapist explained to Anna the importance of carrying out exposure practices in different locations and with different types of dogs. With this in mind, she approached three individuals with dogs that varied in breed and size. She was able to get close to all the dogs and allowed a small dog to jump up onto her legs. The final two steps were to touch the back and face of a large dog on a leash. She asked for the therapist's assistance with these final two tasks. Her therapist modeled the tasks by stroking the back and head of a golden retriever. Anna then touched the dog's back and head a few times and found that her fear decreased.

Over the next few weeks, Anna agreed to continue practicing touching dogs in her neighborhood (always checking first with the owners to make sure the dog was comfortable being touched). She also agreed to visit friends and family members who owned dogs, including a cousin with a friendly German shepherd.

Follow-up visit

A 30-minute follow-up assessment was conducted one month later. At this visit, Anna reported that she was spending time with Michael's pug on a regular basis and had walked him on a few occasions. She reported that she also practiced touching the pug's head and face and was no longer afraid of being that close to a small dog. She had also visited the dog park on a couple of occasions, and visited her cousin (and her German shepherd) once. A final BAT was carried out at the dog park and Anna was able to walk up to many different dogs and touch their heads and faces. The only exception was German shepherds. She had practiced touching a German shepherd on the back, but still had considerable difficulty touching it on the head or face. Anna's symptoms of specific phobia were reassessed using the ADIS-IV and her symptoms no longer met diagnostic criteria for a specific phobia. She agreed to continue exposures to her cousin's German shepherd over the coming weeks. Anna had displayed a solid understanding of principles and procedures of exposure throughout treatment and at one-month follow-up. Furthermore, she had demonstrated that she was able to carry out exposure practices regularly on her own without the assistance of the therapist. Therefore, it was decided that it was not necessary to schedule additional treatment sessions.

Conclusion

In this chapter, we provided an overview of psychological accounts of specific phobia and described a standard protocol for in vivo exposure, the current treatment of choice for specific phobia. There have been a number of important developments in the field that hold promise for improving our theoretical understanding of the disorder and its subtypes, and for enhancing current interventions. One of these developments includes recent research on the role of disgust in the etiology, maintenance, and treatment of specific phobias, challenging the notion that specific phobias are exclusively fear-based conditions. In addition, research on specific phobia is exemplary for its strong integration of methodologies and findings from basic science. Research with animals and humans on the factors that influence the acquisition and retention

of new learning has had a significant influence on experimental investigations of exposure, including research on the effects of the timing and context of sessions, the role of safety behaviors, and other factors on outcome. Finally, recent research on DCS as a potential pharmacologic enhancer for exposure has received considerable attention in the literature. As was noted earlier, there are a number of questions that remain to be answered about the exact mechanisms by which DCS enhances learning during exposure and about the long-term effects of DCS.

Suggested readings

Professional books

Antony MM, Swinson RP. *Phobic Disorders and Panic in Adults: A Guide to Assessment and Treatment.* Washington: American Psychological Association, 2000.

Craske MG, Antony MM, Barlow DH. *Mastering Your Fears and Phobias (Therapist Guide)*, 2nd edn. New York: Oxford University Press, 2006.

Maj M, Akiskal HS, López-Ibor JJ, Okasha A. *Phobias.* Hoboken, NJ: John Wiley and Sons, 2004.

Self-help books

Antony MM, Craske MG, Barlow DH. *Mastering Your Fears and Phobias (Client Workbook)*, 2nd edn. New York: Oxford University Press, 2006.

Antony MM, McCabe RE. *Overcoming Animal and Insect Phobias: How to Conquer Fear of Dogs, Snakes, Rodents, Bees, Spiders, and More.* Oakland, CA: New Harbinger Publications, 2005.

Antony MM, Watling MA. *Overcoming Medical Phobias: How to Conquer Fear of Blood, Needles, Doctors, and Dentists.* Oakland, CA: New Harbinger Publications, 2006.

Antony MM, Rowa K. *Overcoming Fear of Heights: How to Conquer Acrophobia and Live a Life Without Limits.* Oakland, CA: New Harbinger Publications, 2007.

Brown D. *Flying Without Fear.* Oakland, CA: New Harbinger Publications, 1996.

Triffitt J. *Back in the Driver's Seat: Understanding, Challenging, and Managing Fear of Driving.* Tasmania, Australia: Dr. Jacqui Triffitt (www.backinthedriversseat.com.au), 2003.

References

1. American Psychiatric Association. *Diagnostic and Statistical Manual of Mental Disorders*, 4th edn., text revision. Washington, DC: American Psychiatric Association, 2000.

2. Sawchuk CN, Lohr JM, Tolin DF, Lee TC, Kleinknecht RA. Disgust sensitivity and contamination fears in spider and blood-injection-injury phobias. *Behav Res Ther* 2000; **38**: 753–62.

3. Ehlers A, Hofmann SG, Herda CA, Roth WT. Clinical characteristics of driving phobia. *J Anxiety Disord* 1994; **8**: 323–39.

4. Lipsitz JD, Barlow DH, Mannuzza S, Hofmann SG, Fyer JA. Clinical features of four DSM-IV-specific phobia subtypes. *J Nerv Ment Dis* 2002; **190**: 471–8.

5. Antony MM, Brown TA, Barlow DH. Heterogeneity among specific phobia types in DSM-IV. *Behav Res Ther* 1997; **35**: 1089–100.

6. Stinson FS, Dawson DA, Chou SP, *et al.* The epidemiology of DSM-IV specific phobia in the USA: results from the national epidemiologic survey on alcohol and related conditions. *Psychol Med* 2007; **37**: 1047–59.

7. Kessler RC, Berglund P, Demler O, Jin R, Walters EE. Lifetime prevalence and age-of-onset distributions of DSM-IV disorders in the National Comorbidity Survey Replication. *Arch Gen Psychiatry* 2005; **62**: 593–602.

8. Curtis GC, Magee WJ, Eaton WW, Wittchen HU, Kessler RC. Specific fears and phobias: epidemiology and classification. *Br J Psychiatry* 1998; **173**: 212–17.

9. Antony MM, Moras K, Meadows EA, *et al.* The diagnostic significance of the functional impairment and subjective distress criterion: an illustration with the DSM-III-R anxiety disorders. *J Psychopathol Behav Assess* 1994; **16**: 253–62.

10. Pierce KA, Kirkpatrick DR. Do men lie on fear surveys? *Behav Res Ther* 1992; **30**: 415–18.

11. Rowa K, McCabe RE, Antony MM. Specific phobias. In Andrasik F ed. *Comprehensive Handbook of Personality and Psychopathology, Volume 2: Adult Psychopathology.* Hoboken: John Wiley and Sons. 2006, 154–68.

12. Fredrikson M, Annas P, Fischer H, Wik G. Gender and age differences in the prevalence of specific fears and phobias. *Behav Res Ther* 1996; **34**: 33–9.

13. Goisman RM, Allsworth J, Rogers MP, *et al.* Simple phobia as a comorbid anxiety disorder. *Depress Anxiety* 1998; **7**: 105–12.

14. Brown TA, Campbell LA, Lehman CL, Grisham JR, Mancill RB. Current and lifetime comorbidity of the DSM-IV anxiety and mood disorders in a large clinical sample. *J Abnorm Psychol* 2001; **110**: 585–99.

15. Curtis GC, Hill EM, Lewis JA. Heterogeneity of DSM-III-R simple phobia and the simple phobia/agoraphobia boundary: evidence from the ECA study. *Proceedings of the DSM-IV Anxiety Disorders Work-group.* Ann Arbor, MI, University of Michigan, 1990.

16. Öst LG. Blood and injection phobia: background and cognitive, physiological, and behavioral variables. *Behav Res Ther* 1992; **101**: 68–74.

17. Schatzberg AF, Samson JA, Rothschild AJ, *et al.* McLean hospital depression research facility: early-onset phobic disorders and adult-onset major depression. *Br J Psychiatry* 1998; **173**: 29–34.

18. Schwalberg MD, Barlow DH, Alger SA, Howard LJ. Comparison of bulimics, obese binge eaters, social phobics and individuals with panic disorder on comorbidity across the DSM-III-R anxiety disorders. *J Abnorm Psychol* 1992; **101**: 675–81.

19. Lehman CL, Patterson MD, Brown TA, *et al.* Lifetime alcohol use disorders in patients with anxiety or mood disorders. *Proceedings of the Association for Advancement of Behavior Therapy;* 1998, November: Washington DC.

20. Mowrer OH. Stimulus response theory of anxiety. *Psychol Rev* 1939; **46**: 553–65.

21. Davey GCL. Classical conditioning and the acquisition of human fears and phobias: a review and synthesis of the literature. *Advan Behav Res Ther* 1992; **14**: 29–66.

22. Field AP. Is conditioning a useful framework for understanding the development and treatment of phobias? *Clin Psychol Rev* 2006; **26**: 857–75.

23. Rachman S. The conditioning theory of fear-acquisition: a critical examination. *Behav Res Ther* 1977; **15**: 375–87.

24. Rachman S. Neoconditioning and the classical theory of fear acquisition. *Clin Psychol Rev* 1991; **11**: 155–73.

25. Rachman S. The passing of the two-stage theory of fear and avoidance: fresh possibilities. *Behav Res Ther* 1976; **14**: 125–31.

26. Field AP, Lawson J, Banerjee R. The verbal threat information pathway to fear in children: the longitudinal effects on fear cognitions and the immediate effects on avoidance behavior. *J Abnorm Psychol* 2008; **117**: 214–24.

27. Rachman S. The determinants and treatment of simple phobias. *Adv Behav Res Ther* 1990; **12**: 1–30.

28. Cook M, Mineka S. Observational conditioning of fear to fear-relevant versus fear-irrelevant stimuli in rhesus monkeys. *J Abnorm Psychol* 1989; **98**: 448–59.

29. Carver LJ, Vaccaro BG. 12-month-old infants allocate increased neural resources to stimuli associated with negative adult emotion. *Dev Psychol* 2007; **43**: 54–69.

30. Dubi K, Rapee RM, Emerton JL, Schniering CA. Maternal modeling and the acquisition of fear and avoidance in toddlers: Influence of stimulus preparedness and child temperament. *J Abnorm Child Psychol* 2008; **36**: 499–512.

31. Egliston K-A, Rapee R. Inhibition of fear acquisition in toddlers following modeling by their mothers. *Behav Res Ther* 2007; **45**: 1871–82.

32. Seligman MEP Phobias and preparedness. *Behav Ther* 1971; **2**: 307–20.

33. Menzies RG, Clarke JC. A comparison of in vivo and vicarious exposure in the treatment of childhood water phobia. *Behav Res Ther* 1993; **31**: 9–15.

34. Poulton R, Menzies RG. Fears born and bred: toward a more inclusive theory of fear acquisition. *Behav Res Ther* 2002; **40**: 197–208.

35. Poulton R, Menzies RG. Non-associative fear acquisitions: a review of the evidence from retrospective and longitudinal research. *Behav Res Ther* 2002; **40**: 127–49.

36. Mineka S, Ohman A. Born to fear: non-associative versus associative factors in the etiology of phobias. *Behav Res Ther* 2002; **40**: 173–84.

37. Davey GCL. 'Nonspecific' rather than 'nonassociative' pathways to phobias: a commentary on Poulton and Menzies. *Behav Ther Res* 2002; **40**: 151–8.

38. Kleinknecht RA. Comments on non-associative fear acquisition: a review of the evidence from retrospective and longitudinal research. *Behav Res Ther* 2002; **40**: 159–63.

39. Hofmann SG. Cognitive processes during fear acquisition and extinction in animals and humans: implications for exposure therapy of anxiety disorders. *Clin Psychol Rev* 2008; **28**: 199–210.

40. Seligman MEP. On the generality of the laws of learning. *Psychol Rev* 1970; **77**: 406–18.

41. Hettema JM, Neale MC, Kendler KS. A review and meta-analysis of the genetic epidemiology of anxiety disorders. *Am J Psychiatry* 2001 **158**: 1568–78.

42. Fyer AJ, Mannuzza S, Gallops MS, *et al.* Familial transmission of simple phobias and fears. *Arch Gen Psychiatry* 1990; **47**: 252–6.

43. Kendler KS, Karkowski LM, Prescott CA. Fear and phobias: reliability and heritability. *Psychol Med* 1999; **29**: 539–53.

44. Kendler KS, Myers J, Prescott CA, Neale MC. The genetic epidemiology of irrational fears and phobias in men. *Arch Gen Psychiatry* 2001; **58**: 257–65.

45. Skre I, Onstad S, Torgersen S, Lygren S, Kringlen E. The heritability of common phobic fears: a twin study of a clinical sample. *J Anxiety Disord* 2000; **14**: 549–62.

46. Kagan J, Snidman N. Early childhood predictors of adult anxiety disorders. *Biol Psychiatry* 1999; **46**: 1536–41.

47. Pine DS, Cohen P, Brook J. Adolescent fears as predictors of depression. *Biol Psychiatry* 2001; **50**, 721–4.

48. Biederman J, Rosenbaum JF, Hirshfeld DR, *et al.* Psychiatric correlates of behavioral inhibition in young children of parents with and without psychiatric disorders. *Arch Gen Psychiatry* 1990; **47**: 21–6.

49. Goodwin RD, Fergusson DM, Horwood LJ. Early anxious/withdrawn behaviors predict later internalising disorders. *J Child Psychol Psychiatry* 2004; **45**: 874–83.

50. Reiss S, Peterson RA, Gursky DM, McNally RJ. Anxiety sensitivity, anxiety frequency and the prediction of fearfulness. *Behav Res Ther* 1986; **24**: 1–8.

51. Verburg C, Griez E, Meijer JA. 35% carbon dioxide challenge in simple phobias. *Acta Psychiatr Scand* 1994; **90**: 420–3.

52. Valentiner DP, Telch MJ, Petruzzi DC, Bolte MC. Cognitive mechanisms in claustrophobia: an examination of Reiss and McNally's expectancy model and Bandura's self-efficacy theory. *Cognit Ther Res* 1996; **20**: 593–612.

53. Antony MM, Brown TA, Barlow DH. Response to hyperventilation and 5.5% CO_2 inhalation of subjects with types of specific phobia, panic disorder, or no mental disorder. *Am J Psychiatry* 1997; **154**: 1089–95.

54. Öhman A, Flykt A, Esteves F. Emotion drives attention: detecting the snake in the grass. *J Exp Psychol* 2001; **130**: 466–78.

55. Mogg K, Bradley BP. Time course of attentional bias for fear-relevant pictures in spider-fearful individuals. *Behav Res Ther* 2006; **44**: 1241–50.

56. Thorpe SJ, Salkovskis PM. Selective attention to real phobic and safety stimuli. *Behav Res Ther* 1998; **36**: 471–81.

57. Teachman BA, Stefanucci JK, Clerkin EM, Cody MW, Proffitt DR. A new mode of fear expression: perceptual bias in height fear. *Emotion* 2008; **2**: 296–301.

58. Rachman S, Cuk M. Fearful distortions. *Behav Res Ther* 1992; **30**: 583–9.

59. Riskind JH, Kelly K, Moore R, Harman W, Gaines H. The looming danger: does it discriminate focal phobia and general anxiety from depression? *Cognit Ther Res* 1992; **16**: 1–20.

60. Hunt M, Bylsma L, Brock J, *et al.* The role of imagery in the maintenance and treatment of snake fear. *J Behav Ther Exp Psychiatry* 2006; **37**: 283–98.

61. Arntz A, Lavy E, Van den Berg G, Van Rijsoort S. Negative beliefs of spider phobics: a psychometric evaluation of the Spider Phobia Beliefs Questionnaire. *Adv Behav Res Ther* 1993; **15**: 257–77.

62. Dadds MR, Bovbjerg D, Redd WH, Cutmore T. Imagery and human classical conditioning. *Psychol Bull* 1997; **121**: 89–103.

63. Hunt M, Fenton M. Imagery rescripting versus in vivo exposure in the treatment of snake fear. *J Behav Ther Exp Psychiatry* 2007; **38**: 329–44.

64. Choy Y, Fyer AJ, Lipsitz JD. Treatment of specific phobia in adults. *Clin Psychol Rev* 2007; **27**: 266–86.

65. Wolitzky-Taylor KB, Horowitz JD, Powers M, Telch MJ. Psychological approaches in the treatment of specific phobias: a meta-analysis. *Clin Psychol Rev* 2008; **28**: 1021–37.

66. Chambless DL, Baker MJ, Baucom DH, *et al.* Update on empirically validated therapies, II. *The Clinical Psychologist* 1998; **51**(1): 3–14.

67. Swinson RP, Antony MM, Bleau P, *et al.* Clinical practice guidelines: management of anxiety disorders. *Can J Psychiatry* 2006; **51**(8 Suppl 2): 1S–92S.

68. Bandura A, Blahard EB, Ritter B. Relative efficacy of desensitization and modeling approaches for inducing behavioral, affective, and attitudinal changes. *J Pers Soc Psychol* 1969; **13**: 173–99.

69. Öst LG. One-session treatment of specific phobias in youths: a randomized clinical trial. *J Consult Clin Psychol* 2001; **69**: 814–24.

70. Öst LG, Fellenius J, Sterner U. Applied tension, exposure in vivo, and tension-only in the treatment of blood phobia. *Behav Res Ther* 1991; **29**: 561–74.

71. Öst LG, Johansoon J, Jerremalm A. Individual response patterns and the effects of different behavioral methods in the treatment of claustrophobia. *Behav Res Ther* 1982; **20**: 445–60.

72. Hellström K, Öst LG. Prediction of outcome in the treatment of specific phobia: a cross-validation study. *Behav Res Ther* 1996; **34**: 403–11.

73. Rothbaum BO, Hodges L, Kooper R. Virtual reality exposure therapy. *J Psychother Pract Res* 1997; **6**: 219–26.

74. Rothbaum BO, Hodges LF, Smith S, Lee JH, Price L. A controlled study of virtual reality exposure therapy for the fear of flying. *J Consult Clin Psychol* 2000; **68**: 1020–6.

75. Emmelkamp P, Krijin M, Hulsbosch AM, *et al.* Virtual reality treatment versus exposure in vivo: a comparative evaluation in acrophobia. *Behav Res Ther* 2002; **40**: 509–16.

76. Antony MM, Barlow DH. Specific phobias. In Barlow DH, ed. *Anxiety and its Disorders: The Nature and Treatment of Anxiety and Panic*, 2nd edn. New York: Guilford Press. 2002, pp. 380–417.

77. Hofmann SG, Pollack MH, Otto MW. Augmentation treatment of psychotherapy for anxiety disorders with d-cycloserine. *CNS Drug Rev* 2006; **12**: 208–17.

78. Ressler KJ, Rothbaum BO, Tannenbaum L, *et al.* Cognitive enhancers as adjuncts to psychotherapy: use of d-cycloserine in phobic individuals to facilitate extinction of fear. *Arch Gen Psychiatry* 2004; **61**: 1136–44.

79. Davis M. Role of NMDA receptors and MAP kinase in the amygdala in extinction of fear: clinical implications for exposure therapy. *Eur J Neurosci* 2002; **16**: 395–8.

80. Davis M, Walker D, Myers K. Role of the amygdala in fear extinction measured with potentiated startle. *Ann NY Acad Sci* 2003; **985**: 218–32.

81. Hofmann SG. Enhancing exposure-based therapy from a translational research perspective. *Behav Res Ther* 2007; **45**: 1987–2001.

82. First MB, Spitzer RL, Gibbon MM, Williams JBW. *Structured Clinical Interview for DSM-IV Axis I Disorder – Patient Edition (SCID-I/P Version 2.0).* New York: Biometrics Research Department, New York State Psychiatric Institute, 1996.

83. Di Nardo P, Brown TA, Barlow DH. *Anxiety Disorders Interview Schedule for DSM-IV.* New York: Oxford University Press, 1994.

84. Antony MM. Specific phobia: a brief overview and guide to assessment. In Antony MM, Orsillo SM, Roemer L, eds. *Practitioner's Guide to Empirically Based Measures of Anxiety.* New York: Springer, 2001. pp. 127–32.

85. Rowa K, McCabe RE, Antony MM. Specific phobia and social phobia. In Hunsley J, Mash EJ, eds. *A Guide to Assessments that Work.* New York: Oxford University Press. 2008, pp. 207–28.

86. Moscovitch DA, Antony MM, Swinson RP. Exposure-based treatments for anxiety disorders: theory and process. In Antony MM, Stein MB, eds. *Oxford Handbook of Anxiety and Related Disorders.* New York: Oxford University Press, 2009.

87. Foa EB, Jameson JS, Turner RM, Payne LL. Massed vs. spaced exposure sessions in the treatment of agoraphobia. *Behav Res Ther* 1980; **18**: 333–8.

88. Öst LG. One-session group treatment for spider phobia. *Behav Res Ther* 1996; **34**: 707–15.

89. Antony MM, Swinson RP. *Phobic Disorders and Panic in Adults: A Guide to Assessment and Treatment.* Washington: American Psychological Association, 2000.

90. Antony MM, Craske MG, Barlow DH. *Mastering Your Fears and Phobias (Client Workbook), 2nd edn.* New York: Oxford University Press, 2006.

91. Craske MG, Mystkowski JL. Exposure therapy and extinction: clinical studies. In Craske MG, Hermans D, Vansteenwegen D, eds. *Fear and Learning: From Basic Processes to Clinical Implications.* Washington, DC: American Psychological Association. 2006, pp. 217–33.

92. Rachman S, Radomsky AS, Shafran R. Safety behavior: a reconsideration. *Behav Res Ther* 2008; **46**: 163–73.

93. Wolpe J. *Psychotherapy by Reciprocal Inhibition.* Stanford, CA: Stanford University Press, 1958.

94. Lazarus AA. Crucial procedural factors in desensitization therapy. *Behav Res Ther* 1964; **2**: 63–70.

95. Marshall WL. An examination of reciprocal inhibition and counterconditioning explanations of desensitization therapy. *Eur J Behav Anal Mod* 1975; **1**: 74–86.

96. Antony MM, Watling MA. *Overcoming Medical Phobias: How to Conquer Fear of Blood, Needles, Doctors, and Dentists.* Oakland, CA: New Harbinger Publications, 2006.

97. Rachman S. The return of fear: review and prospect. *Clin Psychol Rev* 1989; **9**: 147–68.

98. Mystkowski JL, Craske MG, Echiverri AM. Treatment context and return of fear in spider phobia. *Behav Ther* 2002; **33**: 399–416.

99. Rachman S. The return of fear. *Behav Res Ther* 1979; **17**: 164–5.

100. Bouton ME, King DA. Contextual control of the extinction of conditioned fear: tests for the associative value of the context. *J Exp Psychol Anim Behav* 1983; **9**: 248–65.

101. Rosas JM, Bouton ME. Renewal of a conditioned taste aversion upon return to the conditioning context after extinction in another one. *Learn Motiv* 1997, **28**: 216–29.

102. Craske MG, Kircanski K, Zelikowsky M, *et al.* Optimizing inhibitory learning during exposure therapy. *Behav Res Ther* 2008; **46**: 5–27.

103. Mystkowski JL, Mineka S, Vernon LL, Zinbarg RE. Changes in caffeine states enhance return of fear in spider phobia. *J Consult Clin Psychol* 2003; **71**: 243–50.

104. Otto M, Basden SL, Leyro TM, McHugh RK, Hofmann S. Clinical perspectives on the combination of D-Cycloserine and cognitive-behavioral therapy for the treatment of anxiety disorders. *CNS Spectr* 2007; **12**: 59–61.

105. Antony MM, McCabe RE. *Overcoming Animal and Insect Phobias: How to Conquer Fear of Dogs, Snakes, Rodents, Bees, Spiders, and More.* Oakland, CA: New Harbinger Publications, 2005.

106. McCabe RE, Antony MM. Anxiety disorders: social and specific phobias. In *Psychiatry*, 3rd edn. Tasman A, Kay A, Lieberman JA, First MB, Maj M, eds. Chichester, UK: John Wiley & Sons, Ltd, 2008.

107. Cohen DC. Comparison of self-report and overt behavioral procedures for assessing acrophobia. *Behav Ther* 1977; **8**: 17–23.

108. Radomsky AS, Rachman S, Thordarson DS, *et al.* The Claustrophobia Questionnaire. *J Anxiety Disord* 2001; **15**: 287–97.

109. Stouthard MEA, Mellenbergh GJ, Hoogstraten J. Assessment of dental anxiety: a facet approach. *Anx Stress Coping* 1993; **6**: 89–105.

110. Haug T, Brenne L, Johnsen BH, *et al.* The three-systems analysis of fear of flying: a comparison of a consonant vs. a non-consonant treatment method. *Behav Res Ther* 1987; **25**: 187–94.

111. Marks IM, Mathews AM. Brief standard self-rating for phobic patients. *Behav Res Ther* 1979; **17**: 263–7.

112. Szymanski J, O'Donohue W. Fear of Spiders Questionnaire. *J Behav Ther and Exp Psychiatry* 1995; **26**: 31–4.

113. Geer JH. The development of a scale to measure fear. *Behav Res Ther* 1965; **3**: 45–53.

114. Wolpe J, Lang PJ. A Fear Survey Schedule for use in behaviour therapy. *Behav Res Ther* 1964; **2**: 27–30.

115. Wolpe J, Lang PJ. *Fear Survey Schedule.* San Diego, CA: Educational and Industrial Testing Service; 1969.

116. Wolpe J, Lang PJ. *Manual for the Fear Survey Schedule* (revised). San Diego, CA: Educational and Industrial Testing Service, 1977.

117. Kleinknecht RA, Thorndike RM, Walls MM. Factorial dimensions and correlates of blood, injury, injection and related medical fears: cross validation of the Medical Fear Survey. *Behav Res Ther* 1996; **34**: 323–31.

118. Cutshall C, Watson D. The Phobic Stimuli Response Scales: a new self-report measure of fear. *Behav Res Ther* 2004; **42**: 1193–201.

119. Klorman R, Hastings J, Weerts T, *et al.* Psychometric description of some specific-fear questionnaires. *Behav Ther* 1974; **5**: 401–9.

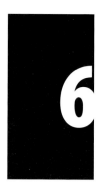

6 Panic disorder and agoraphobia

Jason M. Prenoveau and Michelle G. Craske

Nature of the disorder

Symptoms

Panic disorder is characterized by unexpected panic attacks, anxiety about experiencing future attacks, and avoidance or dread of situations where attacks might occur. Panic attacks are defined as discrete periods of fear that develop abruptly and are accompanied by physical symptoms, cognitive symptoms, or both [1]. Panic attack symptoms include sweating, shortness of breath, heart palpitations, trembling or shaking, chest pain or discomfort, feeling of choking, nausea, fear of dying or going crazy, derealization or depersonalization, chills or hot flushes, numbness, and feeling dizzy, unsteady, or faint.

Diagnostic criteria

The first criterion of panic disorder is the presence of recurrent, unexpected panic attacks [1]. It is required that "unexpected" panic attacks occur, meaning that from the patient's perspective, such attacks seem to occur "out of the blue" or without any obvious causes. This is an important feature when conducting a differential diagnosis, as panic attacks that occur due to other anxiety disorders are situationally bound or situationally predisposed (e.g., panic attacks cued by social situations in social phobia). Although panic disorder patients *may* experience such situationally bound or situationally predisposed panic, in order to meet diagnostic criteria for panic disorder, they *must* experience recurrent, "unexpected" panic attacks. Also, the panic attacks must not be caused by the direct physiological effects of a substance or general medical condition [1].

Experiencing unexpected panic attacks is necessary, but not sufficient, for a diagnosis of panic disorder. The disorder's defining feature is the response to such attacks, specifically, at least one month of one or more of the following: significant behavioral change related to the attacks, persistent worry about recurrence of the attacks, or worry about the consequences of the attacks [1]. Examples of behavioral changes related to panic attacks include avoiding activities that might induce panic-related physiological sensations, or engaging in safety-related behaviors such as carrying a cell phone or medication. Worry about the consequences of attacks might involve fear of having a fatal heart attack or passing out in front of others.

Panic disorder can be diagnosed either with or without the presence of agoraphobia. According to the *Diagnostic and Statistical Manual of Mental Disorders*, agoraphobia is characterized by anxiety about situations where it would be difficult (or embarrassing) to escape, or difficult to get help if one were to experience a panic attack or panic symptoms. Such situations are avoided, endured with extreme distress or anxiety about experiencing panic, or are only attended with a companion [1]. Common agoraphobic situations include waiting in line, crowded places such as malls or movie theaters, being alone, or traveling by bus, train, or car.

Course

Although relatively rare, panic disorder in children and adolescents tends to be chronic [2], and most of those diagnosed in childhood or adolescence will still meet criteria for the disorder as young adults [3]. In adults, longitudinal results from clinical settings indicate that the typical course of panic with agoraphobia is constant, whereas panic without agoraphobia tends to be characterized by periods of remission and relapse [4]. However, persistence of the disorder, as defined by

Cognitive–behavioral Therapy with Adults: A Guide to Empirically Informed Assessment and Intervention, ed. Stefan G. Hofmann and Mark A. Reinecke. © Cambridge University Press 2010.

the 12-month prevalence of the disorder among life-time cases, is not significantly different for panic disorder with (57.4%) or without (62.6%) agoraphobia [5]. This relatively chronic condition results in significant interpersonal and financial impairment and is associated with increased levels of disability and increased emergency room, medical provider, and mental health visits [6].

Epidemiology

A recent epidemiological study, the National Comorbidity Survey –Replication (NCS-R), estimated lifetime prevalence for panic disorder with or without agoraphobia at 4.7%, while 12-month prevalence is estimated at 2.8%; the ratio of females to males is approximately 2 to 1 [5]. The NCS-R also found a median age of onset of 24 years with an interquartile range spanning from age 16 to 40 [7].

Comorbidity

Panic disorder, with or without agoraphobia, typically occurs in combination with other Axis I disorders. When considering lifetime diagnoses in a nationally representative sample, one or more conditions have at some point been diagnosed in 83% of those with panic disorder without agoraphobia and 100% of those with panic with agoraphobia [5]. For panic without agoraphobia, 66% have been diagnosed with another anxiety disorder, 50% with a mood disorder, 47% with an impulse-control disorder, and 27% with a substance use disorder. The most common anxiety disorders co-occurring with panic disorder are specific phobias (34%), social phobia (31%), post-traumatic stress disorder (22%), and generalized anxiety disorder (21%). The most common non-anxiety disorders seen in those with panic disorder include major depression (35%), alcohol abuse or dependence (25%), and conduct disorder (22%).

Review of cognitive models of the condition

Panic disorder is conceptualized as an acquired fear of bodily sensations, specifically those sensations associated with autonomic arousal [8, 9]. After experiencing unexpected panic attacks, those with panic disorder develop anxiety about experiencing such attacks in the future. But why do individuals experience unexpected panic attacks in the first place and what causes some people to develop fear of experiencing future attacks?

From an evolutionary perspective, a fear or panic response is adaptive in the presence of threatening situations. Panic in the absence of threatening stimuli, or unexpected panic, is presumed to be caused by the interaction of stressful life events and psychological and biological vulnerabilities. A tendency to experience negative emotions, often labeled neuroticism or negative affect, is largely inherited [10] and has been shown to be predictive of panic attacks [11]. This inherited temperament likely serves as a biological vulnerability to experience both fear – an immediate alarm reaction characterized by strong sympathetic nervous system arousal – and anxiety – a negative mood state characterized by worry about future events and somatic symptoms of tension. Environmental factors in childhood can play a role in shaping whether or not an individual feels confidence in themselves and their abilities to deal with, or control, future life events. Such a sense of control, or uncontrollability, might serve as a psychological vulnerability to experience fear and anxiety [12]. Stressful life events, such as a new job or death in the family, might interact with biological and psychological vulnerabilities to trigger an emotional fear response, or panic attack. Although increased stress levels caused by stressful life events might contribute to causing a panic attack, an individual could still perceive the attack as being "unexpected" because of the absence of imminent threatening stimuli.

After the occurrence of an unexpected panic attack, the same general vulnerabilities mentioned above likely play a role in determining whether or not an individual then develops "anxious apprehension" about experiencing future attacks. In addition to these general vulnerabilities to experience panic and anxiety, it is believed that there are also specific vulnerabilities that contribute to the development of panic disorder. One example is anxiety sensitivity, which is the belief that anxiety and its symptoms cause harmful physical, social, and psychological consequences outside the physical discomfort of a panic episode [13]. Enhanced awareness of, or ability to detect, bodily sensations of arousal is another proposed psychological vulnerability specific to panic disorder [14]. Experience with medical illnesses in childhood (either personal or parental), specifically those involving respiratory disturbance, might also contribute to a specific psychological vulnerability for panic disorder [15].

Anxiety about future panic attacks is associated with fears of somatic sensations that accompany the attacks. Anxiety focused on bodily sensations of panic is attributed to interoceptive conditioning and catastrophic misappraisals of bodily sensations, two factors posited to maintain panic disorder. Interoceptive conditioning is the process by which low-level, non-panic bodily sensations of arousal come to serve as conditioned stimuli that can trigger increased autonomic arousal through Pavlovian conditioning [16]. Thus, small changes in physiological functioning can lead to conditioned fear or panic as a result of prior pairings of these initial somatic sensations with full blown panic. Catastrophic misappraisals of bodily sensations, such as the idea that sensations will lead to death or permanent loss of control, is another factor believed to contribute to anxiety about bodily sensations of arousal [9]. Whether the result of interoceptive conditioning or catastrophic misappraisals, extreme anxiety about bodily sensations of somatic arousal in panic disorder has been reliably demonstrated using a wide range of paradigms.

Such anxiety about bodily sensations plays a central role in the maintenance of panic disorder. Sensations can be caused by physical activity, chemical compounds such as caffeine, feared environmental stimuli, and anxious thoughts or images. Once the bodily sensations are noticed, they elicit fear in an individual with panic disorder. This fear serves to intensify the sensations, causing an increase in fear, which further enhances the bodily sensations as part of a self-perpetuating cycle of fear and bodily sensations that typically results in a panic attack. Thus, the fear of experiencing bodily sensations of arousal contributes to the development of a full blown panic attack, reinforcing the belief that the sensations should be feared.

Individuals with panic disorder often are unaware that panic attacks can be triggered in this manner (by bodily sensations or preceding internal or external stimuli). This means that for those with panic disorder, panic attacks often are perceived as unexpected and unpredictable. Because they are unable to stop the symptoms of a panic attack once it begins, such attacks are also perceived as uncontrollable. Perceived unpredictability and uncontrollability of panic attacks can amplify chronic anxiety levels. Higher chronic anxiety levels can increase the probability of future panic attacks through enhancing the frequency/intensity of anxiety-related sensations as well as enhancing an individual's awareness of the sensations [8].

Behavioral responses to panic, specifically safety behaviors and avoidance, also serve as maintaining factors of the disorder. As previously mentioned, an individual with panic disorder mistakenly believes that a panic attack will result in catastrophic physical or mental harm, such as having a heart attack, passing out, going crazy, or losing control. Therefore, experiencing panic attacks where none of these things occur should disconfirm these beliefs. However, those with panic disorder may engage in safety behaviors that they believe enable them to escape or avoid the feared outcome. For example, if an individual believes that they will pass out during a panic attack, they might sit down or hold on to an object for support. Engaging in safety behaviors prevents disconfirmation of cognitive misappraisals, thus contributing to the maintenance of panic disorder [17]. Individuals may also engage in safety behaviors designed to prevent panic, or its feared consequences, such as always carrying around anxiolytic medication or traveling with a companion who makes them feel safe.

Another panic-maintaining behavioral response is overt avoidance. Individuals will tend to avoid particular places or situations where they believe there is increased likelihood of developing panic. Avoidance prevents disconfirmation of catastrophic misappraisals, and reinforces the fear that those particular situations are dangerous, increasing the likelihood of panicking in those situations in the future. Furthermore, if an individual avoids those circumstances where they have experienced unexpected panic in the past, future attacks will inevitably occur in new, previously "safe" circumstances. Thus, the arena of safe circumstances shrinks as more of the world becomes a dangerous place where panic is likely to occur. This pattern can enhance both behavioral avoidance as well as chronic levels of anxious apprehension.

Empirical support for efficacy and effectiveness of treatment

Cognitive–behavioral therapy (CBT) is an empirically supported intervention that American Psychiatric Association guidelines "recommend with substantial clinical confidence" for the treatment of panic disorder [18]. Cognitive–behavioral therapy treatments evaluated in clinical trials demonstrate short- and long-term efficacy in both individual [19, 20] and group modalities [21, 22]. A meta-analysis including

22 studies of CBT for panic disorder found that at the end of treatment 63.3% of those who completed treatment had improved while 53.8% of the intent-to-treat sample had improved [23]. When assessed 12 to 23 months after treatment termination, these percentages improved to 75.3% and 71.6%, respectively. When considering panic disorder, a more recent meta-analysis of CBT for adult anxiety disorders found CBT resulted in significantly better outcomes than a placebo condition [24]. In addition to reducing symptoms of anxiety and depression, CBT for panic disorder also produces improvements in quality-of-life indices [25] and has a beneficial impact on physical health [26].

When comparing CBT to pharmacotherapy for the treatment of panic, a recent meta-analysis of 129 studies found that CBT was as effective as pharmacotherapy and demonstrated significantly lower drop-out rates [27]. Meta-analytic findings seem to indicate that compared to CBT alone, combining CBT and pharmacotherapy might improve short-term, but not long-term, outcomes [27, 28]. One large clinical trial found that following medication discontinuation, the group receiving both CBT and medication did not perform as well as those receiving only CBT [19]. Thus, the presence of medication during therapy might serve as a state or context effect, reducing the generalizability of learning that occurs during CBT.

While many controlled trials have demonstrated the efficacy of CBT for panic disorder, far fewer studies on naturalistic implementation of interventions – effectiveness studies – have been conducted. Effectiveness studies typically have fewer exclusionary criteria and broaden the scope of outcome measurement, making their findings more generalizable than those of efficacy studies. Results from primary care settings, where many cases present and are treated, indicate that CBT combined with medication recommendations provides significantly better results on a number of outcome measures than treatment as usual for panic disorder [e.g., 29].

Introduction to a clinical case

The case example described below is used to highlight areas of treatment protocol, difficulties encountered during treatment, and clinical decision making in CBT practice.

Identifying information

Tina was a 19-year-old, single female with no siblings who lived with her parents and was unemployed. She presented to a specialty clinic for assessment and treatment of her symptoms of anxiety and depression.

Presenting problem

Tina reported that she experienced "terrible" episodes several times a week. During these episodes, she would experience shortness of breath, an "uncontrollably" racing heart, trembling, dizziness, tingling in her hands and feet, lightheadedness, and feelings of unreality. Tina indicated that she had gone to the emergency room during her first episode because she thought she was dying. Her physician told her that her physical symptoms would not cause physical harm such as a stroke or heart attack and she believed him. Despite this, she still feared something terrible might happen, such as losing control or fainting.

Tina reported that she constantly feared having another episode and that she never left the house without one of her parents because she felt "unsafe" outside of the house without them. Tina reported that things had been so bad lately that she felt worthless and guilty about "ruining" her parents' lives. She felt sad almost all of the time and was unable to enjoy the few activities she was still able to do, such as watching movies at home. Although she had been nervous and reluctant to talk to somebody about these problems, her parents had insisted when she had started saying things like maybe she would be better off dead. Tina reported that she would never do anything to physically harm herself – she was too afraid of death.

Relevant history

Tina said she has been somewhat anxious and shy for as long as she could remember, but that she did not experience a panic episode until she left home for college. She was feeling particularly anxious around this time because she was concerned about making new friends, living away from home, and whether or not she was smart enough for college. The panic episodes quickly became so frequent, and Tina feared them so much, that she dropped out of college and returned home. She attended community college near home and had a part-time job, but after several unexpected panic episodes in these settings she left both school and work. She was currently being supported by her parents. Since her mother did not have a job, she was able to stay at home with Tina much of the time and accompany Tina when she needed to go out.

Tina reported that she had terrible asthma attacks during her childhood. Although she had outgrown her asthma during high school, she still always carried her inhaler in case her asthma should return. Tina did not report any other current or past medical issues, medications, or alcohol or substance use. She indicated that neither she nor her parents had ever been treated for mental health problems. She said that her mother was "high-strung" and very superstitious.

Diagnostic impressions and treatment recommendations

Tina was diagnosed with panic disorder with agoraphobia and major depression. Individual CBT was recommended and a psychiatric consultation to discuss medication options was offered. Tina agreed to treatment but expressed doubt that it would be helpful for her. She turned down the psychiatric consultation indicating that she refused to take any medication as even aspirin made her "feel funny."

Overview of CBT treatment protocol

Structure of session

Sessions begin with a brief review of material from the prior week, enabling the therapist to assess the client's perception and understanding of previously covered material. Next, the therapist discusses session goals with the client, setting an agenda of what is to be covered in the coming session. The first agenda item is typically to review the past week's homework. Such review reinforces clients' homework completion behavior and provides the therapist an opportunity to assess understanding and provide corrective feedback where needed.

The remainder of the session is spent working on the major components of CBT for panic disorder. As laid out in the session-by-session example below, different components are stressed at different stages of therapy. Early sessions involve psychoeducation and instruction of skills such as breathing retraining and cognitive restructuring. Later sessions involve designing and conducting exposures where clients employ these skills while facing their fears. Before ending each session, feedback is elicited to assess how the client has interpreted the presented material and to determine if there are any questions. Clients are given instructions or asked to write down any between-session assignments. Therapists review these assignments to reinforce their importance and to assess for client questions or concerns about homework.

Therapeutic relationship

When considering CBT for a range of disorders, certain therapist variables, such as empathy, positive regard, and genuineness, are consistently related to positive outcomes, while patients' perception of the therapist as being self-confident, active, and skillful are somewhat related to positive outcomes [30]. In CBT for panic disorder, directive statements and explanations in session 1 have been shown to be associated with poorer outcomes [31]. Also, session 1 empathic statements are associated with better outcomes whereas session 3 empathic statements are associated with poorer outcomes [31]. Such findings indicate that the best outcomes might be achieved by establishing a therapeutic alliance through empathic statements and questioning in the first session, and becoming more directive in later sessions.

Strategies and techniques

The major elements of CBT for panic disorder include psychoeducation, self-monitoring, breathing retraining, cognitive restructuring, and exposure (both interoceptive and in vivo). These elements are used to remedy catastrophic misappraisals and avoidance/fear of bodily sensations and agoraphobic situations; each element is briefly discussed here and their implementation is detailed in the session-by-session example below. Psychoeducation provides information to help correct misconceptions about panic/anxiety, normalize the condition for clients, and let them know that treatments for panic are effective. It also provides a rationale for subsequent treatment activities.

Self-monitoring helps clients objectively observe their emotional responding rather than subjectively judge it. Self-monitoring can lessen distress, increase understanding of emotional reactions, and increase a sense of control. Breathing retraining is introduced as a coping skill for interrupting physiological over-reactivity. The mechanisms by which breathing retraining is effective, and the degree to which it is effective for panic, are still under study [32]. However, it is important that clients do not use it as a means of avoiding negative feelings. Cognitive restructuring is the process of replacing automatic anxious thoughts, or cognitive errors, with more realistic thoughts. This involves teaching the client the typical cognitive errors of anxiety (overestimation of risk and catastrophizing), and how to identify their own automatic anxious thoughts. Next, they are taught how to treat these thoughts as hypotheses and gather evidence to confirm or disconfirm them. Finally, they are encouraged to generate alternative hypotheses that they also gather evidence to confirm or disconfirm.

Repeated exposure to both feared bodily sensations (interoceptive exposure) and feared situations (in vivo exposure) is performed to disconfirm cognitive misappraisals and extinguish conditioned emotional responses to these sensations and situations. Using breathing retraining and cognitive restructuring to face these sensations and situations provides clients with corrective experiences that are not achieved by avoiding or escaping these feared sensations and situations.

Relapse prevention

Therapists can help clients maintain treatment gains and prevent symptomatic relapse after therapy termination by educating them about what to expect after treatment ends and helping them plan for it. A schedule of exposures to be conducted in the months following therapy termination should be established. Booster sessions can be scheduled so the therapist can check the client's progress several months after termination and review coping skills. Clients are informed that despite their best efforts, flare-ups of anxiety or avoidance behavior are likely to occur in the future. It is essential that they do not confuse such lapses with failure. The most important thing to do when symptoms return is to apply their coping skills and practice interoceptive and in vivo exposure. At such times, it might also be beneficial to return to therapy for booster sessions. Clients are informed that such flare-ups are more likely to occur when general life stress increases, such as during a serious illness or loss of a relationship. Also, clients are taught to recognize signs of symptom return (such as subtle avoidance or safety signals), as early identification and corrective action can help control the magnitude of symptom recurrence. If the client has been taking medication during treatment, it is helpful to reinforce the idea that exposure outcomes, and therefore exposure learning, are independent of the medication. This is especially important if the client is using quick-acting benzodiazepine medications, which may block fear responding. If time permits, the possibility of discontinuing the medication during therapy can be explored.

Session-by-session example

Session 1

The goals for the first session are to begin psychoeducation, provide a treatment rationale, and initiate self-monitoring. Psychoeducation involves a description of anxiety disorders and their treatment, informing clients that many people experience such problems and CBT is often successful in helping. The differences between fear and anxiety are explained as well as the adaptive purposes of both: to protect us from threat or danger (whether the threat is real or imagined) that is immediate (fear) and distant (anxiety). The psychophysiology of the fight-or-flight response is detailed, including how it can help to deal with imminent danger, hence contributing to survival. This information is provided to correct common misconceptions about panic symptoms (e.g., they signal that one is going crazy) and to lay the groundwork for developing an alternative conceptual framework for understanding emotional reactions that will compete with the client's catastrophic appraisals.

Next taught are the three major components of fear and anxiety – physical symptoms, thoughts (cognitions), and behaviors – and how they interact contributing to the maintenance of panic disorder. Clients are encouraged to list physical symptoms, thoughts, and behaviors from a recent panic episode and explore how their responses might prolong or intensify each other. For example, when Tina notices her heart beating rapidly, she becomes afraid she will have a panic attack and pass out. This alarming thought results in a more rapid heart-beat and other physical symptoms of anxiety, which in turn enhances her fear of having a panic attack. Her behavior – rushing home where it is "safe" – reinforces her belief that everywhere else is not safe. It is explained that treatment will be aimed at disrupting this negative cycle by addressing the three major anxiety components: changing self-statements or beliefs, controlling physiological reactions, and facing fear-producing objects, situations, and places.

Self-monitoring is taught to help clients objectively observe their emotional responding. For example, Tina's subjective evaluation, "I'm feeling anxious so there's no way I could go shopping" could be objectively described, "My heart is beating harder. One of my thoughts is that I will have a panic episode and pass out if I go to the store." Clients are asked to complete a monitoring form for a recent panic attack detailing physical sensations, thoughts, and behavioral reactions as well as the situation where the attack occurred and their maximal fear rating. Self-monitoring of panic episodes is assigned for the coming week. Clients are also provided with bibliotherapy material about anxiety and fear to read during the coming week.

Session 2

The goals are to reinforce self-monitoring, continue psychoeducation, and introduce coping skills: breathing retraining and cognitive restructuring. As with all sessions, homework is reviewed and corrective feedback is provided. Psychoeducation is continued by explaining Pavlovian conditioning to help clients understand that both external and internal cues can serve as triggers for panic and these cues can generalize in the absence of conscious awareness. Understanding this model helps clients to understand that their panic attacks are explainable and are not random, or "out of the blue."

Breathing retraining is next introduced as a coping skill for interrupting physiological over-reactivity and facilitating corrective thinking and action. The client is taught diaphragmatic breathing: breathing from their abdomen rather than their chest. They are to focus on their breathing by counting to themselves as they inhale ("one") and thinking "relax" as they exhale. For their first week of practice, they are to breathe at their normal volume and rate. After three to five minutes of in-session practice, breathing retraining homework is assigned for the coming week: ten minutes of practice, twice daily in a comfortable, quiet location.

Cognitive restructuring is introduced as a coping skill to change client thinking in anxiety-provoking situations. Clients are reminded that anxious thoughts need to be addressed because they generate anxious behaviors and anxious feelings. It is explained that although anxious thoughts can be "automatic," occurring very rapidly without full awareness, they can still influence feelings and actions. These thoughts tend to be specific in content, and may vary across situations and time. Consequently, it is important to identify the specific content or prediction that is creating anxiety in particular situations.

The client is taught to use the "downward arrow" technique to identify these specific automatic cognitions. This technique involves clients asking themselves what they are afraid of in a given situation, and then identifying what would it mean or what would happen if that were true. The meaning of the second thought is then probed and the process is continued until the core automatic anxious thought is identified. For example, Tina wrote on her monitoring form that while she was driving she became scared when her heart started racing so she pulled over and had her mother drive. To uncover her automatic thought, the therapist might ask what would have happened if her heart had continued beating hard. To Tina's response of "It would have been terrible," he could ask what she imagines might have happened that would have been so terrible. To Tina's reply, "My heart would pound harder, I'd get shaky, and I might get lightheaded," he could ask her what she pictured happening if she experienced those sensations. The therapist would continue this questioning until he arrived at her core anxious belief: that if she did not pull the car over, she would pass out and crash the car, killing herself and her mother. It is explained that identifying automatic thoughts is the first step in cognitive restructuring and should be practiced as part of this week's self-monitoring homework.

Session 3

The goal is to continue developing coping skills. The client is instructed in slowed breathing, which involves counting and *then* inhaling, thinking the word "relax" and *then* exhaling. The pace is about three seconds for inhalation and three seconds for exhalation. After practice, slowed breathing is assigned for homework to be completed twice a day for ten minutes.

Cognitive restructuring is continued by explaining the two major types of cognitive errors in anxiety: overestimating risk and catastrophizing. Overestimating risk involves thinking a negative event is much more likely to occur than it really is; catastrophizing is viewing the event as being beyond one's coping ability. Clients are assisted in identifying their automatic thoughts that involve overestimating risk. Tina is overestimating the risk that she will "lose control" when she has a panic attack. Despite never having lost control during an attack, Tina still thinks the likelihood of doing so is high. Clients make several errors in logic that can perpetuate such misappraisals. They might believe that the more intense the anxiety, the greater the risk of the feared event. Clients may also believe that the negative event has not occurred because of luck or because of a safety behavior (rushing someplace "safe" in Tina's case). It is explained to clients how these are mistaken beliefs.

Next, clients are taught to treat their thoughts as hypotheses rather than facts. Socratic questioning is used to help them gather evidence to determine a more realistic probability. For example, Tina thinks the likelihood of losing control of the car and getting into an accident during a panic attack is close to 100%. She is asked if it has ever happened before and if there is any evidence to suggest that it will, or will not, happen. After obtaining a more realistic probability, clients are assisted in generating alternative thoughts. For Tina, an alternate hypothesis might be: I am just experiencing anxiety and I can drive while experiencing anxious thoughts and bodily sensations of anxiety.

Experiments are designed with clients to enable them to gather evidence to support alternative hypotheses and disconfirm their overestimation of risk appraisal. The specific feared outcome is recorded and tested as homework. For example, Tina's task might be to do an activity, such as getting the mail by herself, while she feels lightheaded. Her specific hypothesis is her overestimation of risk, that she will definitely faint. She is to do the activity in the coming week and record the result from the experiment on a hypothesis testing form.

Session 4

The goal is to continue developing coping skills. Breathing retraining issues are discussed and homework is assigned: mini-practices throughout the day in more distracting, but still not anxiety-provoking, situations. After the hypothesis-testing homework exercise is reviewed, additional tests are generated for the coming week.

Clients are next assisted in identifying catastrophizing errors. An example for Tina might be, "It would be terrible to faint in front of my friends – I could never face them again." The goal for handling these errors is to help clients decatastophize them: imagine the worst happening and then evaluate the severity of that consequence and ways of coping with it. This method can be applied to events that are both likely (panicking in front of friends) and unlikely (passing out due to anxiety) to occur. Decatastrophizing stresses that specific catastrophes are unlikely (e.g., fainting due to excessive anxiety) and symptoms of anxiety and their effects (e.g., embarrassment) are time limited and/or manageable.

Once identified, clients are assisted in challenging catastrophic thoughts by questioning the meaning given to the event, identifying where they are blowing things out of proportion, and generating alternative hypotheses where appropriate. The therapist helps the client to switch from focusing on how bad it would be if the event happened to considering ways of coping with the outcome. For example, Tina feared that if her friends saw her faint they would make fun of her behind her back and she would be unable to face them again. Alternative hypotheses might include: people have fainted before and retained their friends, her friends might be concerned and help her, and when she regained consciousness she could face her friends again. Even if the worst happened, and after generating alternatives Tina realized this was unlikely, it would be possible to cope with losing some friends. She had made new friends in the past and could do so again if necessary. Experiments are designed to test one of the client's catastrophic misappraisals during the coming week. As part of self-monitoring, the client is asked to identify valence errors and go through the above process to decatastrophize them.

Session 5

The goal of this session is to introduce exposure with a focus upon exposure to internal cues and implementation of coping skills. After reviewing the past week's practice, the client is encouraged to use breathing retraining as a coping skill for managing acute fear and anxiety. Breathing retraining is to be used to interrupt the anxious cycle upon first experiencing physical sensations of arousal, enabling cognitive restructuring strategies to be applied.

Client's cognitive restructuring of probability overestimation and catastrophizing errors are reviewed and problems are addressed. For example, clients might complain that cognitive tools are not immediately lessening fear and anxiety. In this case, it is explained that the goal is to shift automatic thinking, which helps interrupt the cycle of anxiety in the long term. Results from hypothesis-testing experiments are next reviewed, and disconfirmation of the client's initial misappraisal is reinforced. A new experiment for the coming week is designed.

Unreinforced exposure to feared stimuli results in reducing fear responding to the stimuli through extinguishing fear associations and promoting new learning. While such exposure to feared stimuli is critical for the success of treatment, it is important to be mindful of how difficult exposure can be for clients. The treatment rationale and clients' newly acquired coping skills are reviewed to enhance motivation and increase commitment to engage in exposure exercises. Interoceptive exposure is first conducted to promote new learning about bodily sensations. Clients are told that they will be inducing physical sensations that elicit distress to learn that the sensations are not harmful and can be tolerated. They are reminded of interoceptive conditioning and how subtle changes in physiology can trigger anxious thoughts and increased physiological arousal due to prior pairings of these sensations with panic. Clients are reminded that avoiding changes in physical state or activities that induce them prevents corrective learning that the physical symptoms are not harmful and can be tolerated. It is explained that avoidance maintains fear; by facing the bodily sensations that bother them, they will learn to no longer fear them.

The client is led through activities (e.g., stair climbing, spinning, hyperventilating, etc.) designed to induce physical sensations they experience during panic. They are to continue the activity for 30 seconds beyond when they first notice the sensations. Next, they record the sensations they felt, how anxious they were, and how similar the sensations were to those experienced during panic. An activity with a mild fear rating and some similarity to naturally occurring panic sensations is used for an in-session interoceptive exercise and assigned for homework (to be practiced three times per day). Clients are instructed that exercises are conducted by: inducing the sensations, making fear ratings, and using breathing retraining and cognitive restructuring coping skills. They are to answer the following questions with each exercise: did the feared catastrophe (e.g., loss of control) occur, did they survive being afraid, and does their fear subside with repetition.

It is then explained that the next type of exposure will be in vivo: exposure to places and situations that clients avoid or enter with apprehension. For homework, clients are to construct a hierarchy of such situations ranked by how much they fear the situation. A driving hierarchy for Tina (with fear ratings in parentheses) might include: sitting in the car (1); driving one mile with mom in the car (3); driving to the local store with mom (4); driving on the highway for five miles with mom (7); driving to the local store alone (8); driving on the highway for five miles alone (10).

Session 6

The goals are to conduct repeated interoceptive exposures and to design an in vivo exposure. An interoceptive exposure activity that elicits slightly more fear than last week's activity is chosen, performed in-session

following the guidelines from last session, and then assigned for homework. Next, clients are reminded of the importance of dealing with situations that induce anxiety, and learning to cope with anxiety in those situations. After review of their hierarchy of feared situations, one is chosen to practice for the coming week. The situation should have a fear rating of about 3 or 4 (on a 0 to 10 scale) and should be one they can practice repeatedly in the coming week. The exposure is typically repeated until fear of it reduces to mild or less (2 or less on the scale). They should practice on at least three occasions in the coming week.

The client is taught to rehearse cognitive restructuring in relation to their in vivo exposure task. Before each exposure, they are to identify their anxious thoughts, generate alternative ways of thinking by considering all evidence, and generate ways of coping. It is particularly helpful to imagine becoming anxious or panicky in the situation and then imagine controlling the fear by slow, abdominal breathing and self-talk. Rehearsing these coping skills in session and prior to exposure will enable clients to better use these skills in the midst of the actual situation. Tina's first in vivo exposure was to drive a mile with mom in the car. In session, she imagined herself in the situation feeling panicky. Although she feared losing control and crashing in such a situation, she reminded herself that she had never lost control while driving and that it was more realistic that she would be able to adequately drive with the sensations of panic. She also imagined herself doing abdominal breathing to reduce her physical sensations of arousal.

Sessions 7 and beyond

The goals for this and subsequent sessions are to continue interoceptive and in vivo exposures with implementation of coping skills to manage and reduce anxiety. Relapse prevention strategies are also explored. Clients continue working up their hierarchy of interoceptive exercises each week. As fear to interoceptive sensations subsides, activities that provoke interoceptive cues in naturalistic settings are introduced. Examples include drinking coffee, watching exciting movies, and exercising. Fear ratings for these are obtained and activities are assigned for homework as was done for interoceptive exercises.

Clients' in vivo exposures are reviewed, with the therapist helping clients to focus on the corrective learning derived from the task. The therapist should assess whether the perceived catastrophe happened, whether fear and anxiety were tolerated, and whether fear and anxiety subsided with repetition. In Tina's case, the therapist might ask if Tina had anxious thoughts and physical sensations while she drove. Then, he or she might ask if she "lost control" and crashed the car. Through Socratic questioning, the therapist reinforces the exposure learning: that Tina could tolerate symptoms of anxiety, that her feared catastrophe did not occur, and that anxiety symptoms lessened with repeated exposure. Each week a more anxiety-provoking in vivo exposure is chosen for homework and troubleshooting is performed as necessary.

Later sessions explore safety signals, which include specific people or objects that make one feel safe from anxiety, loss of control, physical injury, or embarrassment. In Tina's case, her house, parents, and inhaler all served as safety signals. It is explained to the client that safety signal removal improves exposure learning efficacy. By facing situations with safety signals, the client retains the belief that the situations are dangerous, but that the danger is being prevented by the safety signal. Safety signal removal is incorporated into the in vivo exposure hierarchy.

Difficulties encountered during treatment

One reason that CBT treatment of panic disorder fails to produce successful results is clients' premature withdrawal from therapy. For example, a large-scale trial of CBT for panic disorder had one out of five clients prematurely drop out of therapy [33]. Identifying predictors of premature withdrawal could aid in determining those at risk for dropping out as well as providing information about how to retain them in therapy. Education, socioeconomic status, and motivation are all negatively associated with drop-out rates in CBT for panic [33, 34]. Self-reported reasons for drop out typically include dissatisfaction with one or more of the following: therapeutic relationship, type of treatment, treatment procedures, or benefits of therapy [33].

Predictors of withdrawal and reasons given for termination suggest ways for improving client retention. Lower education and socioeconomic status might increase attrition through mechanisms such as increased obstacles to session attendance (cost, available time, reliable means of transportation, etc.) or reduced comprehension of CBT rationale and/or

techniques. Obstacles to attendance, such as the examples given above, could be assessed during intake, providing therapists an opportunity to explore solutions with the client. Therapists could also tailor their material presentation such that it will be understood by the client. As discussed in the treatment protocol above, checking in with the client at the beginning and end of sessions can aid in assessing their understanding. Asking clients to provide examples from their lives that are relevant to material or skills being covered can also help the therapist to assess comprehension.

Motivation can be addressed by helping clients to identify ways in which anxiety is interfering with social, professional, or educational functioning. Highlighting how CBT can be effective in reducing anxiety's interference in these domains can enhance motivation by establishing a connection between therapy and improved life functioning. This connection can be reinforced throughout therapy. A possible way to reduce dissatisfaction with the therapeutic relationship is to ensure that early sessions carefully balance instructions and explanations with empathic reflection and exploration of client problems. As discussed in the section on *Therapeutic relationship* above, session 1 empathic statements and questions were positively related to outcome whereas session 1 directive statements and explanations were negatively related to outcome. It is possible that being too directive and not empathic enough at the beginning of therapy could contribute to dissatisfaction with the therapeutic relationship, increasing the likelihood of drop out.

Failure to complete homework is another problem that can lessen outcomes in CBT for panic disorder. Homework completion is positively correlated with treatment outcomes as indicated by meta-analysis of CBT (not panic specific) and individual studies of CBT for panic disorder [35, 36]. Although not specific to CBT or panic disorder, strategies for improving homework compliance in psychotherapy have been proposed. These strategies include: collaborate with the client to formulate homework, describe the homework in detail, provide a rationale for homework, provide a written description and a sheet for recording their experiences, consider strategies for overcoming difficulties, get a commitment from client, practice in session, review homework in subsequent session, and praise homework completion [37].

More specific to anxiety, clients may avoid homework (such as exposures) because they fear that it will provoke anxiety symptoms and elicit distress. Although this response can be normalized by validating avoidance as a way of minimizing immediate distress, it is important to review how avoidance contributes to distress in the long term. With client input, a less demanding homework task that is more likely to be completed can be designed. Also, the client is to be reassured that repeated exposures will lead to a reduction in distress. In-session exposures can be conducted to help reinforce this point. Observation of client exposure and subsequent fearful response can also help therapists to better understand the obstacles to completing exposure, thus better enabling them to assist the client in overcoming these obstacles.

Chronic life stress, or episodic stressful events, can also interfere with CBT treatment for panic. Relationship problems, job stress, financial hardship, and medical problems are examples of stressful situations that can both exacerbate panic symptoms and make it difficult for clients to engage in therapy [38]. In such cases, it might be necessary to attend to the stressful situation before beginning, or returning to, CBT for panic disorder. This might involve recommending couples or family therapy for those with relationship issues or teaching stress-coping skills for those with particularly stressful life circumstances.

Misdiagnosis can also contribute to poor outcomes in CBT for panic disorder. As mentioned in the section on *Diagnostic criteria* above, panic symptoms must not be caused by a substance or general medical condition. Also, attacks that are perceived as unpredictable can be present in other anxiety disorders. Anxiety symptoms that are the result of a medical condition or disorder other than panic disorder might not respond as well, or at all, to interventions aimed at panic disorder. Therefore, if a medical evaluation has not been conducted, it may be wise to advise clients to undergo a medical evaluation to rule out conditions that might present similarly to panic including thyroid conditions, drug withdrawal, pheochromocytoma, and amphetamine intoxication. It is important to conduct a differential diagnosis to ensure the presence of panic disorder. Semi-structured interviews such as the Anxiety Disorders Interview Schedule – 4th edition can be used to reliably diagnose panic disorder [39].

Other issues that can complicate panic treatment for CBT, such as secondary gain, medication management, and comorbid disorders, are addressed below in the section on *Clinical decision making*.

Clinical decision making: integrating science and practice

When treating panic disorder with CBT, therapists integrate their knowledge of available research, their clinical experience, and their understanding of a client's particular circumstances and characteristics when making clinical decisions. Deciding how to handle cases with comorbid mental disorders is a good example of this. Research informs the therapist that major depression is the most likely non anxiety diagnosis for somebody with panic disorder. The research is mixed with respect to the effects of comorbid depression on CBT outcomes for panic disorder. Cognitive–behavioral therapy for panic appears to be efficacious when major depression is present and even appears to reduce depression symptoms in some cases [40]. However, there is also evidence that patients with primary depression have worse outcomes than those without depression, and that treatment completers are less likely to have comorbid depression than non-completers [40].

Because about one in three people with panic disorder will also have depression, a therapist must be able to integrate the research discussed above with their clinical expertise and the patient's characteristics to determine the best course of treatment. The severity of the comorbid depression (or other condition) should be carefully evaluated at the beginning of therapy. If the comorbid condition is so severe that the therapist believes it will interfere with CBT for panic, then the comorbid condition should be addressed first. Otherwise, panic disorder should be treated first, with the knowledge that successful treatment could result in symptom reduction for comorbid conditions [40]. Symptoms of these comorbid conditions should still be monitored throughout treatment, enabling them to be addressed when necessary. Such monitoring will also help the therapist to deal with any residual symptoms after panic treatment is completed.

Anxiety disorders co-occur at a high rate, meaning that it is likely that a client presenting with panic disorder will also have a comorbid anxiety disorder. Research shows that CBT targeting one anxiety disorder yields positive benefits for co-occurring disorders whereas simultaneously treating multiple anxiety problems can dilute treatment effects [e.g., 41]. Therefore, the therapist should work with the client to identify the anxiety problem that is currently most disabling to them and make that the focus of treatment.

As discussed above, research generally shows that combined treatment with CBT and medication improves short-term outcomes relative to CBT alone, but medication discontinuation post-treatment can actually lead to poorer outcomes than CBT alone. Therapists integrate their clinical expertise and client characteristics with this research when dealing with medication issues. For example, many presenting clients will already be taking medication for their anxiety. The therapist should assess clients' preferences and pre-medication functioning as well as educating them about the risks and benefits of medication use. If, based on client characteristics, the therapist believes the client would be able to successfully complete exposures without medication and the client preferred to be medication free, then they would work with the client and prescribing doctor to discontinue medication use. However, the therapist might delay discontinuation if they believed the client might balk at exposures without medication. Also, they might recommend a psychiatric consultation in those cases where they believed a client might benefit from medication to stay in therapy and complete exposures. In either of these cases, they would be careful to educate clients about safety signals and how the feared outcome was not affected by the presence or absence of the medication. Also, they would carefully monitor client progress to determine when an empirically-supported medication discontinuation plan should be put into effect.

Secondary gain can be an obstacle to successful CBT treatment of panic disorder. For example, secondary gain could be involved in Tina's case described above. Perhaps the positive reinforcement of her parents' financial and emotional support plays a role in maintaining her condition. When secondary gain is believed to be an impediment to therapy, experienced practitioners recommend: conducting a functional assessment to identify the relationship between improvement and its consequences; problem-solve obstacles, incorporating exposure as necessary; and addressing secondary gain with the goal of determining if continued therapy is desired [38]. Depending on the client's circumstances, it might also be beneficial to include significant others for portions of the therapy. For example, Tina's parents could be educated about the reinforcing properties of some of their behaviors and these behaviors could be targeted as part of therapy (e.g., requiring Tina to pay rent, or mom not accompanying Tina in the car).

Decisions about how to implement a CBT technique, or whether to use it at all, can also be influenced by client characteristics and clinical expertise. For example, as mentioned earlier, the literature on the effectiveness of breathing retraining is mixed [32]. In cases where the client relies heavily on distraction as a means of coping with anxiety, the therapist might choose to omit breathing retraining. In such cases, the client might use breathing retraining as just another means of distracting themselves, thus interfering with the corrective learning that is supposed to take place during exposures. Breathing retraining might also be omitted if client characteristics make the therapist wary that breathing retraining will be used solely as a sensation-avoidance technique. As discussed above, it is also desirable to tailor the presentation of CBT skills and psychoeducation so that they will be understandable and acceptable to each client.

Conclusion

Approximately 5% of the population will experience the debilitating effects of panic disorder, a condition that is relatively chronic if left untreated. Cognitive–behavioral treatments for panic disorder are highly effective; most clients who undergo CBT for panic disorder show significant reductions in symptoms of panic disorder and comorbid conditions as well as improvements in health and quality-of-life indices. These improvements are seen as early as the end of a twelve-week treatment and continue to be seen over years of follow-up. However, these treatments are not always successful. Approximately 20% of clients will prematurely withdraw from treatment and about 25% of those who do complete treatment will not show meaningful improvements relative to baseline functioning.

These attrition and failure rates highlight the importance of continued research to identify CBT components that are necessary for the successful treatment of panic, to identify the components' mechanisms of change, to determine how to optimally implement these components, and to determine how they could be better individualized. These attrition and failure rates also highlight how important it is for therapists to integrate the available research evidence with clinical expertise and their understanding of patient characteristics when conducting CBT for panic disorder. As discussed in detail above, CBT techniques must be thoughtfully tailored for each individual client in order to achieve optimal outcomes. For scientist-practitioners, the results observed from integrating existing research, clinical expertise, and client characteristics in therapeutic practice should be used as a basis to develop and refine hypotheses for future research. Through this process, such integration will benefit current clinical outcomes as well as research into improving these outcomes in the future.

References

1. American Psychiatric Association. *Diagnostic and Statistical Manual of Mental Disorders*, 4th edn., text revision. Washington, DC: APA, 2000.

2. Biederman J, Faraone SV, Marrs A, *et al*. Panic disorder and agoraphobia in consecutively referred children and adolescents. *J Am Acad Child Adolesc Psychiatry* 1997; **36**: 214–23.

3. Newman DL, Moffitt TE, Caspi A, *et al*. Psychiatric disorder in a birth cohort of young adults: prevalence, comorbidity, clinical significance, and new case incidence from ages 11 to 21. *J Consult Clin Psychol* 1996; **64**: 552–62.

4. Yonkers KA, Bruce SE, Dyck, IR, Keller, MB. Chronicity, relapse, and illness – course of panic disorder, social phobia, and generalized anxiety disorder: findings in men and women from 8 years of follow-up. *Depress Anxiety* 2003; **17**: 173–9.

5. Kessler RC, Chiu WT, Jin R, *et al*. The epidemiology of panic attacks, panic disorder, and agoraphobia in the National Comorbidity Survey Replication. *Arch Gen Psychiatry* 2006; **63**: 415–24.

6. Roy-Byrne PP, Stein MB, Russo J. Panic disorder in the primary care setting: comorbidity, disability, service utilization, and treatment. *J Clin Psychiatry* 1999; **60**: 492–9.

7. Kessler RC, Berglund P, Demler O, *et al*. Lifetime prevalence and age-of-onset distributions of DSM-IV disorders in the National Comorbidity Survey Replication. *Arch Gen Psychiatry* 2005; **62**: 593–602.

8. Barlow DH. *Anxiety and its Disorders: The Nature and Treatment of Anxiety and Panic*, 2nd edn. New York, NY: Guilford Press, 2002.

9. Clark DM. A cognitive approach to panic. *Behav Res Ther* 1986; **24**: 461–70.

10. Hettema JM, Neale MC, Myers JM, Prescott CA, Kendler KS. A population-based twin study of the relationship between neuroticism and internalizing disorders. *Am J Psychiatry* 2006; **163**: 857–64.

11. Hayward C, Killen JD, Kraemer HC, Taylor CB. Predictors of panic attacks in adolescents. *J Am Acad Child Adolesc Psychiatry* 2000; **39**: 1–8.

12. Chorpita BF, Barlow DH. The development of anxiety: the role of control in the early environment. *Psychol Bull* 1998; **124**: 3–21.

13. Reiss S, Silverman WK, Weems CF. Anxiety sensitivity. In Vasey MW, Dadds MR, eds. *The Developmental Psychopathology of Anxiety*. New York, NY: Oxford University Press. 2001, pp. 92–111.

14. Zoellner LA, Craske MG. Interoceptive accuracy and panic. *Behav Res Ther* 1999; **37**: 1141–58.

15. Craske MG, Poulton R, Tsao JCI, Plotkin D. Paths to panic disorder/agoraphobia: an exploratory analysis from age 3 to 21 in an unselected birth cohort. *J Am Acad Child Adolesc Psychiatry* 2001; **40**: 556–63.

16. Bouton ME, Mineka S, Barlow DH. A modern learning-theory perspective on the etiology of panic disorder. *Psychol Rev* 2001; **108**: 4–32.

17. Salkovskis PM, Clark DM, Hackmann A, Wells A, Gelder MG. An experimental investigation of the role of safety-seeking behaviours in the maintenance of panic disorder with agoraphobia. *Behav Res Ther* 1999; **37**: 559–74.

18. American Psychiatric Association. Practice guideline for the treatment of patients with panic disorder. *Am J Psychiatry* 1998; **155**(5 suppl): 1–34.

19. Barlow DH, Gorman JM, Shear MK, Woods SW. Cognitive-behavioral therapy, imipramine, or their combination for panic disorder: A randomized controlled trial. *JAMA* 2000; **283**: 2529–36.

20. Craske MG, Brown TA, Barlow DH. Behavioral treatment of panic disorder: a two-year follow-up. *Behav Ther* 1991; **22**: 289–304.

21. Dannon PN, Gon-Usishkin M, Gelbert A, Lowengrub K, Grunhaus L. Cognitive behavioral group therapy in panic disorder patients: the efficacy of CGBT versus drug treatment. *Ann Clin Psychiatry* 2004; **16**: 41–6.

22. Craske MG, DeCola JP, Sachs AD, Pontillo DC. Panic control treatment of agoraphobia. *J Anxiety Disord* 2003; **17**: 321–33.

23. Westen D, Morrison K. A multidimensional meta-analysis of treatments for depression, panic disorder, and generalized anxiety disorder: an empirical examination of the status of empirically supported therapies. *J Consult Clin Psychol* 2001; **69**: 875–99.

24. Hofmann SG, Smits JAJ. Cognitive-behavioral therapy for adult anxiety disorders: a meta-analysis of randomised placebo-controlled trials. *J Clin Psychiatry* 2008; **69**: 621–32.

25. Telch MJ, Schmidt NB, Jaimez L, Jacquin K, Harrington, P. The impact of cognitive-behavioral therapy on quality of life in panic disorder patients. *J Consult Clin Psychol* 1995; **63**: 823–30.

26. Schmidt NB, McCreary BT, Trakowski J, *et al*. Effects of cognitive-behavioral treatment on physical health status in patients with panic disorder. *Behav Ther* 2003; **34**: 49–63.

27. Mitte K. A meta-analysis of the efficacy of psycho- and pharmacotherapy in panic disorder with and without agoraphobia. *J Affect Disord* 2005; **88**: 27–45.

28. Furukawa TA, Watanabe N, Churchill R. Psychotherapy plus antidepressant for panic disorder with or without agoraphobia: systematic review. *Br J Psychiatry* 2006; **188**: 305–12.

29. Roy-Byrne PP, Craske MG, Stein MB, *et al*. A randomized effectiveness trial of cognitive-behavioral therapy and medication for primary care panic disorder. *Arch Gen Psychiatry* 2005; **62**: 290–8.

30. Keijsers GPJ, Schapp CPDR, Hoogduin CAL. The impact of interpersonal patient and therapist behavior on outcome in cognitive-behavior therapy. *Behav Modif* 2000; **24**: 264–97.

31. Keijsers GPJ, Schapp CPDR, Hoogduin CAL, Lammers, MW. Patient-therapist interaction in the behavioral treatment of panic disorder with agoraphobia. *Behav Modif* 1995; **19**: 491–517.

32. Meuret AE, Wilhelm FH, Ritz T, Roth WT. Breathing training for treating panic disorder. *Behav Modif* 2003; **27**: 731–54.

33. Keijsers GPJ, Kampman M, Hoogduin CAL. Dropout prediction in cognitive behavior therapy for panic disorder. *Behav Ther* 2001; **32**: 739–49.

34. Grilo CM, Money R, Barlow DH, *et al*. Pretreatment patient factors predicting attrition from a multicenter randomized controlled treatment study for panic disorder. *Compr Psychiatry* 1998; **39**: 323–32.

35. Kazantzis N, Deane FP, Ronan KR. Homework assignments in cognitive and behavioral therapy: a meta-analysis. *Clin Psychol Sci Prac* 2000; **7**: 189–202.

36. Schmidt NB, Woolaway-Bickel K. The effects of treatment compliance on outcome in cognitive-behavioral therapy for panic disorder: quality versus quantity. *J Consult Clin Psychol* 2000; **68**: 13–18.

37. Scheel MJ, Hanson WE, Razzhavaikina TI. The process of recommending homework in psychotherapy: a review of therapist delivery methods, client acceptability, and factors that affect compliance. *Psychotherapy: Theory, Research, Practice, Training* 2004; **41**: 38–55.

38. Sanderson WC, Bruce TJ. Causes and management of treatment-resistant panic disorder and agoraphobia: a survey of expert therapists. *Cogn Behav Pract* 2007; **14**: 26–35.

39. Di Nardo P, Brown TA, Barlow DH. *Anxiety Disorders Interview Schedule-Fourth Edition (ADIS-IV)*. New York, New York: Oxford University Press, 1994.

40. Mennin DS, Heimberg RG. The impact of comorbid mood and personality disorders in the cognitive-behavioral treatment of panic disorder. *Clin Psychol Rev* 2000; **20**: 339–57.

41. Craske MG, Farchione TJ, Allen LB, *et al*. Cognitive behavioral therapy for panic disorder and comorbidity: more of the same or less of more? *Behav Res Ther* 2007; **45**: 1095–109.

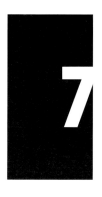

7 Obsessive–compulsive disorder

Maureen L. Whittal and Melisa Robichaud

Nature of the disorder

Definition

Obsessive–compulsive disorder (OCD) is characterized by the presence of obsessions and/or compulsions. Obsessions are defined as persistent thoughts, images, or impulses that intrude into the mind unbidden and cause marked distress. Compulsions, by contrast, involve repetitive behaviors or mental acts that reduce feelings of distress or are completed to prevent a feared event. As such, obsessions are unwanted and involuntary mental intrusions that cause anxiety, whereas compulsions are deliberate acts performed to relieve anxiety. According to DSM-IV-TR criteria, an OCD diagnosis is warranted if the obsessions or compulsions are sufficiently time consuming (i.e., greater than one hour a day), cause marked distress, or significantly interfere in daily life activities [1]. To meet diagnostic criteria, the symptoms must be recognized by the individual as excessive, inappropriate, and unreasonable (although this criterion is waived for children and a specifier of "poor insight" can be given with adults). Obsessive–compulsive disorder is differentiated from other disorders by the diagnostic stipulation that obsessions cannot solely consist of excessive worries about real-life problems (as is characteristic of generalized anxiety disorder, GAD), and that the obsessional content is not restricted to a particular theme more suggestive of another disorder (e.g., preoccupation with appearance as seen in body dysmorphic disorder, preoccupation with a serious illness as seen in hypochondriasis).

Symptoms

Despite its relatively succinct diagnostic criteria, OCD presents as a heterogeneous disorder, as there is significant diversity in its presentation. Obsessions can involve unwanted aggressive thoughts, images, or impulses to harm one's self or others (e.g., pushing someone into oncoming traffic, fear of causing a fire if home appliances are not turned off), sexual and religious/blasphemous intrusions (e.g., thoughts of inappropriately touching a stranger, urge to curse in church), persistent thoughts of doubt (e.g., "Did I turn off the stove?"), and fears of being harmed or contaminated by germs or dirt (e.g., "What if I get AIDS from touching a public toilet?"). Obsessive–compulsive disorder compulsions range from excessive cleaning or washing of the self and/or inanimate objects (e.g., ritualized washing of hands, cleaning of the kitchen counter), excessive checking (e.g., doors, stove, windows), counting / tapping /touching rituals, ordering/arranging, hoarding behavior, and mental rituals (e.g., repeating prayers). Rasmussen and Tsuang reported that 49% of OCD individuals reported multiple obsessional themes and 41% reported multiple rituals [2] (e.g., contamination/washing as well as doubting/checking). Moreover, compulsions are often combined in an idiosyncratic manner, such as the repetition of a prayer for a specified number of counts, or washing one's hands in a specific order (e.g., washing the left hand before the right, starting from the thumb). The motivation, or underlying fear, for these acts can also differ substantially according to the individual. For example, some OCD sufferers might engage in ordering/arranging compulsions out of a fear that the non-occurrence of the behavior would cause harm (e.g., "If I don't align my socks in the drawer correctly, my mother will die"), whereas others are concerned with alleviating a feeling that "it does not feel right" if items are incorrectly arranged.

Cognitive–behavioral Therapy with Adults: A Guide to Empirically Informed Assessment and Intervention, ed. Stefan G. Hofmann and Mark A. Reinecke. © Cambridge University Press 2010.

Prevalence and course

Once viewed as a rare disorder, epidemiological studies estimate the lifetime prevalence of OCD between 1.6 and 2.5% [3–5]. The gender distribution for OCD is roughly equal, with women only slightly outnumbering men [2], although boys outnumber girls at a 2:1 ratio in childhood [6]. This latter finding is consistent with the modal age of onset for OCD, which appears to develop at 13 to 15 years of age for males, compared to 20 to 24 years for females [7].

Obsessive–compulsive disorder is described as a chronic disorder with a waxing and waning course [1]. If left untreated, retrospective studies suggest that most OCD sufferers will maintain their symptoms, with a minority (5 to 10%) displaying a worsening of symptoms over time [2, 8]. In two prospective studies assessing the course of the disorder, approximately half of individuals with an OCD diagnosis continued to display symptoms at five-year [9], and at 40-year follow-up [10]. In the latter research, most participants were found to display improvements in their symptoms over time, however only a fifth were fully recovered, substantiating the assertion that OCD is a chronic and largely unremitting disorder.

Comorbidity

Mood and anxiety disorder diagnoses most frequently co-occur with OCD, with some studies suggesting that approximately 30% meet criteria for depression, and up to 40% merit an additional anxiety disorder diagnosis [2, 3, 11]. Specific phobia, social anxiety disorder, GAD, and panic disorder are the most common comorbid anxiety conditions, ranging from 25 to 60% [5]. Eating disorders and body dysmorphic disorder are also associated with OCD, typically co-occurring in approximately 10% of OCD cases. In addition, Tourette's disorder with tics has been associated with OCD. Despite a high incidence of OCD among individuals with Tourette's, only a small proportion of OCD clients report Tourette's (4 to 7%; see [12] for review).

Cognitive and behavioral models of OCD

Dollard and Miller adapted Mowrer's two-stage theory to explain the development and maintenance of OCD [13, 14]. However, as support for two-stage theory is mixed and fails to explain the origin of obsessions,

subsequent theories focused on cognitive factors. Carr is credited with the first cognitive formulation of OCD [15]. The theory focused on overestimating the probability of threat and the associated consequences. Given a perception of greater likelihood and negative impact of potential threats, a wide variety of situations could elicit anxiety, which would then be decreased through the execution of compulsive behaviors. McFall and Wollersheim expanded upon this conceptualization with the introduction of a cognitive mediation theory [16]. Specifically, it was proposed that individuals with OCD hold a number of erroneous beliefs, such as the belief that one should be perfect and that certain thoughts are unacceptable and could have catastrophic consequences. This primary appraisal of intrusions leads to increased perceptions of threat and anxiety. Compulsions are subsequently performed in response to a secondary appraisal process of individual perceptions of coping (e.g., rituals can prevent danger and are easier than confronting feared thoughts). Although these early theories were novel with respect to the introduction of cognitions into our understanding of OCD, they were criticized for their inability to differentiate between anxiety disorders and an over-reliance upon psychoanalytic constructs such as preconscious and unconscious cognitions [17, 18].

Although there are now a number of contemporary cognitive theories, (e.g., [19–21]), most are derived from the seminal cognitive conceptualization developed by Salkovskis and are based upon the same underlying principle [17]. Specifically, contemporary cognitive formulations begin with the premise that the experience of unwanted thoughts is virtually universal. In community and analogue samples over 90% of participants endorsed the presence of unwanted thoughts, images, or impulses, including urges to harm or attack someone and thoughts of sexually inappropriate acts [22, 23]. Moreover, the thought content of both non-clinical and OCD participants was similar, suggesting that the presence of intrusive and inappropriate thoughts is not the trigger in the development of OCD.

Rather, it is the *appraisal* of the thought that fuels OCD, wherein sufferers view intrusions as meaningful and catastrophic; it is this interpretation that leads to anxiety and distress. For example, many individuals might experience the unwanted thought of pushing someone down a flight of stairs, but most would interpret this as a meaningless thought and dismiss it without any associated anxiety. An individual with OCD, on the other hand, might view this thought as revelatory of their character and potentially dangerous, which would necessarily cause significant feelings of distress. In response to these feelings, individuals with OCD engage in a variety of neutralizing acts (e.g., compulsions) that are designed to reduce the distress and subvert any feared catastrophic consequences engendered by the unwanted thought. As noted by Salkovskis [17], these neutralizing acts serve to maintain OCD in a variety of ways. Given its ability to reduce feelings of distress, neutralization can become a coping mechanism for stress, thereby increasing the probability of subsequent neutralizing. In addition, given the non-occurrence of feared consequences following neutralization, the absence of negative outcomes becomes reinforcing and can be construed as evidence for the validity of obsessional beliefs. Thus, faulty appraisals are maintained by a failure to adequately evaluate alternatives.

Obsessive–compulsive disorder-related beliefs

Several beliefs are posited to contribute to distorted appraisals in OCD. Salkovskis suggested that an *exaggerated sense of responsibility* would negatively interact with intrusive thoughts. It includes the belief that failing to prevent harm [17] (i.e., "sin of omission") is as bad as deliberately causing harm ("sin of commission"), and failing to take action on an intrusive thought (i.e., neutralizing) is the same as wanting a negative event to occur. For example, the intrusive thought "Did I turn off the stove?" would lead to feelings of distress and an urge to check the stove if an individual held the belief that one would be wholly to blame if a fire developed, that a fire is preventable, and not checking the stove suggests that one actually wants to harm others.

Overimportance of thoughts

The overimportance of thoughts is also implicated in the misinterpretation of obsessions, in which the mere presence of a thought provides evidence of its status. Several forms of this belief have been identified. Distorted Cartesian reasoning involves the circular logic "It must be important because I think about it, and I think about it because it is important" [24]. Another manifestation of overimportance of thoughts

is thought–action fusion (TAF; [25]), and it comprises two related components: (1) likelihood TAF is the belief that thinking about something increases the likelihood of its occurrence (e.g., "If I think about harm coming to a loved one, then it is more likely to happen"); and (2) moral TAF, which reflects the belief that having an unacceptable thought is morally equivalent to carrying out the unacceptable act (e.g., "Thinking about harming someone is as bad as actually harming them"). Implicit in these beliefs is the self-blame and accountability that individuals hold for their thoughts, which would be expected to strengthen the meaning given to intrusions and the resultant urge to neutralize.

Other beliefs implicated in the development and maintenance of OCD include the *need to control thoughts* [19], the *need for certainty* or *perfection* [26], and an *overestimation of threat* [18]. For example, Clark and Purdon suggested that individuals with OCD excessively monitor their thoughts for the presence of intrusions [19], and believe that one must have absolute control over thought content to prevent feared outcomes resulting from the intrusions. Several researchers also identified the tendency to overestimate the likelihood and severity of harm in OCD. For example, Foa and Kozak suggested that individuals with OCD display errors in epistemological reasoning [27], wherein they view situations as dangerous unless proven safe despite the fact that most people assume the opposite.

Given the variety in the type of obsessions and compulsions present in OCD, these beliefs are not expected to be mutually exclusive, but rather may often present in combinations according to the particular intrusion and resultant appraisal [28]. For example, thoughts of doubt about having turned off all appliances in the home may involve overestimations of danger, TAF, and exaggerated responsibility.

Although there is a significant amount of research into the various beliefs that are posited to lead to distorted appraisals, less is known about what predisposes individuals to develop OCD. Barlow suggested that both biological and psychological vulnerabilities may contribute to the onset of OCD symptoms [12]. For example, it has been proposed that developmental experiences, such as the encouragement of a broad sense of responsibility in childhood and rigid codes of conduct or duty in school or religious teachings may predispose individuals to OCD [29]. Stressful experiences and negative mood states appear to also play a role, as OCD symptoms can develop in women during pregnancy and childbirth [30], and intrusive thoughts occur with greater frequency during anxious or depressed mood [31]. Given the heterogeneity of the disorder, it is not surprising that multiple etiological and predisposing factors would be involved in the genesis of OCD.

Empirical support for the efficacy and effectiveness of treatment

Exposure and response prevention (ERP) is the psychological treatment of choice for mild to moderate OCD, and a combination of medication and ERP is recommended for moderate to severe forms of the disorder [32]. A recent meta-analysis of randomized trials that included an ERP condition reported an average Yale–Brown Obsessive–Compulsive Scale (YBOCS) decline of 43.5% and an aggregate effect size (ES) of $d = 1.50$ [33]. Contemporary cognitive treatments also demonstrate efficacy (see [34, 35]), resulting in effect sizes that do not significantly differ from traditional ERP. Abramowitz *et al.* reported an aggregate ES of $d = 0.07$ when comparing CT/CBT to ERP randomized trials [33]. For those who make gains during acute treatment, the improvements tend to be retained over a long-term follow-up. Whittal, Robichaud, Thordarson and McLean followed treatment completers for two years following group and individual cognitive therapy (CT) and ERP and reported relapse rates of less than 10% and recovery rates of 50% [36]. Excluding participants randomized to group CT, which appeared to not be as effective, recovery rates increased to 56% two years following treatment. Despite these encouraging results, a substantial number of participants remain on medication or seek out additional services. Whittal *et al.* reported 58% of treatment completers continued to be on medication at two-year follow-up and 40% sought out additional OCD treatment [36]. However, the latter did not impact recovery status at follow-up, which may be suggestive of a treatment-resistant sample or the need for maintenance treatment to prevent relapse. Future developments should focus on increasing the acceptability of OCD treatments, as refusal and drop-out rates are higher compared to other anxiety disorders. Moreover, as improvement rates have reached a plateau in the past 20 years, the disorder is in need of a fresh analysis.

Introduction to a clinical case

"Ryan"[1] is a 35-year-old married man who is employed part time in a professional job. He describes his marriage as supportive but recently strained secondary to the OCD. By choice, he does not have children secondary to his concern that he is a danger around children and that he will not be a good father. He reported that he had been having OCD symptoms for 15 years although he remembers fears of fire and home security as early as ten years of age.

Ryan was interviewed using the YBOCS, which is the gold standard measure to quantify severity, and qualitatively describe, obsessions and compulsions [37]. As is typical for people with OCD [8], Ryan reported multiple symptom themes including doubting/checking, contamination/washing, and egodystonic sexual obsessions. The doubting/checking was equally distressing and time consuming as the sexual obsessions, followed by the contamination/washing. Ryan reported unwanted thoughts and images of sexually molesting children for the past ten years. They began shortly after after he was married. He and his wife began discussing in earnest having children and began sitting his wife's infant niece. While changing a diaper, Ryan thought about sexually touching his niece, which repulsed him. He was not able to be alone with his niece until recently, as she is now a teenager and therefore "old enough" to speak up if Ryan were inappropriate. Ryan knows that these intrusions are characteristic of OCD but he also believes that he is a danger to children and society in general. He believes that if he does not continue to avoid situations where he might see a child, and does not monitor his thoughts, that he will act on his thoughts. Occasionally an unwanted sexual thought or image makes Ryan feel contaminated and is associated with a variety of cleansing compulsions (e.g., showering) that are typically unsuccessful. Although Ryan told his wife about the OCD, he continues to conceal the sexual obsessions. He is concerned that she will think he is a "monster" and initiate divorce proceedings.

In addition to the mental contamination noted above, Ryan also experiences more traditional contact contamination. His primary feared consequence is acquiring a serious disease (e.g., AIDS, hepatitis) and

---

1 "Ryan" is a compilation of many patients; however, the information presented in the tables and figures represents the work of actual patients in our clinic.

passing it on to his loved ones. Triggering situations include coming into contact with people he considers dirty, handling money, touching wet or sticky surfaces, and touching anything used by the general public (e.g., railings, bus poles, pens to sign cheques, etc.). Ryan engages in a number of behaviors to keep him and others safe. Upon returning home, Ryan admitted to removing his clothes in the foyer, putting them in the laundry and having a 30-minute shower. Until recently he required the same of his wife but the strain to his marriage became unmanageable and Ryan relented on the need for a shower. He continues to ask his wife to change her clothes immediately upon coming home. Food preparation is particularly difficult. Although he is able to eat food prepared by his wife, Ryan repeatedly asks her to wash her hands while cooking and to decontaminate the kitchen counter and cutting boards especially if she is preparing chicken. Ryan sits in only one kitchen chair and one living room chair and asks that neither is used by anyone else.

Ryan's fears of being responsible for a fire or break-in are equally as distressing and time consuming as his repugnant obsessions. Prior to going to bed and leaving the house, Ryan engages in an elaborate checking routine. He checks items in the kitchen and living room in a particular order, and if interrupted he must start again. His wife is required to go to bed prior to the start of his checking lest she interfere or use an item that was previously checked. Items checked include the stove/oven, taps, lights, windows, doors, and that appliances such as the coffee pot and toaster oven are unplugged. The checking routine varies between 30 to 60 minutes and is much longer if he and his wife are leaving for extended periods (e.g., vacation). If Ryan is leaving the house alone and his wife is inside, he does not feel the need to check. However, if they are leaving together, Ryan can not allow his wife to lock the door as he must do it himself.

The only comorbid condition as identified by a semi-structured clinical interview is dysthymia of mild to moderate severity. He denied suicidality but reported dysphoric affect, anhedonia, restless sleep, and impaired concentration. The depression began approximately ten years ago shortly after the onset of the sexual obsessions. Ryan considers the depression to be the result of his repetitive thoughts of abusing children and his belief that he is a pedophile in waiting.

Overview of the treatment protocol

Session structure

Although it varies according to severity, initial sessions in our clinic are once a week for an hour. In more severe cases initial sessions can be massed, but this does depend upon practical issues such as therapist and patient availability. However, Abramowitz, Foa and Franklin reported no differences in treatment outcome with daily sessions or twice-weekly sessions [38]. The final appointments are spaced out to every two or three weeks, again depending upon availability. The goal with intermittent appointments is to allow time to consolidate information and treatment gains and to assist the patient with the task of becoming their own therapist.

Therapeutic relationship

Like all cognitive–behavioral treatments, the therapeutic relationship is a collaborative one. The therapist does not purport to have the answers nor tell the patient the way s/he is thinking is incorrect. Rather, alternative interpretations to unwanted intrusions are developed during treatment and patients are encouraged to test them out between sessions. They are also encouraged to assess the practical utility of these alternative interpretations (e.g., does it improve their ability to function in their lives). Similar to CBT for other anxiety disorders, treatment for OCD involves behavior change, which is typically anxiety provoking. A strong therapeutic alliance can offset some of the perceived risks associated with behavior change.

Non-judgmental assessment of symptoms may aid in the development of therapeutic alliance. The comprehensiveness of the YBOCS checklist can be normalizing and provides a platform for patients to discuss topics that are typically private. It is not uncommon for patients to hide their symptoms for years from friends, family, and colleagues. Newth and Rachman identified concealment as a potential maintaining factor for primary obsessions [39]. Reasons for concealment can be encapsulated as a fear that others will view the obsessional as they view themselves (i.e., "mad, bad or dangerous") and abandon the individual. Secondary to these concerns, therapists should also recognize that concealment may extend to the assessment and to part or potentially all of the treatment. Although there is no empirical literature to

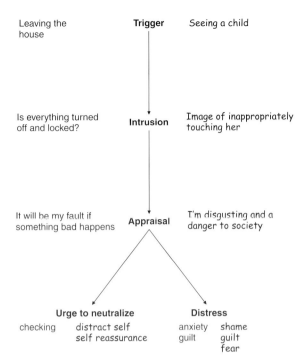

| Leaving the house | **Trigger** | Seeing a child |

Figure 7.1 The basic CBT model for two of Ryan's OCD concerns

guide increasing honest reporting of symptoms, we routinely ask patients to be upfront despite their discomfort as it will ultimately improve their outcome. We also make clear the ease we have in differentiating egodystonic from syntonic thought, images, and impulses. When working with people who have strong religious backgrounds that factor into their OCD, it is our practice to discuss religion prior to starting treatment. We indicate that it is not our intention to be disrespectful but we will provide alternative interpretations that may at times be at odds with their religious teachings. All that we ask of the patient is that s/he considers the alternative and not immediately rejects it.

Strategies and techniques

Psychoeducation

Following assessment of symptoms and a review of social history, treatment moves to psychoeducation. The goal of these initial sessions is to differentiate between obsessions and compulsions, and presentation of an idiosyncratic model to account for the maintenance of OCD. The model derived for Ryan's intrusive sexual thoughts and doubting/checking is

presented in Figure 7.1. The ubiquity of unwanted intrusions is reviewed with emphasis on the importance of the appraisal [22] (i.e., the meaning of the intrusive thought). Consistent with contemporary cognitive models, the presence of the intrusion is de-emphasized but the meaning attributed to it is identified as the target for treatment. To underscore the importance of appraisals, Ryan was given a list of intrusions experienced by people with OCD [22]. He identified infrequent intrusions that *did not* produce much distress. Invariably, associated appraisals were neutral and/or not personally relevant (e.g., 'It's just a thought'; 'I won't do it'). The emotional distress is likewise minimal and the urge to neutralize the intrusion is typically not present. This relatively non-anxiety provoking example is compared and contrasted to an example from the patient's OCD. When Ryan compared his own benign example to an OCD example, the differences in the appraisals were clear. The way in which an intrusion is appraised is analogous to a fork in the road. A personally-relevant appraisal is associated with anxiety or other negative emotions, and efforts to control and/or neutralize the intrusion. A neutral appraisal is associated with little distress and few control efforts.

If possible, patients also involve confidantes in a survey regarding their own intrusive thoughts. Specifically, friends and family are asked to share with patients their own unwanted intrusive thoughts and associated appraisals. The goal of the latter is to normalize the presence of unwanted intrusions and the importance of neutral appraisals. If the patient completely concealed the OCD or if a supportive person is unavailable, the survey is delayed and possibly not completed. If possible, utilizing clinic co-workers to anonymously complete the survey is an alternative. Normalizing the presence of unwanted intrusions is the foundation of treatment. Occasionally it is necessary to revisit these points as some patients are not initially convinced.

Psychoeducation is emphasized in the first one to two sessions, but continues throughout treatment. The cognitive strategies aimed at Ryan's repugnant obsessions and checking will be discussed first, followed by traditional ERP for his contamination.

Overimportance of and the need to control thoughts

Thought–action fusion and the self-propelling nature of thought, frame a discussion of the overimportance of thoughts. It is common for patients to wonder why an intrusive thought occurred and assume that it has meaning simply because it occurred, leading to further dwelling on the thought and subsequent increases in the importance of the thought.

A number of strategies exist to challenge TAF including thought and alternating day experiments and a morality continuum. Ryan exhibited extensive likelihood and moral TAF. The presence of sexual thoughts about children was as abhorrent as engaging in such an action. He also believed that the thoughts were a precursor to action; why would they otherwise occur and be so frequent. He attributed the non-occurrence of the event to his hypervigilance toward his thoughts (i.e., a thought does not have the opportunity to "sneak" up on him) and to his avoidance of children. Thought experiments were introduced to address Ryan's likelihood TAF. Ryan was instructed to pick a person with whom he has regular contact (e.g., his therapist) and think about something untoward occurring. The event is meant to be uncommon but not rare. The goal with thought experiments is to address the power of thought to cause action. If a high (e.g., getting the flu in the winter) or low (e.g., getting smallpox) base rate event is chosen, it will not provide useful information about the power of thoughts. For some patients thought experiments are not anxiety provoking as they are too artificial. However, Ryan's thought experiment was sufficiently anxiety provoking (his therapist spraining her ankle). He thought about it daily and was somewhat surprised that his therapist was not on crutches at the following session. Thought experiments continue with the potential consequences becoming increasingly dire and the "target" of the thoughts someone who is closer to the patient.

One method of challenging moral TAF is to do a continuum. Ryan's completed moral continuum is demonstrated in Figure 7.2. He initially identified people at each anchor point (i.e., worst/best person) and then placed himself (Ryan #1) on the continuum. The therapist provided various scenario pairs purposely separating intention as well as thought from

action (e.g., while driving hitting and killing someone in the act of committing suicide versus manslaughter versus using your car as a weapon; engaging in a sexual fantasy versus having an affair, etc.). Ryan placed each on the morality continuum. Although it varies, patients are typically able to separate thought from action for others, thus establishing a double standard. The therapist pointed out Ryan's double standard and asked, given that he had never engaged in any unacceptable sexual behavior, if he deserved to be placed near the "worse person ever." Based upon his actions Ryan repositioned himself closer to the middle of the continuum. Ryan #2 is where he repositioned himself.

The need to control thoughts is closely related to the overimportance of thoughts (i.e., if a thought is not important there is no need to control it). As discussed by Purdon and Clark and others [40], the frequency of thoughts and images increases subsequent to efforts to control. The futility of attempting to control thoughts is illustrated in session with a "pink elephant" exercise. Ryan was asked to get a clear image of a pink, polka-dotted elephant. Once this image was formed he was instructed to think about anything except the elephant. If the image intruded he was to remove it as soon as possible but to note its occurrence on a pad of paper. Thought suppression is contrasted with allowing thoughts of the elephant to intrude. The duration of each condition is typically between one to two minutes. As is typical, thought suppression resulted in an increased frequency of elephant images for Ryan. For some patients the effect of thought suppression is not noticeable. However, these patients typically notice that thought suppression requires more effort than allowing thoughts to naturally occur.

To carry forward the in-session work on the paradox of thought control and to focus it on his obsessional intrusions, Ryan completed an alternating day experiment. Depending upon the intent, an alternating day exercise may take a variety of forms. As the name suggests, patients alternate between two different strategies depending upon the goal of the exercise. The

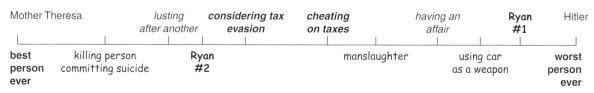

Figure 7.2 A continuum to challenge moral TAF

Table 7.1 Subjective probability = 70%

Item	Probability
1. Stove left on	1/100
2. Flammable object near stove	1/20
3. Item catches on fire	1/5
4. Smoke alarm does not go off	1/1000
5. Nobody at home	1/5
6. Fire spreads	1/2
7. Major fire	

$$\text{Logical probability} = \frac{1 \times 1 \times 1 \times 1 \times 1 \times 1}{100 \times 20 \times 5 \times 1000 \times 5 \times 2}$$
$$= \frac{1}{100,000,000} = 0.000001\%$$

"On duty" (for noticing and fighting thoughts)	"Off duty"

Monday
1. OCD severity (0–10) 8
2. Anxiety (0–10) 8
3. Extent of responsibility
   for the thoughts (0–10) 8
4. % of the day engaging in the
   strategy of the day 90%
	Tuesday
	1. 6
	2. 5
	3. 5
	
	4. 50%

Wednesday 1. 8 2. 8 3. 8 4. 90%	Thursday 1. 5 2. 4 3. 5 4. 75%
Friday 1. 8 2. 8 3. 7 4. 90%	Saturday 1. 4 2. 5 3. 5 4. 80%
Sunday 1. 7 2. 8 3. 8 4. 60%	Monday 1. 4 2. 3 3. 4 4. 90%

Figure 7.3 Results from an alternating day experiment where Ryan was asked to switch between being "on duty" for his thoughts (his usual stance) with "off duty" when he was instructed to let thoughts come and go and he was not not responsible for the presence of the unwanted thoughts

duration of each varies according to patient's ability to tolerate the two conditions. In Ryan's case he was encouraged to alternate daily between his usual stance of being "on duty" (i.e., hypervigilant for his thoughts and fighting with them when they occur) and going "off duty" (i.e., letting thoughts come in and letting them leave of their own accord/not fighting the thought). At the end of each day Ryan was asked to make brief ratings of anxiety and OCD severity and his level of success in using the strategy of the day (i.e., was he "on duty" during the appropriate times). Ryan predicted that "off duty" would result in more anxiety and more OCD. Figure 7.3 revealed that when Ryan was able to be "off duty" it resulted in less OCD and less anxiety.

The role of attention in the paradox of thought control is illustrated through a behavioral exercise. Patients are asked to recall the number of occasions in which they recalled seeing a meaningless item (e.g., a for sale sign, a particular make of vehicle). Typically this number is zero or close to it but it increases several-fold following the instruction to attend to the item and count the occurrences of it. Once something has meaning we notice it more (e.g., couples who are pregnant typically notice more pregnant women; people who purchase a new vehicle notice more of them). The same is true of unwanted thoughts. By trying to not think a thought, Ryan was inadvertently paying more attention to his thoughts, which resulted

in him noticing them more. However, Ryan interpreted the higher frequency of sexual thoughts as evidence he was becoming more dangerous and as such he needed to watch himself even closer.

Inflated responsibility and overestimation of danger

Estimations of danger and responsibility are inextricably linked [41]. As such both are typically addressed in OCD treatment. There are a variety of avenues to address overestimations of danger. Two avenues to correct overestimations of danger are accomplished by discussing logical probabilities and behavioral experiments. Ryan's tendency to overestimate danger is typical of many OCD patients. For example, he thought there was a 70% chance that if he didn't check the stove upon leaving the house that it would be on and result in a major fire. Ryan identified all the events and the associated probabilities that would need to occur prior to the final feared consequence (i.e., a large-scale fire) (see Table 7.1). The probability of the final feared consequence is the multiplicative product of the prior steps (i.e., if there are two steps and each has a one-in-ten chance of occurring, the final probability is one in a hundred). The logical probability identified in Table 7.1 (0.000001%) is compared to the subjective probability identified by the patient (70% in Ryan's case).

Targeted behavioral experiments can also be helpful in decreasing overestimations of danger and would be appropriate to address Ryan's doubting and his contamination fears. Prior to engaging in a behavioral exercise, a hypothesis regarding outcome is developed. For example, Ryan predicted that leaving a stove burner on high would start a fire (i.e., the heat from the burner would ignite the paint on the wall next to the stove). Various iterations of this exercise were repeated and included watching the burner while it was on for 15 minutes, remaining in the kitchen but not looking for 30 minutes, remaining in the next room for 15 to 30 minutes, and finally stepping out of the house for brief periods of time. If patients do not believe that sufficient time elapsed to test their prediction, duration of the experiment should be extended. The longest period of time that our patients left burners on is two hours and ovens left on low (with nothing inside) overnight. The key to threat experiments is to identify the feared consequence and then design the experiment to maximize the disconfirmation.

Pie-charting is a main method for challenging inflated responsibility. Much like wearing blinders, patients often have a difficult time looking beyond their own actions in accounting for a situation. For example, if Ryan's house was burgled, he would allot

himself 75% of the responsibility because he did not do a sufficient job of securing it. Figure 7.4 represents the collaborative effort between Ryan and his therapist to identify other people and situations that also factor into the event. Once Ryan considered the other possibilities, his responsibility reduced to 15%. With time, the goal of pie-charting is to have patients identify other sources of responsibility in the moment and to recognize that responsibility is not absolute but is rather a shared phenomenon.

Transfers of responsibility are another possible avenue to sharing responsibility. As Ryan's wife must go to bed before the initiation of the nightly checking routine, Ryan clearly has difficulty in sharing responsibility. If Ryan were avoiding responsibility (e.g., purposely leaving his wife to lock up when they leave the house or retire for the evening), then a transfer would not be appropriate. In this case a transfer of responsibility, psychological and actual, to Ryan's wife is indicated. Ryan asked his wife if she would be willing to assume the safety and security of the home for the upcoming week. The decision to check was her responsibility. Ryan agreed to not ask his wife if she checked and not do it himself. A slight modification to this exercise can incorporate an element of threat overestimation. Specifically, Ryan's wife could be asked to check half the time but not tell Ryan which days until the end of the week. Ryan's task is to examine the house each morning and upon returning from an outing looking for breaches of safety and security. At the end of the week Ryan and his wife would compare

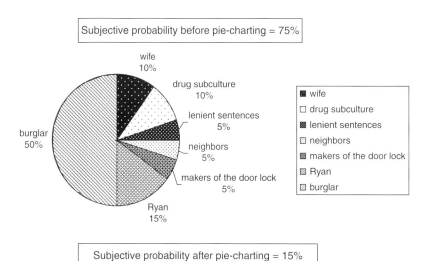

Subjective probability before pie-charting = 75%

wife
10%

drug subculture
10%

lenient sentences
5%

burglar
50%

neighbors
5%

makers of the door lock
5%

Ryan
15%

■ wife
□ drug subculture
▨ lenient sentences
▨ neighbors
▨ makers of the door lock
▨ Ryan
▨ burglar

Subjective probability after pie-charting = 15%

Figure 7.4 Clinical example of pie-charting for addressing exaggerated responsibility beliefs: "How much would Ryan be responsible if his house was robbed and who/what else plays a role in addition to Ryan?"

Table 7.2 Fear of AIDS/hepatitis hierarchy

Items	SUDS
1. Using a pen found in the waiting room of the anxiety clinic[1]	30
2. Using a pen from general hospital admission	40
3. Handling brochures from the AIDS clinic	50
4. Stepping on red spots of unknown origin	60
5. Walking by AIDS Vancouver brushing the side of the building with his hand	70
6. Reading a magazine from the blood draw laboratory	75
7. Sitting in the lobby of AIDS Vancouver ensuring that hands and body are in contact with the seat	80
8. Using a pen from AIDS Vancouver	85
9. Shaking hands with a staff member at AIDS Vancouver	90
10. Handling a vacucontainer of non-contaminated blood	95
11. Shaking hands with an AIDS patient	95
12. Holding a vacucontainer from a person with confirmed AIDS	100

[1] Each item is typically followed by full response prevention (i.e., elimination of all behaviors [mental and physical]) associated with a precipitous drop in anxiety

Table 7.3 Fear of contamination (from distal sources)

Item	SUDS
1. Touch light switches in non-hospital buildings	20
2. Using railings and doorknobs in non-hospital buildings	30
3. Touching railings, doorknobs, light switches in the hospital	40
4. Touching bus poles	45
5. Touching bathroom doorknobs (entry and not exit)	50
6. Handling money	55
7. Handling money while eating finger food	65
8. Touching wet surfaces, near the sink in a public bathroom	70
9. Touching bathroom doorknob (exit)	75
10. Touching toilet handle	85
11. Touching the base of the toilet (i.e., the porcelain)	90
12. Lifting public toilet seat	100

notes where Ryan would typically see that checking was independent from making mistakes.

Contamination and cleaning

Ryan exhibited mental and contact contamination. It is only recently that the two forms of contamination were distinguished [42]. As cognitive methods to challenge mental contamination are in development, Ryan's need to wash following an unacceptable thought was addressed using ERP. However, continuing to ask patients about the presence of mental contamination will be useful. Rachman lists interview questions [43].

Preliminary data from our laboratory indicate that cognitive strategies are not as effective for OCD themes of contamination and washing, perhaps secondary to the amount of associated avoidance [43]. As such, Ryan's contamination concerns were addressed using ERP. The fine points of hierarchy development and conducting exposure-based treatments will not be discussed herein as ample references are available

[44, 45]. However, two of the hierarchies developed for Ryan's contamination fears are presented in Tables 7.2 and 7.3. As is typical in contamination fears, the triggers initially identified are the veritable tip of the iceberg. As such the items listed in the hierarchies are only a representative sample of feared stimuli. However, similar to other contaminators, Ryan experienced a natural generalization during ERP. Specifically, after his fear to the first few items extinguished, he tackled other triggers at a similar level without talking to the therapist.

In building a hierarchy and initiating ERP, it is important to begin with an item that produces relatively little anxiety and one in which the patient is quite confident of successfully completing. Subsequent steps are gradual, analogous to going up stairs one at a time as opposed to multiple steps at once. Consistency is the second key to successful ERP. The greater the number of exposures to a feared situation, barring sensitization, the quicker the fear declines. Although there are a variety of ways to do exposure, therapist modeling and full response prevention is associated with the highest effect sizes [44]. However, recent theorizing regarding the judicious use of safety behaviors provides an interesting, although as yet unexplored, alternative to traditional full response prevention [46]. In Ryan's case he was permitted limited use of hand sanitizer in specific situations (e.g., after going into a hospital, visiting the doctor, and handling money) as these were particular difficult triggers. The use of this safety behavior is viewed as a temporary measure to assist with decreasing avoidance and increasing a sense of control (i.e., he knew he could use it if necessary). Ryan's therapist built in a delay in the use of the hand sanitizer and Ryan ultimately faded it out on his own and did not become dependent upon it.

Difficulties encountered during treatment

One of the biggest hurdles occurs before treatment begins. Deciding to access services requires courage. With the exception of those with poor insight, a hallmark of OCD is the recognition that the intrusions as well as the compulsions are excessive and unnecessary. Although shame and embarrassment are part of most mental disorders, the discrepancy between "knowing" that the intrusions are false but struggling with the residual "what if" promotes a sense of incompetence. For a subset of people with OCD, the content provides an additional barrier to acquiring help. Although it is not common, for the unfortunate ones with repugnant obsessions previous attempts at obtaining help are sometimes met with their worst fears. Examples include the egodystonic sexual obsessive who was assumed to be a sexual predator and treated as such, obtaining a previous incorrect diagnosis of schizophrenia and unwanted aggressive intrusions taken as an indicator of homicidal intent.

Common reasons for treatment failure

Treatment failure is relative in OCD. As indicated earlier, the majority of people who complete treatment receive benefit although inclusion of drop-outs and treatment refusers in randomized trials would negatively impact success rates [44]. The factors that play into treatment failure are probably the same as those that result in attenuated treatment gains. There are no consistent predictors of short- and long-term outcome in randomized trials. However, overvalued ideation (OVI), severe depression, and homework compliance are implicated in some studies.

Patients with extreme OVI can hold their beliefs with delusional intensity (e.g., a male patient who was 100% convinced that he had a sexually transmitted disease and would pass it along to his young daughter if she were to sit on his lap even if they were both fully clothed). The intensity of his belief could not be shifted after several sessions, and treatment was discontinued. He remained unwilling to take the risk associated with exposure. Another example is of a devoutly religious woman who experienced unwanted sexual images of her father. She firmly believed that if she did not work to get the image out of her head as soon as it arrived that she committed serious sin and would go to hell as a result. Despite a course of cognitive therapy, one second longer than necessary remained too long and it resulted in a mutual decision to terminate treatment. It is our clinical observation that patients with OVI who are not in randomized trials may have improved outcomes if the number of treatment sessions are extended. Provided these individuals are willing to engage in treatment and consider alternative interpretations, change can occur albeit it at a slower rate.

As discussed by Franklin and Foa attenuated outcomes or treatment failures associated with fixed beliefs may be mediated by treatment compliance [44]. Non-compliance may be associated with a number of factors including feared consequences associated with exposure or behavioral experiments and personality characteristics. In our clinic patients are told that if an assignment is too difficult, there is always a way to make it easier. Although previous research indicates that full response prevention is preferable over partial response prevention [44], it is only true if patients are able to comply. We routinely incorporate partial measures if patients are unable to complete a particular exercise (e.g., rinsing hands as opposed to washing with soap). We make it clear that these measures are temporary and that patients will ultimately be asked to refrain from engaging in these behaviors. Although the empirical work is yet to be conducted, the judicious use of safety behaviors may prove to be useful for patients who are functionally limited secondary to avoidance [46] (e.g., the contaminator who can not make her own food or use public transportation).

Similarly, the need for control for some patients is readily apparent, which can be reflected in compliance with homework assignments. For example, we recently completed treatment with a patient who readily admitted that his need for control was paramount. His OCD was characterized by multiple themes, the most apparent of which were contamination and checking. Mutually agreed upon behavioral exercises that he predicted would be relatively easy (i.e., predicted anxiety of 40/100) were more difficult than anticipated and were not completed. After a few weeks of similar outcomes the therapist put the control back into the patient's hands by asking him to choose the exercise and combine it with a little less compulsive behavior than he felt he ought to. For example, if he chose a contamination exercise it would be associated with a little less washing/cleaning than his OCD would normally dictate. This strategy combined with specific threat exercises (e.g., leaving a burner unattended for 15 minutes) allowed this patient to move more quickly through his hierarchies.

Severe and multiple comorbidities can also contribute to treatment failure. Abramowitz *et al.* demonstrated that severe comorbid depression attenuates OCD treatment outcome as well as maintenance of gains [47]. Anhedonia and lethargy associated with depression may contribute to initiation difficulties with homework assignments. It also may contribute to beliefs about the self (e.g., the sexual obsessive who is severely depressed may be more willing to believe that the presence of the thoughts makes her an evil person). Depending upon the severity of the comorbidity and the extent to which it is interfering with the OCD treatment, it may be appropriate to switch direction and treat the comorbid condition.

Clinical decision making

When developing a treatment plan for OCD patients, a number of factors need to be considered. First, given the varied presentation of the disorder an idiographic assessment of subtype themes is warranted. Although there is no definitive consensus to date, researchers have identified several classification schemes, most of which are derived from the YBOCS [38, 48]. An understanding of the different OCD themes is not only important from an empirical standpoint but also for treatment, as it brings coherence to a multiplicity of troubling thoughts and behaviors. In Ryan's case, he displayed contamination/washing concerns, thoughts of doubt and associated checking, as well as sexual obsessions. Of note, although the majority of his excessive washing is related to his fear of contamination, he also reports showering on occasion when experiencing unwanted sexual thoughts. This behavior would be better understood, and as a consequence

treated, within the framework of primary obsessions and an associated feeling of mental pollution or contamination, even though it is a washing compulsion [42].

Similarly, some OCD patients report obsessive fears of harming others. However, to devise an appropriate CBT plan, an understanding of the underlying reasons behind this fear is recommended. For example, clients may report obsessions of harming as a result of carelessness or as a result of deliberate intention. The former case is illustrated by a fear of making others ill secondary to improper hygiene while cooking, compared to obsessions of purposely poisoning others (e.g., adding bleach to food). Although both obsessions involve harm to others, accidental harm fears are better accounted for by doubts/checking, while deliberate harm is an example of an unwanted aggressive obsession. When devising a cognitive treatment plan, therapeutic strategies for doubting obsessions would differ from those used for aggressive intrusive thoughts. For example, interventions aimed at altering perceptions of inflated responsibility and overestimations of danger would be used for doubting fears, whereas challenging beliefs about the overimportance of thoughts and the need to control thoughts would be most appropriate for primary obsessions. As such, a further consideration of OCD symptom themes according to the beliefs that drive them can assist in establishing a treatment plan, and has in fact been investigated as a classification system for OCD subtypes [48].

As with most patients presenting with heterogeneous symptoms, a clinical decision about which OCD theme to target first is also required. This decision is often not a simple one, as there are multiple considerations, including OCD-theme severity, degree of interference in the patient's life, the expectation of initial treatment success, and, rather importantly, client preference. For many clients, the first target of treatment is typically the symptom constellation that leads to the greatest distress or interference in their lives. In Ryan's case, this might be his sexual obsessions or doubting/checking. In both cases, the severity of Ryan's symptoms is exacerbated by the apparent strain being placed upon his relationship with his wife. In particular, Ryan's wife is made to change her clothes when returning home, wash her hands frequently while cooking, and go to bed prior to her husband as Ryan cannot trust her with the responsibility of home security. It is not uncommon for the significant others' of OCD clients to become complicit in the performance of rituals. This enlisted participation in compulsions can lead to significant distress within the family, such that treatment interventions involving family members have some success (see [49] for a review).

Assuming primary impairment from one or more OCD themes, the choice of where to place treatment emphasis first can be based on both the patients' distress tolerance and flexibility for a particular fear theme, and the expectation of maximal treatment gains early on. In Ryan's case, his fear of being responsible for harming a child, for example, may be so strong that conducting any behavioral exposures might be perceived as overwhelmingly difficult. As a consequence, his adherence to ERP and the reduction in his symptoms would be minimal, rendering it a less than ideal starting point for treatment. Conversely, he may be more willing to conduct behavioral experiments involving his doubts about the safety and security of his home. If he were willing to conduct transfer of responsibility experiments with his wife, and he reported a strong likelihood of being able to tolerate the distress these experiments would generate, then this would be a preferable starting point. As a result, Ryan would likely demonstrate early treatment success that would both enhance his motivation for treatment and increase his confidence. Moreover, by involving his wife in the experiments, he would further benefit by potentially enhancing his marital relationship.

Conclusions

In this chapter we provided a brief overview of the empirical literature for OCD and its treatment. As OCD is idiographic in presentation, treatment of it is likewise idiographic, which can make it difficult to learn from reading written accounts. Moreover, some of what we do in treatment is not guided by empirical literature but rather our clinical judgment and experience (e.g., using primarily cognitive methods to address obsessions and exposure-based treatments for contamination). In our section on clinical decision making we attempted to highlight how we use the information provided to guide our treatment decisions. Fortunately, the foundation of treatment, exposure to anxiety-provoking situations, is straightforward and the effect is robust. The rest comes with practice and listening to our patients. Although the behaviors may seem illogical on the surface, with sufficient questioning they will make sense given the belief system. Understanding the feared consequences will assist in designing useful exposures and behavioral experiments.

In the absence of treatment people with OCD may suffer a tremendous burden. In the past decade cognitively focused treatments have demonstrated efficacy and provide an alternative or adjunct to the existing gold standard ERP. Despite these improvements the psychological treatments described herein continue to be largely restricted to specialized centers. Moreover, patients must continue to tolerate tremendous amounts of anxiety, making treatment unacceptable for some. Future areas of research must address these issues by focusing on dissemination and increasing acceptability while continuing to strive for improvements in efficacy and durability.

Internet resources: educational and therapeutic information

Anxiety Disorders Association of America. Treat it, don't repeat it: break free from OCD. www.adaa.org/treatOCD/index.html

Anxiety Disorders Association of British Columbia. Adult self-help section. www.anxietybc.com/resources/introduction.php

Obsessive Compulsive Foundation. www.ocfoundation.org

References

1. American Psychiatric Association. *Diagnostic and Statistical Manual of Mental Disorders, 4th edn., text revision*. Washington, DC: APA, 2000.

2. Rasmussen SA, Tsuang MT. Clinical characteristics and family history in DSM III obsessive-compulsive disorder. *Am J Psychiatry* 1986; **143**: 317–82.

3. Karno MG, Golding M, Sorensen SB, Burnam, A. The epidemiology of OCD in five U.S. communities. *Arch Gen Psychiatry* 1988; **45**: 1094–9.

4. Kessler RC, Berglund P, Demler O, *et al.* Lifetime prevalence and age-of-onset distributions of DSM-IV disorders in the national comorbidity survey replication. *Arch Gen Psychiatry* 2005; **62**: 593–602.

5. Weissman MM, Bland R, Canino G, *et al.* The cross-national epidemiology of obsessive compulsive disorder. *J Clin Psychiatry* 1994; **55**: 5–10.

6. Hanna GL. Demographic and clinical features of obsessive compulsive disorder in children and adolescents. *J Am Acad Child Adolesc Psychiatry* 1995; **34**: 19–27.

7. Rasmussen SA, Eisen JL. Epidemiology of obsessive-compulsive disorder. *J Clin Psychiatry* 1990; **51**: 10–14.

8. Rasmussen SA, Eisen JL. Phenomenology of obsessive-compulsive disorder: clinical subtypes, heterogeneity, and coexistence. In Zohar J, Insel J, Rasmussen S, eds. *Psychobiology of Obsessive–compulsive Disorder*. New York: Springer-Verlag. 1991, pp. 743–58.

9. Steketee G, Eisen J, Dyck I, Warshaw M, Rasmussen S. Predictors of course in obsessive-compulsive disorder. *Psychiatry Res* 1999; **89**: 229–38.

10. Skoog G, Skoog I. A 40-year follow-up of patients with obsessive-compulsive disorder. *Arch Gen Psychiatry* 1999; **56**: 121–7.

11. Brown TA, Campbell LA, Lehman CL, Grisham JR, Mancill RB. Current and lifetime comorbidity of the DSM-IV anxiety and mood disorders in a large clinical sample. *J Abnorm Psychol* 2001; **110**: 49–58.

12. Barlow DH. *Anxiety and its Disorders,* 2nd edn. New York: Guilford Press, 2002.

13. Dollard J, Miller NL. *Personality and Psychotherapy: An Analysis in Terms of Learning, Thinking and Culture.* New York: McGraw-Hill, 1950.

14. Mowrer, OH. A stimulus–response analysis of anxiety and its role as a reinforcing agent. *Psychol Rev* 1939; **46**: 553–65.

15. Carr AT. Compulsive neurosis: a review of the literature. *Psychol Bull* 1974; **81**: 311–18.

16. McFall ME, Wollersheim JP. Obsessive-compulsive neurosis: a cognitive-behavioral formulation and approach to treatment. *Cognit Ther Res* 1979; **3**: 333–48.

17. Salkovskis PM. Obsessional-compulsive problems: a cognitive-behavioural analysis. *Behav Res Ther* 1985; **23**: 571–83.

18. van Oppen P, Arntz A. Cognitive therapy for obsessive-compulsive disorder. *Behav Res Ther* 1994; **32**: 79–88.

19. Clark DA, Purdon C. New perspectives for a cognitive theory of obsessions. *Aust Psychol* 1993; **28**: 161–7.

20. Rachman, S. A cognitive theory of obsessions. *Behav Res Ther* 1997; **35**: 793–802.

21. Rachman, S. A cognitive theory of obsessions: elaborations. *Behav Res Ther* 1998; **36**: 385–401.

22. Rachman S, de Silva P. Abnormal and normal obsessions. *Behav Res Ther* 1978; **16**: 233–48.

23. Salkovskis PM, Harrison J. Abnormal and normal obsessions: a replication. *Behav Res Ther* 1984; **22**: 549–52.

24. Freeston MH, Ladouceur R, Rhéaume J, Letarte H. Images and doubts in intrusive cognitive activity. *Behav Cogn Psychother* 1994; **22**: 189–98.

25. Shafran R, Thordarson DS, Rachman S. Thought-action fusion in obsessive-compulsive disorder. *J Anxiety Disord* 1996; **10**: 379–91.

26. Rhéaume J, Freeston MH, Dugas M, Letarte H, Ladouceur R. Perfectionism, responsibility and obsessive compulsive symptoms. *Behav Res Ther* 1995; **33**: 785–94.

27. Foa EB, Kozak MJ. Emotional processing of fear: exposure to corrective information. *Psychol Bull* 1986; **99**: 20–35.

28. Freeston MH, Rhéaume J, Ladouceur R. Correcting faulty appraisals of obsessional thoughts. *Behav Res Ther* 1996; **34**: 433–46.

29. Salkovskis P, Shafran R, Rachman S, Freeston MH. Multiple pathways to inflated responsibility beliefs in obsessional problems: possible origins and implications for therapy and research. *Behav Res Ther* 1999; **37**: 1055–72.

30. Diaz SF, Grush LR, Sichel DA, Cohen LS. Obsessive-compulsive disorder in pregnancy and the puerperium. In Dickstein LJ, Riba MB, Oldham JM, eds. *Review of Psychiatry (Vol. 16)*. Washington, DC: American Psychiatric Press, 1998.

31. Rachman S, Hodgson RJ. *Obsessions and Compulsions.* Englewood Cliffs, NJ: Prentice-Hall, 1980.

32. March J, Frances A, Carpenter D, Kahn D. The expert consensus guideline series: treatment of obsessive–compulsive disorder. *J Clin Psychiatry* 1997; **58** (Suppl. 4): 1–16.

33. Abramowitz JS, Franklin ME, Foa EB. Empirical status of cognitive-behavioral therapy for obsessive-compulsive disorder: a meta-analytic review. *Rom J Cogn Behav Psychother* 2002; **2**: 89–104.

34. Whittal ML, Thordarson DS, McLean PD. Treatment of obsessive-compulsive disorder: cognitive behavior therapy vs. exposure and response prevention. *Behav Res Ther* 2005; **43**: 1559–76.

35. van Oppen P, de Haan E, van Balkom AJLM, *et al.* Cognitive therapy and exposure in vivo in the treatment of obsessive compulsive disorder. *Behav Res Ther* 1995; **33**: 379–90.

36. Whittal ML, Robichaud M, Thordarson DS, McLean PD. Group and individual treatment of OCD using cognitive therapy and exposure plus response prevention: a two-year follow-up of 2 randomized trials. *J Consult Clin Psychol* 2008; **76**: 1003–14.

37. Goodman WK, Price LH, Ramussen SA, *et al.* The Yale–Brown Obsessive-Compulsive Scale: I. Development, use and reliability. *Arch Gen Psychiatry* 1989; **46**: 1006–11.

38. Abramowitz JS, Foa EB, Franklin ME. Exposure and ritual prevention for obsessive-compulsive

disorder: effects of intensive versus twice-weekly sessions. *J Consult Clin Psychol* 2003; **71**: 394–8.

39. Newth S, Rachman S. The concealment of obsessions. *Behav Res Ther* 2001; **39**: 457–64.

40. Purdon C, Clark D. A. The need to control thoughts. In Frost RO, Steketee G, eds. *Cognitive Approaches to Obsessions and Compulsions: Theory, Assessment and Treatment.* Oxford: Elsevier. 2002, pp. 29–44.

41. Rachman S. A cognitive theory of compulsive checking. *Behav Res Ther* 2002; **40**: 625–39.

42. Rachman S. *Fear of Contamination: Assessment and Treatment.* Oxford: Oxford University Press, 2006.

43. McLean PD, Whittal ML, Thordarson DS, *et al.* Cognitive versus behavior therapy in the group treatment of obsessive-compulsive disorder. *J Consult Clin Psychol*, 2001; **69**: 205–14.

44. Franklin ME, Foa EB. Obsessive-compulsive disorder. In Barlow DH, ed. *Clinical Handbook of Psychological Disorders: A Step-by-step Treatment Manual.* New York: Guildford, 2008.

45. Himle MB, Franklin ME "The more you do it, the easier it gets": Exposure and response prevention for OCD. *Cogn Behav Pract* 2009; **16**: 29–39.

46. Rachman SJ, Radomsky AS, Shafran R. Safety behaviour: a reconsideration. *Behav Res Ther* 2008; **46**: 163–73.

47. Abramowitz JS, Franklin ME, Street GP, Kozak MJ, Foa EB. Effects of comorbid depression on response to treatment for obsessive-compulsive disorder. *Behav Ther* 2000; **31**: 517–28.

48. Calamari JE, Cohen RJ, Rector NA, *et al.* Dysfunctional belief-based obsessive-compulsive disorder subgroups. *Behav Res Ther* 2006; **44**: 1347–60.

49. Renshaw KD, Steketee G, Chambless DL. Involving family members in the treatment of OCD. *Cogn Behav Ther* 2005; **34**: 164–75.

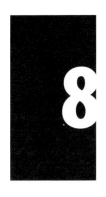

8 Post-traumatic stress disorder

Tiffany Fuse, Kristalyn Salters-Pedneault, and Brett T. Litz

Cognitive–behavioral therapy for post-traumatic stress disorder

Post-traumatic stress disorder (PTSD), which is characterized by intrusive memories, marked avoidance of trauma reminders, affective numbing, and hyperarousal following a traumatic experience was introduced into the diagnostic nomenclature in 1980 with the publication by the American Psychiatric Association of DSM-III [1]. Since then, a large body of research on the presentation and treatment of PTSD has been assembled. A number of efficacious cognitive–behavioral therapies (CBTs) are now offered, such as prolonged exposure [2] and cognitive processing therapy (CPT; [3]), and the rates of successful treatment in a variety of populations are improving [4, 5].

The nature of PTSD

Symptoms and diagnostic criteria

In the DSM-IV-TR [1], there are six diagnostic criteria (Criterion A–F) that must be present for a diagnosis of PTSD. First, the individual must have experienced a traumatic event (Criterion A) during which: (1) the person experienced or witnessed an event or events that involved actual threatened death or serious injury, or a threat to the physical integrity of oneself or others; and (2) the person's reaction involved intense fear, helplessness, or horror (in children this may present as agitated or disorganized behavior). Examples of traumatic events include serious threats to life or physical integrity such as military combat, sexual assault, motor vehicle accidents, physical assault, natural or human-made disasters, or witnessing violence or severe human suffering.

The symptoms of PTSD are categorized into three clusters in DSM-IV (Criterion B, C, and D): intrusive recollection, avoidance and numbing, and hyper arousal symptoms. Intrusive recollection (Criterion B) refers to recurrent re-experiencing of the traumatic event(s) through either intrusive memories, distressing dreams, flashbacks (a sense of actually reliving the trauma), and intense distress in response to trauma cues. Avoidance and numbing symptoms (Criterion C) refer to avoidance of stimuli reminiscent of the trauma and general unresponsiveness (particularly to positive stimuli). Avoidance symptoms include efforts to avoid thoughts, feelings, or conversations related to the trauma; efforts to avoid activities, places, or people reminiscent of the trauma; and difficulty remembering an important aspect of the traumatic event. Numbing symptoms include markedly diminished interest or participation in significant activities, feelings of detachment from others, restricted range of affect, and a sense of a foreshortened future. Hyperarousal (Criterion D) pertains to persistent increased arousal, as evidenced by sleep difficulties, irritability or outbursts of anger, concentration difficulties, hypervigilance, and exaggerated startle response. At least one Criterion B, three Criterion C, and two Criterion D symptoms must be present for at least one month (Criterion E) at clinical levels (Criterion F; e.g., causing significant impairment or distress) to warrant a diagnosis of PTSD.

Course

Among the general population, PTSD-like symptoms are very common immediately following a traumatic event. For example, after a sexual assault, 94% of women report symptoms consistent with PTSD [6]. However, for most individuals these symptoms decline

Cognitive–behavioral Therapy with Adults: A Guide to Empirically Informed Assessment and Intervention,
ed. Stefan G. Hofmann and Mark A. Reinecke. © Cambridge University Press 2010.

sharply in the days following the trauma (see [7] for a review). For this reason, PTSD cannot be diagnosed until at least one month after the trauma. Individuals with clinically significant symptoms seeking treatment before a month has elapsed post-trauma are instead diagnosed with acute stress disorder [1].

Post-traumatic stress disorder tends to be a chronic condition once sustained symptoms are evident [8]. Research examining the course of PTSD from baseline to 34 to 50 months follow-up in a sample of adolescents and young adults living in a German community revealed that approximately 52% of participants with PTSD at baseline remitted during the follow-up period whereas 48% did not [9]. Post-traumatic stress disorder is also relatively resistant to treatment; the gold standard treatments for PTSD produce far lower rates of high-end state functioning than are seen in treatments for most other anxiety disorders [10].

Epidemiology

In the United States about 8 to 9% of individuals will meet criteria for PTSD over the course of their lifetime [11]. One epidemiological study of trauma exposure and PTSD among 1,007 young adults living in the Detroit, MI area found that 39% of the sample was exposed to trauma over the course of their lifetime [12]. However, these same authors found that only about 23.6% of the trauma victims developed PTSD.

The likelihood of developing PTSD after a trauma is related to both individual factors and trauma-related variables. The results of a recent meta-analysis examining findings from 68 studies indicate that peri-traumatic experiences such as dissociation, perceived life threat, and emotionality strongly predict the development of PTSD [13]. Furthermore, Brewin, Andrews, and Valentine [14] found perceived social support to buffer against the development of PTSD in adults exposed to trauma. Overall, Ozer and her colleagues found that pre-trauma individual factors such as prior history of trauma, prior psychological adjustment, and demographic variables (age, race, education, gender, education, and socioeconomic status), were weaker predictive factors of PTSD in comparison to peri-traumatic psychological factors [13].

Comorbidity

Exposure to trauma is linked with both PTSD and other psychological disorders [15]. Results from the National Comorbidity Study suggest that PTSD typically precedes the development of additional psychological problems [11]. Kessler and his colleagues found that individuals with PTSD had higher rates of alcohol abuse (52% of men, 28% of women), drug abuse (35% of men, 27% of women), major depressive disorder (48% of men, 49% of women), social phobia (11% of men, 14% of women), agoraphobia (4% of men, 8% of women), generalized anxiety disorder (3% of men, 6% of women), and panic disorder (2% of men, 4% of women). However, PTSD does not appear to be comorbid with all mental disorders. Research examining the relationship between PTSD and obsessive–compulsive disorder (OCD) found that OCD was not more common among individuals diagnosed with PTSD, as compared to controls [16].

In addition to an increased risk of psychological problems, research suggests a significant comorbidity between PTSD and overall worse physical health [17]. Post-traumatic stress disorder has also been linked to specific medical issues, such as cardiovascular and autoimmune disorders [18]; respiratory, neurologic, gastrointestinal problems; and non-sexually transmitted infections [19], as well as tinnitus [20].

Cognitive–behavioral theories of PTSD

The first cognitive–behavioral theories of PTSD were introduced more than two decades ago [21]. Since that time, models of PTSD have become more sophisticated in response to the rapid expansion of the research literature. Now, most cognitive–behavioral theories of PTSD point to conditioning and information processing phenomena to explain the development and maintenance of the disorder.

Conditioning theories of PTSD, which assume that PTSD develops through associative and operant learning processes (see Mowrer's two-factor theory [22]), were among the earliest psychological models of the disorder. For example, Keane and colleagues' conditioning model (e.g., [21, 23]) described PTSD as resulting from classically conditioned fear and fear generalization processes. In this theory, the traumatic event, which by definition elicits intense emotion (including fear, terror, or horror), serves as an unconditioned stimulus. During the course of a trauma, a number of explicit and contextual cues, which are not inherently dangerous, are paired with the unconditioned stimulus and form conditioned stimuli. Thus, the strong fear response triggered by exposure to these trauma-related cues after a trauma is considered a conditioned version of the original response to the event. Over the course of time, the fear becomes generalized through higher order conditioning and stimulus generalization, and is maintained through avoidance of trauma-related conditioned stimuli.

Although theories of PTSD that relied strictly on conditioning accounts of the disorder were criticized for their limitations in describing the full range of posttraumatic symptoms and sequelae (e.g., emotional numbing, dissociation), fear conditioning remains one of the most widely accepted aspects of modern cognitive–behavioral models of PTSD. The theoretical role of conditioned fear and avoidance forms one rationale for the use of exposure-based therapies that employ principles of extinction learning in the treatment of PTSD, and outcome data from exposure-based CBT trials support the role of causal learning processes in successful treatment. Researchers continue to explore the role of fear learning and extinction in PTSD [24], with promising results.

Modern information processing theories of PTSD propose that the disorder is the result of dysfunctional cognitive processing of traumatic events, including disrupted encoding, storage, and retrieval of traumatic memories, unconscious attentional biases, and maladaptive beliefs (although most also acknowledge the central role of classical conditioning in the development of trauma-related fear). Dominant current information processing theories of PTSD include Foa's emotional processing theory [25], Brewin's dual representation theory [26], and Ehlers and Clark's cognitive theory [27]. In particular, most of these theories posit that traumatic memories, because they are encoded under extraordinary circumstances, may behave somewhat differently than normal memories.

Foa and colleague's emotional processing theory [2, 28, 29] is an extension of Lang's bioinformational theory of emotion [30], which understands emotion as an action tendency, which resides in a network of information including stimulus, response, context, and meaning elements. Foa [28] theorizes that because trauma memories are created under circumstances of extreme distress and fear, the trauma–fear network has particularly strong response elements (e.g., physiological arousal), and strong associations with a variety of environmental cues and contexts. Further, memories resulting from traumatic events may be poorly elaborated (e.g., may include gaps, be disjointed, or overly simplistic). Foa proposes that avoidance of content or

responses in the trauma–fear network would maintain PTSD symptoms, and that repeated imaginal exposure to all elements of the trauma memory network (and in vivo exposure to external cues/contexts) produces habituation of fear and allows the individual to incorporate safety information into the network. In addition, exposure creates a more fully elaborated trauma memory that becomes integrated into the rest of memory and then functions more like a "normal" memory.

Brewin's theory [26] proposes that aspects of the trauma memory that are consciously attended to during the event are stored in a "verbally accessible memory" (VAM) system, whereas material that is not consciously attended to but is encoded nonetheless is stored in a "situationally accessible memory" (SAM) system. The VAM system maintains memories that can be intentionally accessed and reflected on, including the individual's thoughts and beliefs before and after the event. In contrast, the SAM system records information that is processed at a lower, perceptual level, and is recalled only through situational reminders (e.g., trauma cues). For example, flashbacks and physiological responses are thought to reside in the SAM system. Because these memories cannot be intentionally accessed they are experienced as uncontrollable, unpredictable, and distressing. Brewin [31] proposes that the VAM and SAM systems must be targeted with different treatment strategies. The VAM system is amenable to cognitive methods (e.g., cognitive restructuring) in which beliefs or thoughts about the trauma (e.g., "I am responsible for this event") are accessed and directly modified through verbal exchanges in therapy. Elements of trauma in the SAM system must be addressed through the production of new SAMs in which trauma-related cues are associated with reduced arousal and negative affect (e.g., through exposure and habituation).

Ehlers and Clark [27] also proposed that trauma memories are encoded differently than other types of memories. Specifically, they suggest that due to peritraumatic factors such as dissociation, emotional numbing, and overwhelmed cognitive resources, trauma memories may be recorded without coherent elaboration or adequate contextual information. This accounts for difficulties retrieving complete accounts of traumatic events, and difficulty placing traumatic images in time and place (e.g., re-experiencing symptoms that are experienced as happening "now"). These memories may also not be integrated well into the store of general memory, making them difficult to understand and connect with other relevant information. Ehlers and Clark also posit a role of negative appraisals in PTSD, including negative thoughts about the self, the future, and other people, and overgeneralized thoughts about danger or threat. Thus, treatment of PTSD involves explicit cognitive techniques that target negative or maladaptive appraisals and aim to more fully elaborate trauma memories and integrate these memories into the rest of the autobiographical memory system.

While modern cognitive–behavioral theories differ in terms of the precise processes involved in the development and maintenance of PTSD, there are several underlying principles that are shared. For example, all cognitive–behavioral theories of PTSD propose that avoidance of trauma memories, and cues and contexts associated with the trauma, plays a role in the maintenance of symptoms. Thus, successful treatment must always involve accessing the trauma memory in some fashion (including imaginal or in vivo exposure to trauma-related memories/stimuli, cognitive restructuring of trauma-related thoughts or beliefs, or narrative structuring of trauma accounts). Further, most theories propose that maladaptive beliefs about the trauma (e.g., overgeneralized beliefs about threat) maintain the disorder and must be addressed either by direct cognitive restructuring or through cognitive processing that occurs in the course of trauma-focused work (e.g., exposure). Finally, cognitive–behavioral models generally presume that the trauma memory must be integrated into the larger body of autobiographical memory, either through narrative elaboration, imaginal exposure and processing, or some other technique.

Efficacy and effectiveness of CBT for PTSD

There is now evidence from roughly two dozen randomized controlled trials to support the use of CBT for PTSD [32]. Cognitive–behavioral therapy yields large effect sizes [33], and is considered the gold standard of care for PTSD by the International Society for Traumatic Stress [34], the American Psychiatric Association [35], and the Departments of Veterans Affairs and Defense [36]. However, despite the advantages of CBT for PTSD over other treatment modalities, there is significant room for improvement. Approximately half of patients show no improvement post-treatment [32], and attrition is high: about 25% of CBT patients drop out in randomized controlled trials [37], and many more (roughly

70%) fail to complete treatment in clinical settings [38]. Also, despite relative success in civilian contexts, the efficacy of CBT with veterans is unclear. Some research found only modest effects [39]; whereas a second trial of CBT for combat veterans was more encouraging [40].

Most evidence-based CBT protocols involve some combination of exposure to trauma-related memories, in vivo exposure to feared contexts, implicit or explicit cognitive processing and restructuring, and stress management or emotion regulation skills-building [10]. At present, there is no single CBT package that is clearly more efficacious or well tolerated than any other. Theoretical disadvantages of exposure therapy relative to other forms of CBT (e.g., stress inoculation training), including acute symptom exacerbation and attrition, have not been supported by research [37, 41]. There is some evidence that exposure-based interventions may lead to more rapid change than other forms of therapy (e.g., relaxation training or eye-movement desensitization and reprocessing; [41]), but this needs to be explored further.

Given the support for the use of CBT, many researchers have moved to the next stage of clinical research: dissemination and effectiveness studies. A number of recent trials have examined the effectiveness of CBT for PTSD when delivered by non-experts in purely clinical contexts. Foa and colleagues [42] examined the outcomes of prolonged exposure (PE) and PE plus cognitive restructuring in an academic setting (with doctoral-level expert therapists) or a community clinic (with masters-level non-expert therapists), and found equivalent or better outcomes in patients treated in the community clinic. Gillespie and colleagues similarly found that cognitive therapy for PTSD was comparably effective when delivered in a community setting [43]. A recent study by Schulz *et al.* suggests that CPT for PTSD is effective when delivered in a community setting to a diverse population with the use of interpreter services [44].

Unfortunately, despite its superiority to other treatment approaches and evidence for its successful use outside of research settings, CBT for PTSD is extraordinarily under-utilized [45, 46]. Clearly, more work is needed to: (1) demonstrate that CBT, and especially exposure-based CBT, can be effective in a variety of settings; and (2) tackle the professional barriers that likely exist, including lack of familiarity or comfort with exposure procedures and beliefs that exposure interventions are poorly tolerated [47].

A case study of CBT for PTSD

Mr. B was a 46-year-old, never-married Navy veteran who was referred by his psychiatrist to the National Center for PTSD (NC-PTSD) Behavioral Science Division for treatment of PTSD symptoms. The client was living in a half-way house with other veterans and had recently begun a part-time job at a hardware store. Mr. B reported having a very strained relationship with his family, mostly due to his history of substance use and legal troubles related to his substance dependence. Despite a history of difficulties in romantic relationships, he had good relationships and regular contact with his two teenage daughters.

Mr. B's medical chart revealed a long history of depression, multiple suicide attempts, polysubstance abuse, and PTSD symptomatology. The client had been clean and sober for about a year (submitting to weekly drug tests), and was actively involved in formal group substance abuse counseling and Alcoholics Anonymous (AA)/Narcotics Anonymous (NA). The client's last suicide attempt was about one year prior to beginning treatment for PTSD.

The client presented as extremely guarded, refusing to provide details about the traumatic event(s) associated with his PTSD symptoms. However, Mr. B did acknowledge experiencing a very violent physical assault during his military service, as well as an instance of sexual abuse by an older neighbor when he was about five years old. Mr. B was most evasive, uncomfortable, and irritable when discussing his military history. He reported that he had been extremely idealistic when he enlisted in the Navy – desiring to serve his country and visit exotic places. Mr. B was stationed on a ship off the east coast of Africa for approximately six months. He reported that during this time he was singled out by a group of several sailors and physically attacked when he declined a sexual advance made by one of them. Mr. B reported that afterward he experienced severe dissociative symptoms, began drinking heavily, and eventually was medically discharged from the Navy.

The client's symptom presentation included severe re-experiencing symptoms (intrusive memories, nightmares, distress in response to traumatic reminders), extreme avoidance of trauma-related stimuli, feelings of detachment from others, restricted range of affect, sleep difficulties, irritability, and hypervigilance. The client initially associated these symptoms with both his history of childhood sexual abuse and the physical attack he sustained when he was in the Navy.

Mr. B presented with severe functional impairment: he experienced extreme and incapacitating distress when exposed to trauma reminders and went to extraordinary lengths to avoid these cues. Additionally, he reported that his avoidance and detachment from others led to the break up of several intimate relationships. The client's long history of substance abuse appeared to be a form of avoidance: prior to becoming abstinent he would respond to trauma cues by abusing substances. He would generally be so desperate to avoid thoughts and feelings associated with his traumatic experiences that he would use whatever substance was most readily available – hence his polysubstance dependence. The client's symptom presentation included prominent depressive symptoms. In particular, Mr. B complained of severe depressed mood, anhedonia, and feelings of worthlessness. His depression was the result of significant ruminating about his history.

Overview of the treatment approach

Assessment

The first several meetings between Mr. B and the therapist consisted of assessment sessions in which the client completed a structured interview designed to assess the frequency and severity of PTSD symptoms and was asked to provide details about his life history and traumatic experiences. After several assessment sessions Mr. B anxiously confessed that the physical assault he reported initially was actually an extremely violent rape, and that this incident was the true source of his PTSD symptoms.

Case conceptualization and treatment choice

During the assessment process Mr. B frequently made self-denigrating comments and displayed a tendency to view the world inflexibly (e.g., "If I try to get close to someone they will reject me once they know the real me"). Mr. B's therapist hypothesized that maladaptive cognitions played a central role in the maintenance of his PTSD symptoms. The therapist conceptualized Mr. B's avoidance of trauma cues as a second factor maintaining his PTSD, preventing him from obtaining corrective feedback from the environment about the validity of his thoughts and beliefs (Mr. B avoided close relationships and he did not have the opportunity to test his belief that if he opened up to others they would automatically reject him). Mr. B's therapist selected CBT because this treatment approach addresses both maladaptive thoughts and beliefs, and avoidance.

In a hierarchical approach to CBT for PTSD, the most pressing or immediate treatment needs are met well before any trauma-focused treatment is attempted. These needs may include crisis management (e.g, managing imminent threat of suicidal or homicidal behavior or violence), elimination of therapy-destroying behaviors, such as non-compliance [48], or treatment of more pressing comorbid conditions, including severe depression, substance use disorders, active psychosis or mania, or serious self-harming behaviors. If the patient is in a current situation that puts them at a high risk of revictimization, this must also be addressed prior to embarking on trauma-focused work [2]. Other concerns, such as homelessness, legal, or occupational problems may also need to be addressed. While below we focus on the core, trauma-focused portion of CBT for PTSD, it is important to note that in many cases this portion of treatment will need to be preceded or augmented by attention to a variety of other issues (see also the discussion of clinical decision making below).

Cognitive processing therapy is an empirically supported therapy for PTSD that consists of 12 or 13 structured sessions [49–51]. Originally developed for the treatment of PTSD related to sexual victimization, it has been used successfully to treat combat-PTSD as well as PTSD associated with other traumatic events. Cognitive processing therapy has been successfully administered in both individual and group formats. Regular assessment and monitoring of PTSD symptoms is an important component of CPT. The client completes a PTSD checklist (PCL; [52]) on a weekly basis, and the therapist maintains a record of the client's PCL scores. At the end of each session the clinician checks-in with the client about his or her reactions to the session and to material covered in the session. In this way misunderstandings or confusion can be addressed immediately. Psychoeducation about PTSD, cognitive restructuring, and exposure are key components of CPT. Each will be discussed below.

Psychoeducation

The first session of the therapy focused on introducing Mr. B to the CPT protocol and educating him in PTSD. Issues such as PTSD symptomatology, natural

recovery from trauma, and cognitive theory of the etiology of PTSD were covered. Mr. B and his therapist discussed the role of maladaptive beliefs (termed "stuck points" in CPT), and avoidance, in the maintenance of PTSD. Stuck points were explained to Mr. B as automatic thoughts related to his interpretation of the rape. A frank discussion of avoidance of therapy, and the importance of compliance were also covered. Mr. B was anxious about fully engaging in treatment and not relying on avoidance as a coping strategy. However, he acknowledged that years and years of avoidance had not brought about any improvement in his symptoms, but had only made his life more difficult. Therefore, Mr. B made a commitment to attend all therapy sessions and fully participate in treatment.

An important element of cognitive theory that the therapist taught Mr. B about is the impact that traumatic events have on beliefs. Mr. B and the therapist discussed the process of assimilation, in which a survivor alters his or her interpretation of the event to match pre-existing beliefs. For example, Mr. B believed that the rape was his fault and that he was responsible for what happened because he "didn't do enough to stop it." This interpretation fit in with his belief that men should always be in control of every situation. Discussion also focused on the opposing process, accommodation, in which a survivor changes his or her existing beliefs to accommodate the new experience of the trauma. While this is often a positive outcome, some individuals may over-accommodate (change their beliefs in an extreme fashion). For example, after the rape Mr. B believed that he could not trust anyone, and that people were out to get him. This belief system caused Mr. B to be suspicious and guarded in his social relationships, leading to the break-up of an eight-year romantic relationship with the mother of his daughters, severely strained relationships with family members, and the client having no true friendships.

Examining meaning elements

During the first session Mr. B was asked to write an "impact statement," or brief narrative describing his beliefs about the traumatic event. In the next session, Mr. B and the therapist focused on uncovering the meaning of the traumatic event. Mr. B was asked to read his "impact statement." During the reading, the therapist listened for "stuck points." While the impact statement is read, the therapist attempts to identify instances of assimilation, accommodation, and over-accommodation (e.g., that the attack was his fault, and a sign that he was not a "real man"). This provides information about the root of the PTSD, and allows the client and therapist to discuss connections between events, cognitions, and emotions.

In his impact statement, Mr. B revealed his belief that his intense feelings of depression were directly caused by the rape. The therapist explained the role that his thoughts play in his emotional responses: Mr.B's thoughts such as "I am not a real man because I let the rape happen to me" led to feelings of guilt and shame that fueled his symptoms. To enable Mr. B to become more aware of these connections, the therapist introduced him to a basic monitoring sheet in which an event, the client's thoughts/interpretations of the event, and the resulting emotions, are recorded. Mr. B was asked to complete at least one such sheet per day about the rape for homework.

In the next session, Mr. B and the therapist reviewed his homework sheets and focused on identifying thoughts and feelings associated with the trauma and distinguishing between the two. Mr. B had some difficulty distinguishing between thoughts and feelings, tending to label thoughts as feelings. For example, Mr. B wrote "stupid" and "weak" down as feelings. The therapist taught the client that "I am stupid" was a thought that led to a feeling of sadness.

The therapist then employed Socratic questioning to challenge Mr. B's maladaptive cognitions about the trauma. For example, the therapist challenged Mr. B's thought that a "real man" could avoid rape under any circumstances. She pushed the client to consider the validity of this statement. The client acknowledged that the circumstances of his rape included multiple (at least four) armed assailants versus him (unarmed, alone, and taken off guard by the assault), and realized that even "the strongest man in the world" would be unable to prevent a rape under such circumstances.

Trauma exposure

After the cognitive skills groundwork was laid, Mr. B was instructed to write a detailed account of his most traumatic incident for homework. The therapist explained that this account is different than the impact statement, and should detail the specifics of the trauma, including physical sensations, thoughts, and feelings. As outlined in the treatment manual, trauma-focused

exposure narratives of this type should be hand-written because hand-written accounts tend to be more emotionally evocative [53]. The therapist stressed that spelling, grammar, and handwriting are unimportant, so long as the account is legible. Mr. B was asked to complete the account as soon as possible and to read it daily until the next session. Mr. B and the therapist discussed the importance of real engagement with the account during each reading; Mr. B was asked to be careful to not engage in any avoidance behaviors when writing or reading the account, but to allow himself to fully feel the emotions associated with the traumatic event. Mr. B acknowledged considerable anxiety surrounding this, but also displayed a remarkable willingness to tolerate the discomfort for the purpose of long-term reduction of PTSD symptoms. Clear and comprehensive psychoeducation about the role of avoidance in the maintenance of PTSD lays the groundwork for the client's willingness to tolerate temporary discomfort in service of long-term treatment gains.

Mr. B was asked to read the trauma account in session. Mr. B expressed considerable emotion as he read, frequently crying at some points and shaking with anger at other moments. The therapist did not attempt to comfort him, but encouraged his expression of emotion. Afterward she asked him if there were any parts he omitted. Mr. B acknowledged that he left an important detail out of his account – that at one point during the rape he got one of his hands free, but was still unable to end the attack. The therapist explored with Mr. B why this point was particularly difficult for him. He stated that he interpreted this as evidence that he "could have stopped the rape, but didn't." The therapist utilized further Socratic questioning to challenge this "stuck point" with the client.

Integrating cognitive skills and trauma processing

As the client becomes more skilled at challenging his or her maladaptive thoughts, the focus of therapy becomes a more clear integration of the trauma-exposure work and the cognitive-skills work. In this case, the fifth session began with Mr. B reading the second trauma account out loud in session. It is important to listen for and note differences between the first and second renditions. The differences between Mr. B's first and second accounts were remarkable. His first trauma account included statements such as "I let it happen, I am a punk," and "They took away my soul." His second account was very different. He clearly placed the blame for the attack where it belonged – with the perpetrators. He even wrote "I had the mistaken thought I had 'caused it.'" Although Mr. B's narrative did contain some statements of self-blame, he was able to challenge his own thoughts. To further encourage this behavior the client was given a worksheet of generic questions that can be used to challenge maladaptive thoughts. Mr. B was instructed to select "stuck points" each day and use this worksheet to challenge them.

The worksheets were reviewed in subsequent sessions, and Mr. B and the therapist continued to address the "stuck points" that emerged. For example, Mr. B brought up the belief that "nobody can be trusted." The therapist challenged this, and through Socratic questioning the client eventually acknowledged that although some people cannot be trusted, others can be trusted. Other tools to facilitate cognitive restructuring, including a worksheet listing common patterns of problematic thinking, were introduced. In this case Mr. B was overgeneralizing the lack of trustworthiness of the assailants to all people. The therapist noted that Mr. B also had a strong tendency to disregard important aspects of the traumatic event. For example, Mr. B continued to blame himself somewhat for the rape, believing that he should have been able to stop it. However, he was disregarding the fact that there were multiple assailants, and they had a weapon. During the course of completing exposure exercises the client remembered an additional fact – that he had been wearing flip-flops during the rape (which occurred on a wet floor) whereas the rapists were wearing heavy boots. This made it even more difficult for him to fight back. Mr. B and the therapist discussed the need to consider the actual traumatic context when making decisions about self-blame, and talked about how to generate alternative, competing thoughts based on the available evidence.

The final four sessions (sessions 8 to 12) of the CPT protocol focus on specific issues that are often problematic for trauma survivors. These issues include safety, trust, power/control, esteem, and intimacy. Each may apply to both the self and others. For example, trust can refer to either trusting oneself and one's own judgment or trusting other people. Each topic is discussed in session, and handouts are provided with more details about how that week's theme relates to reactions to trauma. The client and therapist relate the week's topic to the client's own experiences, and, if this is a relevant area for the client, homework (e.g., cognitive restructuring) is assigned in relation to beliefs about that topic.

At this point in treatment Mr. B continued to have some issues trusting his own judgment. Specifically, he believed that he used poor judgment by joining the Navy in the first place. After enlisting in the Navy, Mr. B discovered that his assailants had raped several other men on the ship, and that his attackers frequently raped local women when the ship was in port. The client insisted that he "should have known" this would happen to him and should have joined another branch of the military instead. Mr. B and the therapist worked to challenge this belief, replacing it with statements such as "There is no reasonable way that I could have known there would be rapists aboard the ship ahead of time. This does not mean that my judgment is bad."

Trust issues, as well as issues of power and control, were also addressed with Mr. B. As traumatic experiences often involve a loss of control, some trauma survivors may focus on attempting to control everything in their current environment. Alternatively, they may go to the other extreme and believe that because they were powerless during the trauma, they will always be powerless. Such clients may present as extremely passive and refuse to take responsibility in their lives. The clinician's goal is to assist the client in forming a balanced view of control.

Mr. B had great difficulty accepting that he did not have control during the attack. He insisted that as a man he *should have been* in complete control at all times, and therefore been able to stop the rape. However, as he continued to process the trauma Mr. B was able to adopt a more balanced perspective, realizing that nobody, regardless of their gender, can be in complete control of any situation. This conversation led nicely into a discussion of esteem issues. Mr. B often struggled with thoughts that he was "worthless" because he was a rape survivor. Mr. B held on to the belief that he was raped because of some feature related to him as a person. Through Socratic questioning Mr. B was able to assign the blame for the attack where it belonged – on the rapists and not on him. Mr. B completed homework to challenge his current beliefs related to esteem issues. He was also instructed to practice behavioral changes related to esteem, including giving and receiving complements each day, and doing nice things for himself.

The final session of CPT addresses intimacy issues and making meaning of the trauma. Mr. B had difficulty with self-intimacy, or the capacity to engage in adaptive self-soothing without relying on harmful external means (such as substance abuse). He identified his history of poly-substance dependence as such (the client continued to maintain his sobriety throughout the duration of the treatment). Mr. B was encouraged to utilize his new coping skills in place of substances.

Treatment outcome

This final session focused on reading a final impact statement and discussing the meaning of the trauma. The client's final rendition of his impact statement was remarkably different from his original. First, Mr. B clearly placed the blame for the rape on the perpetrators, and not on himself. Second, in his final impact statement Mr. B described the impact the attack had on his thoughts and beliefs in the past tense (e.g., "For many years I thought the rape was my fault"), as compared to his original impact statement where he stated "I was raped because I was a punk who didn't do anything to stop it." Mr. B was startled when his therapist showed him his original impact statement, stating "I can't believe I used to think like that." In his final impact statement, Mr. B continued to express some feelings of shame, but he was better able to challenge his own thoughts on this matter. Importantly, Mr. B's PCL scores dropped considerably over the course of treatment (63 at the beginning of treatment, a high of 68, to 41 following treatment).

Difficulties encountered during treatment

One of the most common reasons for treatment failure is avoidance. The clinician should anticipate this, as avoidance is one of the hallmark features of PTSD. An important facet of treatment for PTSD is psychoeducation about the nature of avoidance and the role that avoidance plays in the development and maintenance of PTSD. Such psychoeducation should occur early on in treatment, preferably during the first session. As discussed above, avoidance is conceptualized as playing a key role in the etiology of PTSD [54]. This is communicated to the client both verbally during session and through written materials provided to the client. Treatment adherence in CPT is evidenced by attendance and completion of homework assignments. It is paramount that clients attend all sessions and

complete all homework assignments on time, in order to benefit the most from treatment. Clients should be made aware that this treatment requires considerable effort on their part.

Prior to embarking on treatment, the client must agree to give up his or her old patterns of avoidance. Avoidance can take multiple forms, including but not limited to client attempts to change the subject when the trauma is discussed, dissociation, failing to complete homework assignments, substance abuse or other addictive behaviors, arriving late to session, self-harm behaviors, or anger and aggression. It is extremely important for the therapist to identify avoidance and confront the client about engaging in avoidance behaviors. Therapists' inadvertent collusion with client avoidance behaviors is a common cause of treatment failure. During CPT the therapist comes to label behaviors that interfere with treatment as avoidance behaviors for the client. For example, if the client arrives to session without having completed her homework, the therapist would re-assign the same homework task, along with the next homework assignment (according to the protocol). If the client complains that they do not have a place to complete the assignment the therapist would schedule a time and place at the clinic for the client to come in and finish their homework.

One particularly harmful form of avoidance is premature withdrawal from treatment. Often the most effective method for combating this unfortunate event is careful planning prior to initiating treatment. Exposure-based treatment for PTSD, such as CPT, is not always suitable for clients. If a client is unwilling or unable to dedicate themselves to the treatment for 12 weeks, CPT may need to be postponed until the client's life circumstances are more conducive to active and full participation in treatment. It is important that clients have a solid understanding of what treatment will entail. The therapist should acknowledge and fully inform the client that this type of treatment is very difficult and requires a significant amount of time and energy on the part of the client. It should be stressed that participation is voluntary.

Sometimes clients withdraw from treatment due to serious obstacles to completing the protocol. For example, a client may lose his or her housing during the course of treatment and not have a private place to complete homework assignments. In such cases the therapist should help the client problem solve to find strategies for addressing obstacles. In this example, the client could be instructed to complete their assignment at a local library, or the therapist could arrange for the client to use a private location in the clinic for this purpose.

Some obstacles may be overcome by the clinician altering the protocol to meet the needs of the client. This should be done if it can be accomplished without sacrificing the integrity of the protocol. For example, psychoeducation materials can be modified and simplified to make them more understandable for a client with low intelligence.

One difficulty commonly encountered in treatment is crisis management. Clients may initiate treatment and then present with a crisis situation that requires the therapist's immediate attention. In some cases this may reflect avoidance behavior, whereas other times the client may be experiencing a legitimate emergency. If the client becomes actively suicidal or homicidal, or suffers a substance abuse relapse, the therapist may need to suspend treatment until the client is more stable. For clients who are in immediate danger, such as those who are suicidal or in abusive relationships, treatment should focus on safety planning. However, treatment may resume once the clinician and client are both satisfied that the client has been stabilized.

Clinical decision making

Post-traumatic stress disorder is a remarkably heterogeneous condition, and patients may arrive for treatment with very different circumstances. For this reason, there is no prescriptive approach tied to the diagnosis. Rather, conceptualization of a PTSD case must include thorough consideration of the patient's skill sets, comorbid conditions, resources, etc. While a flexible, hierarchical approach to treatment is the most likely to garner success, this type of approach also requires a great deal of responsive and individualized clinical decision making. Some of the clinical decisions made in CBT for PTSD have an empirical basis; others are based on anecdotal information or clinical experience. Clearly, much more work is needed to fully understand clinical decision making in CBT for PTSD, including choices about how to best prepare the patient for exposure-based elements of treatment, how to match the patient with the exposure-focused treatment that is most likely to produce good outcome, how to time treatment elements, when to stop trauma-focused work, and how to handle relapse.

Preparation for exposure-based CBT

One of the first decisions a therapist will face is whether the patient will require a course of work focused on preparation for trauma-focused therapy. Again, given the diverse presentations of patients with PTSD, the elements included in this aspect of treatment can vary greatly. Some patients may require a single session of psychoeducation about PTSD and the rationale for exposure-based treatment. Others may require many sessions of preparatory training before they are able to approach highly distressing trauma-related content.

There are several factors to consider when choosing the types of preparation that the patient will need before engaging in trauma-focused work. For example, theory suggests that the ability to fully engage, all elements of the trauma-related fear network (including physiological and emotional response to the event), is necessary for habituation to occur and thus related to treatment outcome [25]. The patient must be able to access emotional responses, such as fear (including subjective response and somatic arousal) of the traumatic material, and to tolerate that affect without suppressing or otherwise avoiding it [55, 56]. Patients who are unwilling or unable to access intense fear, sadness, guilt, or anger, may require preparatory training to improve their chances of success. For example, a patient with difficulty accessing intense affect (e.g., an alexithymic patient), may require skills training focused on observing and maintaining contact with emotion (e.g., mindfulness or acceptance-based skills training may be necessary; see [57]).

It may be that the patient does not have the necessary skill set to regulate the emotions that will arise from trauma-focused work. If insufficient regulatory strategies are present, or if the patient tends to rely on destructive regulation practices (e.g., self-harming behavior or substance use), a course of emotion regulation skills training may be necessary. Some CBT protocols have been developed which incorporate this first step [58]. Or, skills training techniques from other sources, e.g., dialectical behavior therapy [48], may be incorporated.

Research has demonstrated that anger may interfere with symptom reduction in exposure-based treatments [59, 60]. While the mechanism of this effect has not been explored deeply, it may be that anger interferes with access to the trauma-related fear network [55]. Patients with significant anger may benefit from anger management training prior to or following exposure, or, depending on the function of the anger, may need training to access primary emotional responses.

Finally, as discussed above, patient motivation is likely critical to the success of a trauma-focused therapy. Theoretically, drop out from exposure could lead to sensitization rather than habituation (although this has not been examined empirically). If there are indications that the patient is likely to drop out of therapy (e.g., has dropped out of therapy frequently in the past, has communicated strong ambivalence about engaging in treatment), it may make sense to engage in a motivation-building intervention before trying exposure or other emotionally-evocative work.

It is important to note that some patients may never complete the preparatory stage and move into trauma-focused work. There are some boundary conditions that the patient may not be able to meet or are not amenable to training. For example, the patient will need to have a clear memory of at least a large part of the trauma to engage in exposure-based CBT (although, inability to remember some elements of the trauma may be acceptable). Of note, other factors that had been previously thought to predict treatment outcome, such as pre-existing traumatic events and chronicity of trauma [61], have been shown to have no substantial impact on response [62, 63], and thus should not be considered exclusionary criteria for exposure-based CBT.

Treatment matching

While there is no empirical basis to choose one type of trauma-focused CBT over another, patient factors may lead the clinician to select a particular treatment package. For example, a trauma-focused CBT including imaginal exposure elements (e.g., prolonged exposure; [2]) will require the ability to image. Patients who cannot image well may be better suited for a more verbal–linguistic based type of trauma-focused work, such as the narrative accounting approach taken in CPT. Alternatively, patients who have difficulty writing (or who dislike writing) may prefer a treatment approach such as PE.

Timing of treatment elements

The therapist must consider the best timing to initiate trauma-focused work, and when to stop this work and move on to other elements. For example, the patient may experience an exacerbation of re-experiencing symptoms for a day or two after each exposure session [64]; if they have an important work project or family event happening during a particular time, it may make sense to schedule exposures so as to reduce disruption of outside activities as much as possible. Also, some patients may require more or fewer sessions of exposure than is prescribed by a particular protocol. Some patients may achieve habituation and symptom reduction in just a few sessions, and may feel that further exposures are boring or redundant. Other patients, particularly those with multiple traumas, may require several courses of exposure-based treatment focusing on different traumatic events (particularly if there are events with no or little overlapping content). In these cases, it can be difficult to know when learning has sufficiently generalized to all trauma-related fear networks, but symptom reduction is a good metric to examine. In making decisions about treatment timing and termination, the therapist must be attuned to both the patient's (and possibly also the therapist's) sometimes subtle or obvious impulses to avoid.

Therapist variables in clinical decision making

In addition to patient factors, therapist variables cannot be overlooked. It may be that the patient is willing and able to engage in exposure, and every patient-related variable prognosticates success. But, if the therapist does not have the necessary training to competently deliver exposure, or does not confidently believe that exposure-based therapy will be helpful, it is unlikely that the treatment will have the desired outcome. Any therapist delivering CBT for PTSD should have received training and supervision in the provision of these types of therapies; the use of therapy manuals to guide treatment without previous experience is not recommended. Further, the therapist must be able to tolerate strong affect to deliver these therapies effectively. Any wavering on the part of the therapist about the patient's ability to handle strong affect could destroy a patient's sense of security in the therapy. Finally, the therapist must be confident about the rationale for cognitive–behavioral techniques. Because emotional material is instinctively avoided, the patient will almost inevitably question the wisdom of exposing themselves to the trauma. If the therapist has any doubts about the rationale for exposure, it will be evident to the patient and will jeopardize treatment completion. The therapist may need to consider referring the patient to a clinician with expertise in exposure-based CBT for PTSD if there is an indication that the current therapist is not well suited for this work.

Conclusion

There is a wealth of evidence to support the successful use of exposure-based CBT for PTSD. Due to a great deal of heterogeneity within PTSD , the treatment approach is not as prescriptive or clear cut as is the case in other anxiety disorders, but there are clear indications for the efficacy and effectiveness of a variety of cognitive behavioral treatments for PTSD. Careful assessment of PTSD and co-occurring conditions, as well as patient strengths, limitations, values, and context are critical to successful implementation of treatment. The cognitive–behavioral techniques employed should be based on a careful conceptualization of the case and an evaluation of learning and information-processing factors implicated in the development and maintenance of the disorder. A flexible, hierarchical approach to therapy, in which pressing or therapy-destroying concerns are addressed first, followed by preparation for and completion of trauma-focused work, is most likely to garner success in more complex cases of PTSD.

Suggested readings

Readings

Foa EB, Hembree EA, Rothbaum BO. *Prolonged Exposure Therapy for PTSD: Emotional Processing of Traumatic Experiences*. Oxford: Oxford University Press, 2007.

Foa EB, Rothbaum BO. *Treating the Trauma of Rape*. New York: Guilford Press, 1998.

Follette VM, Ruzek JI. *Cognitive-behavioral Therapies for Trauma*, 2nd edn. New York, NY: Guilford Press, 2006.

Resick PA, Schnicke M. *Cognitive Processing Therapy for Rape Victims: A Treatment Manual*. Newbury Park, CA: Sage Publications, Inc, 1993.

Online resources

National Center for PTSD www.ncptsd.va.gov

International Society for Traumatic Stress Studies www.istss.org

Association for Behavioral and Cognitive Therapies www.abct.org

References

1. American Psychiatric Association. (2000). *Diagnostic and Statistical Manual of Mental Disorders*, 4th edn., text revision. Washington, DC: APA.

2. Foa EB, Hembree EA, Rothbaum BO. *Prolonged Exposure Therapy for PTSD: Emotional Processing of Traumatic Experiences: Therapist Guide*. New York, NY: Oxford University Press, 2007.

3. Resick PA, Schnicke M. *Cognitive Processing Therapy for Rape Victims: A Treatment Manual*. Newbury Park, CA. Sage Publications, Inc, 1993

4. Follette VM, Ruzek JI. *Cognitive-behavioral Therapies for Trauma*, 2nd edn. New York, NY: Guilford Press, 2006.

5. Litz BT, Bryant R. Early intervention for trauma in adults: cognitive-behavioral therapy. In Foa E, Friedman M, Keane T, Cohen J, eds. *Effective Treatments for PTSD: Practice Guidelines from the International Society for Traumatic Stress Studies*, 2nd edn. New York: Guilford Press. 2008, pp. 117–35.

6. Rothbaum BO, Foa EB, Riggs DS, Murdock T, Walsh W. A prospective examination of post-traumatic stress disorder in rape victims. *J Trauma Stress*, 1992; **5**(3): 455–75.

7. Bonanno GA. Loss, trauma, and human resilience: have we underestimated the human capacity to thrive after extremely aversive events?*Am Psychol* 2004; **59**(1): 20–8.

8. Zlotnick C, Warshaw M, Shea MT, *et al.* Chronicity in posttraumatic stress disorder (PTSD) and predictors of course of comorbid PTSD in patients with anxiety disorders. *J Trauma Stress* 1999; **12**(1): 89–100.

9. Perkonigg A, Pfister H, Stein MB, *et al.* Longitudinal course of posttraumatic stress disorder and posttraumatic stress disorder symptoms in a community sample of adolescents and young adults. *Am J Psychiatry* 2005; **162**(7): 1320–7.

10. Foa EB, Davidson JRT, Frances A, *et al.* The expert consensus guideline series: treatment of posttraumatic stress disorder. *J Clin Psychiatry* 1999; **60**(Suppl 16): 4–76.

11. Kessler RC, Sonnega A, Bromet E, Hughes M, Nelson CB. Posttraumatic stress disorder in the National Comorbidity Survey. *Arch Gen Psychiatry* 1995; **52**(12): 1048–60.

12. Breslau N, Davis GC, Andreski P, Peterson E. Traumatic events and posttraumatic stress disorder in an urban population of young adults. *Arch Gen Psychiatry* 1991; **48**(3): 216–22.

13. Ozer EJ, Best SR, Lipsey TL, Weiss DS. Predictors of posttraumatic stress disorder and symptoms in adults: a meta-analysis. *Psychol Bull* 2003; **129**(1): 52–73.

14. Brewin CR, Andrews B, Valentine JD. Meta-analysis of risk factors for posttraumatic stress disorder in trauma-exposed adults. *J Consult Clin Psychol* 2000; **68**: 748–66.

15. Kilpatrick DG, Ruggiero KJ, Acierno R, *et al.* Violence and risk of PTSD, major depression, substance abuse/dependence, and comorbidity: results from the National Survey of Adolescents. *J Consult Clin Psychol* 2003; **71**(4): 692–700.

16. Grabe HJ, Ruhrmann S, Spitzer C, *et al.* Obsessive-compulsive disorder and posttraumatic stress disorder. *Psychopathology* 2008; **41**(2): 129–34.

17. Mallik K, Reeves RJ, Dellario DJ. Barriers to community integration for people with severe and persistent psychiatric disabilities. *Psychiatr Rehabil J* 1998; **22**(2): 175–80.

18. Boscarino JA. Posttraumatic stress disorder and physical illness: results from clinical and epidemiologic studies. *Ann N Y Acad Sci* 2004; **1032**: 141–53.

19. Davidson JR, Hughes D, Blazer DG, George LK. Post-traumatic stress disorder in the community: an epidemiological study. *Psychol Med* 1991; **21**(3): 713–21.

20. Fagelson MA. The association between tinnitus and posttraumatic stress disorder. *Am J Audiol* 2007; **16**(2), 107–17.

21. Keane TM, Kaloupek DG. Imaginal flooding in the treatment of a posttraumatic stress disorder. *J Consult Clin Psychol* 1982; **50**(1): 138–40.

22. Mowrer OH. *Learning Theories and Behavior.* New York: Wiley, 1960.

23. Keane TM, Zimering RT, Caddell JM. A behavioral formulation of posttraumatic stress disorder in Vietnam veterans. *Behavior Therapist* 1985; **8**(1): 9–12.

24. Orr SP, Milad MR, Metzger LJ, *et al.* Effects of beta blockade, PTSD diagnosis, and explicit threat on the extinction and retention of an aversively conditioned response. *Biol Psychol* 2006; **73**(3): 262–71.

25. Foa EB, Huppert JD, Cahill SP. Emotional processing theory: an update. In B. O. Rothbaum, ed. *The nature and treatment of pathological anxiety.* New York: Guilford. 2006, pp. 3–24.

26. Brewin CR. Cognitive processing of adverse experiences. *Int Rev Psychiatry* 1996; **8**(4); 333–9.

27. Ehlers A, Clark DM. A cognitive model of posttraumatic stress disorder. *Behav Res Ther* 2000; **38**(4): 319–45.

28. Foa EB, Steketee G, Rothbaum BO. Behavioral/cognitive conceptualizations of post-traumatic stress disorder. *Behav Ther* 1989; **20**(2): 155–76.

29. Foa EB, Rothbaum BO. *Treating the Trauma of Rape: Cognitive-behavioral Therapy for PTSD.* New York, NY: Guilford Press, 1998.

30. Lang PJ. A bio-informational theory of emotional imagery. *Psychophysiology* 1979; **16**: 495–512.

31. Brewin CR. Cognitive change processes in psychotherapy. *Psychol Rev* 1989; **96**: 379–94.

32. Bradley R, Greene J, Russ E, Dutra L, Westen D. A multidimensional meta-analysis of psychotherapy for PTSD. *Am J Psychiatry* 2005; **162**(2): 214–27.

33. Butler AC, Chapman JE, Forman EM, Beck AT. The empirical status of cognitive-behavioral therapy: a review of meta-analyses. *Clin Psychol Rev* 2006; **26**(1): 17–31.

34. Foa EB, Keane TM, Friedman MJ. *Effective Treatments for PTSD: Practice Guidelines from the International Society for Traumatic Stress Studies.* New York, NY: Guilford Press, 2000.

35. Ursano RJ, Sonnenberg SM, Lazar SG. *Concise Guide to Psychodynamic Psychotherapy: Principles and Techniques of Brief, Intermittent, and Long-term Psychodynamic Psychotherapy.* Washington, DC: American Psychiatric Publishing, 2004.

36. Mojtabai R, Rosenheck RA, Wyatt RJ, Susser ES. Use of VA aftercare following military discharge among patients with serious mental disorders. *Psychiatr Serv* 2003; **54**(3): 383–8.

37. Hembree EA, Foa EB, Dorfan NM, *et al.* Do patients drop out prematurely from exposure therapy for PTSD? *J Trauma Stress* 2003; **16**(6): 555–62.

38. Zayfert C, DeViva JC, Becker CB, *et al.* Exposure utilization and completion of cognitive behavioral therapy for PTSD in a "real world" clinical practice. *J Trauma Stress* 2005; **18**(6): 637–45.

39. Schnurr PP, Friedman MJ, Foy DW, *et al.* Randomized trial of trauma-focused group therapy for posttraumatic stress disorder: results from a Department of Veterans Affairs cooperative study. *Arch Gen Psychiatry* 2003; **60**(5): 481–9.

40. Monson CM, Schnurr PP, Resick PA, *et al.* Cognitive processing therapy for veterans with military-related posttraumatic stress disorder. *J Consult Clin Psychol. Special Issue: Benefit-Finding* 2006; **74**(5): 898–907.

41. Taylor S, Thordarson DS, Maxfield L, *et al.* Comparative efficacy, speed, and adverse effects of three PTSD treatments: exposure therapy, EMDR, and relaxation training. *J Consult Clin Psychol* 2003; **71**(2): 330–8.

42. Foa EB, Hembree EA, Cahill SP, *et al.* Randomized trial of prolonged exposure for posttraumatic stress disorder with and without cognitive restructuring: outcome at academic and community clinics. *J Consult Clin Psychol* 2005; **73**(5): 953–64.

43. Gillespie K, Duffy M, Hackmann A, Clark DM. Community-based cognitive therapy in the treatment

of post-traumatic stress disorder following the Omagh bomb. *Behav Res Ther* 2002; **40**(4): 345–57.

44. Schulz PM, Resick PA, Huber LC, Griffin MG. The effectiveness of cognitive processing therapy for PTSD with refugees in a community setting. *Cogn Behav Pract* 2006; **13**(4): 322–31.

45. Rosen CS, Chow HC, Finney JF, *et al*. VA practice patterns and practice guidelines for treating posttraumatic stress disorder. *J Trauma Stress* 2004; **17**(3): 213–22.

46. Becker CB, Zayfert C, Anderson E. A survey of psychologists' attitudes towards and utilization of exposure therapy for PTSD. *Behav Res Ther* 2004; **42**(3): 277–92.

47. Astin MC, Rothbaum BO. Exposure therapy for the treatment of posttraumatic stress disorder. *National Center for PTSD Clinical Quarterly*, 2000; **9**: 49–54.

48. Linehan MM. *Skills Training Manual for Treating Borderline Personality Disorder*. New York, NY: Guilford Press, 1993.

49. Owens GP, Pike JL, Chard KM. Treatment effects of cognitive processing therapy on cognitive distortions of female child sexual abuse survivors. *Behav Ther* 2001; **32**(3): 413–24.

50. Resick PA, Nishith P, Griffin MG. How well does cognitive-behavioral therapy treat symptoms of complex PTSD? An examination of child sexual abuse survivors within a clinical trial. *CNS Spectr* 2003; **8**(5): 351–5.

51. Resick PA, Nishith P, Weaver TL, Astin MC, Feuer CA. A comparison of cognitive-processing therapy with prolonged exposure and a waiting condition for the treatment of chronic posttraumatic stress disorder in female rape victims. *J Consult Clin Psychol* 2002; **70**(4): 867–79.

52. Weathers F, Litz L, Huska J, Keane T. *PTSD Checklist (PCL) for DSM-IV*. Boston, MA: National Center for PTSD – Behavioral Science Division, 1994.

53. Resick PA, Monson CM, Chard KM. *Cognitive Processing Therapy: Veteran/Military Version*. Washington, DC: Department of Veterans Affairs, 2007.

54. Keane TM, Barlow DH. Posttraumatic stress disorder. In Barlow DH, ed. *Anxiety and its Disorders*. New York: Guilford Press. 2002; pp. 418–53.

55. Foa EB, Riggs DS, Massie ED, Yarczower M. The impact of fear activation and anger on the efficacy of exposure treatment for posttraumatic stress disorder. *Behav Ther* 1995; **26**(3): 487–99.

56. Pitman RK, Orr SP, Altman B, Longpre RE. Emotional processing and outcome of imaginal flooding therapy in Vietnam Veterans with chronic posttraumatic stress disorder. *Compr Psychiatry* 1996; **37**(6): 409–18.

57. Hayes SC, Strosahl KD, Wilson KG. *Acceptance and Commitment Therapy: An Experiential Approach to Behavior Change*. New York, NY: Guilford Press, 1999.

58. Cloitre M, Heffernan K, Cohen L, Alexander L. *STAIR/MPE: A Phase-based Treatment for the Multiply-traumatized*. Unpublished manual, 2001.

59. Forbes D, Creamer M, Hawthorne G, Allen N, McHugh T. Comorbidity as a predictor of symptom change after treatment in combat-related posttraumatic stress disorder. *J Nerv Ment Dis* 2003; **191**(2): 93–9.

60. Forbes D, Bennett N, Biddle D, *et al*. Clinical presentations and treatment outcomes of peacekeeper veterans with PTSD: preliminary findings. *Am J Psychiatry* 2005; **162**(11): 2188–90.

61. Litz BT, Blake D, Gerardi R, Keane TM. Decision making guidelines for the use of direct therapeutic exposure in the treatment of Post-Traumatic Stress Disorder. *The Behavior Therapist* 1990; **13**: 91–3.

62. Tarrier N, Sommerfield C, Pilgrim H, Faragher B. Factors associated with outcome of cognitive-behavioural treatment of chronic post-traumatic stress disorder. *Behav Res Ther* 2000; **38**(2): 191–202.

63. Jaycox LH, Foa EB, Morral AR. Influence of emotional engagement and habituation on exposure therapy for PTSD. *J Consult Clin Psychol* 1998; **66**(1): 185–92.

64. Foa EB, Zoellner LA, Feeny NC, Hembree EA, Alvarez-Conrad J. Does imaginal exposure exacerbate PTSD symptoms? *J Consult Clin Psychol* 2002; **70**(4): 1022–8.

9 Eating disorders

Zafra Cooper and Christopher G. Fairburn

Introduction

Eating disorders, such as anorexia nervosa and bulimia nervosa, are the source of substantial physical and psychosocial impairment among adolescent girls and young women. These disorders begin in adolescence and, once established, they are difficult to treat. The eating disorders provide one of the strongest indications for cognitive–behavioral therapy (CBT). This bold claim arises from two sources: first, the fact that eating disorders are essentially cognitive disorders; and, second, the demonstrated effectiveness of CBT in the treatment of bulimia nervosa, which has led to the widespread acceptance that CBT is the treatment of choice [1]. Eating disorders are essentially cognitive disorders as they have as their distinctive core feature an overevaluation of shape and weight and their control. This overevaluation, which results in those with eating disorders judging their self-worth largely or exclusively in terms of their shape and weight and their ability to control them, is shared across anorexia nervosa and bulimia nervosa and occurs in most cases of those who fall within the DSM residual category, eating disorder not otherwise specified. In addition to being the treatment of choice for bulimia nervosa, CBT is also widely used to treat anorexia nervosa although this application has not been adequately evaluated [2]. Recently, its use has been extended to eating disorder NOS, a diagnosis that applies to over 50% of outpatient cases [3], and emerging evidence suggests that it is just as effective with these cases as it is with cases of bulimia nervosa [4]. In this chapter, we describe the psychopathology of the eating disorders and a cognitive–behavioral account of the mechanisms that maintain them. We then describe a "transdiagnostic" cognitive–behavioral treatment designed to disrupt these maintaining mechanisms and discuss its implementation with patients with any form of eating disorder.

Classification and diagnosis

The DSM scheme for classifying and diagnosing eating disorders recognizes two specific disorders, anorexia nervosa and bulimia nervosa. In addition, there is a residual category termed "eating disorder not otherwise specified" (eating disorder NOS) [5].

In essence, three features need to be present to make a diagnosis of anorexia nervosa:

1. The overevaluation of shape and weight; that is, judging self-worth largely, or even exclusively, in terms of shape and weight. This is often expressed as a strong desire to be thin combined with an intense fear of gaining weight and becoming fat.
2. The active maintenance of an unduly low body weight (for example, maintaining a body weight less than 85% of that expected or a body mass index $\leq 17.5^{1}$).
3. Amenorrhoea (in post-pubertal females).

Three features also need to be present to make a diagnosis of bulimia nervosa:

1. The overevaluation of shape and weight, as in anorexia nervosa.
2. Recurrent binge eating. A "binge" is an episode of eating during which an objectively large amount of food is eaten and there is a sense of loss of control at the time.

---

1 Body mass index (BMI) is a widely used way of representing weight adjusted for height. It is weight (in kg) divided by height squared (in m) (i.e., Wt/Ht^{2}). The healthy range for adults (of either gender) is 20.0 to 25.0.

Cognitive–behavioral Therapy with Adults: A Guide to Empirically Informed Assessment and Intervention, ed. Stefan G. Hofmann and Mark A. Reinecke. © Cambridge University Press 2010.

3. Extreme weight-control behavior, such as strict dietary restriction, recurrent self-induced vomiting, or marked laxative misuse.

In addition, there is an exclusionary criterion, namely that the diagnostic criteria for anorexia nervosa should not be met.

There are no diagnostic criteria for eating disorder NOS. Rather, it is a residual category for eating disorders of clinical severity that do not meet the diagnostic criteria for anorexia nervosa or bulimia nervosa. Eating disorder NOS is the most common eating disorder diagnosis, constituting about half the cases seen in outpatient settings, with bulimia nervosa constituting about a third, and the remainder being cases of anorexia nervosa [6] and around 75% of the cases found in the community [7]. In inpatient settings, the great majority of cases are either underweight forms of eating disorder NOS or anorexia nervosa [8].

In DSM-IV a new provisional eating disorder diagnosis was proposed termed "binge eating disorder." This disorder is characterized by recurrent binge eating in the absence of extreme weight-control behavior and currently remains an example of eating disorder NOS.

Clinical features

As noted, anorexia nervosa, bulimia nervosa, and most cases of eating disorder NOS are united by a distinctive core psychopathology: patients overevaluate the importance of their shape and weight, and their ability to control them. This psychopathology is specific to the eating disorders (and body dysmorphic disorder). Whereas most people evaluate themselves on the basis of their perceived performance in a variety of domains of life, people with eating disorders judge themselves primarily in terms of their shape and weight, and their ability to control them. Most of their other clinical features can be understood as stemming directly from this "core psychopathology."

In anorexia nervosa there is a sustained and successful pursuit of weight loss, which results in patients becoming severely underweight. Neither the weight loss nor its pursuit is seen as a problem and often patients have little desire to change. Some patients engage in a driven type of exercising, which contributes to their weight loss. Self-induced vomiting and other extreme forms of weight control (the misuse of laxatives or diuretics) are practiced by a subgroup of these patients and an overlapping group have episodes of loss of control over eating although the amount eaten

may not be objectively large. Depressive and anxiety features, irritability, lability of mood, impaired concentration, loss of sexual appetite, and obsessional symptoms are also frequently present. Typically these features worsen with weight loss and improve with weight regain. Interest in the outside world also wanes and patients become socially withdrawn and isolated.

The eating habits of those with bulimia nervosa resemble those seen in anorexia nervosa. The main distinguishing feature is that the attempts to restrict food intake are interrupted by repeated episodes of binge eating. In most cases, each binge is followed by compensatory self-induced vomiting or laxative misuse but there is a subgroup of patients who do not "purge" (non-purging bulimia nervosa). The weight of most patients with bulimia nervosa is in the healthy range (BMI between 20 and 25) reflecting a balance between undereating and overeating. Depressive and anxiety features are prominent, and there is a subgroup who engage in substance misuse or self-injury or both. This subgroup, also present among those with anorexia nervosa who binge eat, often attracts the diagnosis of borderline personality disorder.

The psychopathology of eating disorder NOS resembles that seen in anorexia nervosa and bulimia nervosa and is of comparable duration and severity [9]. Patients with binge eating disorder (a subgroup of eating disorder NOS), report recurrent binge eating, much as in bulimia nervosa, but their eating habits outside the binges are quite different in that they also tend to overeat at other times. Self-induced vomiting, laxative misuse, and overexercising are not present. Most patients are overweight or meet criteria for obesity (BMI $\geq$ 30.0).

Development and course

Anorexia nervosa typically starts in mid-teenage years with dietary restriction, which becomes progressively more extreme. In its early stages the disorder may be self-limiting and treatment responsive. In between 10 and 20% of cases, it proves intractable. Residual features are common (particularly concerns about shape, weight, and eating) even in those who recover. About half the cases progress to full bulimia nervosa. Anorexia nervosa is associated with a raised mortality rate, the standardized mortality ratio over the first ten years from presentation being about ten.

Bulimia nervosa has a slightly later age of onset, typically in late adolescence or early adulthood. It also usually begins with dietary restriction and in about a quarter of cases the diagnostic criteria for anorexia nervosa are met for a time. Eventually episodes of binge eating interrupt the dietary restriction and body weight increases to normal levels. Patients often present with an unremitting history of eight or more years of disturbed eating, and five to ten years after presentation, between a third and a half still have an eating disorder of clinical severity although in many cases it is eating disorder NOS.

Available evidence suggests that patients with eating disorder NOS present in their adolescence or twenties with a comparable duration of disorder as in bulimia nervosa. Between a quarter and a third have had a history of anorexia nervosa or bulimia nervosa [9].

Most patients with binge eating disorder are middle aged and a third or more are male. Clinical experience suggests that its course is episodic. Few report a history of anorexia nervosa or bulimia nervosa, but rather a tendency to overeat and gain weight.

The cognitive–behavioral theory of the maintenance of eating disorders

Although the DSM-IV scheme for classifying eating disorders encourages the view that anorexia nervosa and bulimia nervosa are distinct clinical states, consideration of their clinical features and course over time does not support this [10]. As noted, patients with anorexia nervosa, bulimia nervosa, and eating disorder NOS have many features in common, and studies of their course indicate that most patients migrate between these diagnoses over time [11]. This temporal movement, together with the fact that the disorders share the same distinctive psychopathology, has led to the suggestion that common "transdiagnostic" mechanisms are involved in the persistence of eating disorder psychopathology [12]. If correct, this view suggests that a treatment that is successful in addressing these shared mechanisms should be effective for all forms of eating disorder.

The transdiagnostic cognitive–behavioral view of Fairburn and colleagues is concerned with the processes that maintain eating disorder psychopathology rather than those responsible for its initial development. It is an extension of the original cognitive–behavioral theory of bulimia nervosa [13] and highlights the fact that the eating disorders have much in common. According to

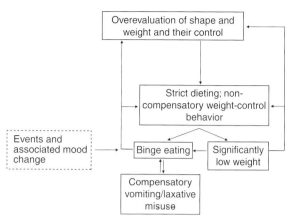

Figure 9.1 The composite transdiagnostic formulation (reproduced with permission from Fairburn CG. *Cognitive Behavior Therapy and Eating Disorders*. New York: Guilford Press, 2008 [24]).

the theory, central to the maintenance of these disorders is the dysfunctional scheme of self-evaluation shared by these patients. As noted, most of their other clinical features can be understood as stemming directly from their overevaluation of the importance of shape and weight and their control, including the extreme weight-control behavior (i.e., the dieting, self-induced vomiting, laxative misuse, and overexercising), the various forms of body checking and avoidance, and the preoccupation with thoughts about eating, shape, and weight. Figure 9.1 provides a "transdiagnostic" representation (or "formulation") of the main processes involved in the maintenance of eating disorders.

The only feature that is not obviously a direct expression of the core psychopathology is binge eating, which is present in all cases of bulimia nervosa, many cases of eating disorder NOS, and some cases of anorexia nervosa. The cognitive–behavioral theory proposes that binge eating is largely a product of attempts to adhere to multiple extreme, and highly specific, dietary rules. The tendency of these patients to react in a negative and extreme fashion to the (almost inevitable) breaking of these rules results in even minor dietary slips being interpreted as evidence of poor self-control. Patients respond to this perceived lack of self-control by temporarily abandoning their efforts to restrict their eating. This produces a highly distinctive pattern of eating in which attempts to restrict eating are repeatedly interrupted by episodes of binge eating. The binge eating maintains the core psychopathology by intensifying patients' concerns about their ability to control their eating, shape, and weight. It also encourages further dietary restraint, thereby increasing the risk of further binge eating.

Three further processes also maintain binge eating. First, difficulties in the patient's life and associated mood changes increase the likelihood that they will break their dietary rules. Second, binge eating temporarily ameliorates such mood states and distracts patients from their difficulties and so can become a way of coping with such problems. Third, patients' mistaken belief in the effectiveness of compensatory vomiting and laxative misuse undermines a major deterrent against binge eating. They do not realize that purging has little effect on energy absorption.

Patients with anorexia nervosa share the core psychopathology of those with bulimia nervosa and atypical disorders. The major distinctive feature lies in the fact that in anorexia nervosa undereating predominates and therefore patients become extremely underweight. This has certain physiological and psychological consequences that contribute to patients continuing to undereat. For example, delayed gastric emptying results in a sense of fullness even after eating modest amounts of food, and secondary social withdrawal magnifies patients' isolation from the influence of others.

The composite "transdiagnostic" formulation shown in Figure 9.1 represents the core processes that maintain any eating disorder. The specific maintaining processes operating in any patient depend upon the nature of the eating disorder psychopathology present, and thus the precise form of the formulation differs from patient to patient. In some cases only certain processes are active (for example, in most cases of binge eating disorder), but in others (for example, cases of the binge eating/purging subtype of anorexia nervosa) most are operating. The formulation highlights the maintaining processes that need to be addressed in treatment, thereby allowing the clinician to design a bespoke treatment to fit the individual patient's psychopathology. Thus, evidence-based treatment procedures can be integrated with clinical judgment and expertise.

Research on treatment

Consistent with the current way of classifying eating disorders, the research on their treatment has focused on the particular disorders in isolation. This research has been reviewed by Wilson, Grilo and Vitousek [14] and an authoritative meta-analysis has been conducted by the UK National Institute for Health and Clinical Excellence (NICE) [15]. The findings indicate that there is a clear leading treatment for bulimia nervosa, a specific form of cognitive–behavioral therapy (CBT-BN)[16]. However, at best, half the patients who start treatment make a full and lasting response. Interpersonal psychotherapy is a potential alternative to CBT-BN, but it takes eight to twelve months longer to achieve a comparable effect. Antidepressant medication (especially fluoxetine) also has a beneficial effect but this is not as great as that obtained with CBT-BN, and the limited evidence available suggests it is often not sustained. Combining CBT-BN with antidepressant medication conveys little, if any, advantage over CBT-BN alone.

There has been much less research on the treatment of anorexia nervosa, with no treatment being supported by robust research evidence. In this case, most of the work has focused on adolescents, and much of it has been concerned with a highly specific form of family-based treatment [17]. To date, there is little evidence that it has a specific beneficial effect [18].

Various approaches have shown promise for the treatment of binge eating disorder, with most support for an adaptation of CBT-BN. While this treatment has a marked effect on the binge eating, it has little effect on body weight, which is typically raised. Until recently there has been no research on the treatment of other forms of eating disorder NOS, but, as noted earlier, emerging evidence suggests that an "enhanced" transdiagnostic cognitive–behavioral treatment derived from CBT-BN may be used with these patients and that it achieves results similar to those obtained with bulimia nervosa.

Enhanced CBT

This transdiagnostic form of CBT is designed for the full range of clinical eating disorders seen in adults. It was derived from CBT-BN [19] and is based on the transdiagnostic theory outlined above. The treatment, "enhanced" CBT (CBT-E), is described as enhanced since it uses a variety of new strategies and procedures designed to improve treatment adherence and outcome, and since the "broad" version of the treatment has modules designed to address certain obstacles to change that are "external" to the core eating disorder, namely clinical perfectionism, low self-esteem, and interpersonal difficulties. Thus there are two forms of CBT-E, a focused form (CBT-F) that focuses exclusively on eating disorder psychopathology, and a broad form (CBT-B) that also addresses these three external obstacles to change. The treatment also exists in two lengths, a 20-week version for patients who are not significantly underweight, defined as having a BMI over 17.5, and 40-week version for patients with a BMI of 17.5 or below, a commonly used threshold for anorexia nervosa.

Enhanced CBT is an outpatient-based treatment designed to be delivered on an individual basis. The indications for the treatment are the presence of an eating disorder of clinical severity. It is not appropriate for those whose psychiatric state, general physical health, or degree of weight loss is such that they cannot safely be treated on an outpatient basis. The remainder of this chapter is devoted to the 20-week focused version of CBT-E [20]. This form of treatment is suitable for the great majority of adult outpatients. Limitations on space preclude the description of the 40-week variant for patients who are significantly underweight, the broad version of the treatment that also addresses the three "external" maintaining mechanisms [21], the version for inpatients [22], and how it is modified for younger patients [23]. Readers wanting to learn more about the treatment and its implementation are referred to the complete account of the treatment and its various forms [24].

Assessing patients and preparing them for treatment

The initial assessment interview has two interrelated goals. The first is to put the patient at ease and begin to forge a positive therapeutic relationship. The goal is that the assessment interview is a collaborative enterprise, ending with the clinician being able to give the patient an expert opinion as to the nature of his or her problems and, if indicated, the treatment options. The patient should also have ample opportunity to ask questions.

The other goal is to establish the diagnosis. Apparent eating disorders may, for example, turn out to be an anxiety disorder (e.g., difficulty eating with others due to a social phobia), a presentation of a mood disorder (e.g., severe weight loss resulting from a clinical depression), or simple overeating in cases of obesity. It is therefore critical to evaluate the problem thoroughly to decide what would be the most appropriate next step.

Toward the end of the interview patients should be weighed and have their height measured. This is an extremely sensitive matter for most patients and some are resistant to it. We explain that we *have* to check their weight in order to complete the assessment. At this point we do not insist upon patients knowing their weight if they prefer not to, but do tell them their BMI when discussing the outcome of the assessment.

In our view, seeing patients twice as part of the assessment process is valuable. On the second occasion there is the opportunity to pursue in greater detail matters that require particularly careful exploration (for example, the nature and extent of any comorbid depressive features) and to discuss treatment options fully.

Patients are routinely asked to complete certain questionnaires prior to the initial appointment, which provide standardized information on the nature and severity of the patient's problem. The two questionnaires used are the Eating Disorder Examination Questionnaire (EDE-Q) [25] and the Clinical Impairment Assessment (CIA) [26]. The EDE-Q provides a measure of current eating disorder features, and the CIA assesses the impact of this psychopathology on psychosocial functioning. In addition, an established measure of general psychiatric features is useful.

By the end of the second appointment it should be possible to decide on the best treatment options. If the problems are minor and likely to be self-limiting it may not be appropriate to offer treatment or it may be best to observe for a period of time. For patients whose BMI is below 14.0 and for those whose physical state is not stable, more intensive treatment (i.e., day-patient or inpatient treatment) is most appropriate. As noted CBT-E is appropriate for the vast majority of patients with an eating disorder who have a BMI between 15.0 and 40.0. However, there may be certain contraindications to embarking upon CBT-E straightaway. They have in common the effect of substantially undermining the patient's concentration, motivation (which in any case may be a problem in some patients), or their ability to work on treatment between sessions. The main contraindications are a comorbid clinical depression, persistent substance abuse, and major life crises. Other co-occurring forms of psychopathology (e.g., anxiety disorders, personality disorders) are not contraindications to CBT-E. In the case of both clinical depression and substance abuse it is best to address these difficulties first and then begin CBT-E, as both may severely undermine the patient's ability to utilize treatment. In the case of major life crises treatment is best deferred until the crisis has resolved (see Fairburn,

Cooper and Waller [27] for a more detailed discussion of "complex cases" and comorbidity).

Clinical case: assessment and preparation for treatment

Patient A was a 22-year-old college senior referred by her primary care physician for the treatment of an eating disorder. Initial assessment indicated that she was suffering from an eating disorder that met DSM diagnostic criteria for bulimia nervosa. She had been dissatisfied with her weight since early adolescence and began dieting to lose weight during her final year at high school. Initially, she lost about 14 lbs (6 kg) in weight but then found it more difficult to stick to her diet and began binge eating and inducing vomiting. At assessment, the patient described her daily food intake as consisting of a very small bowl of cereal for breakfast and a small salad for lunch. She often tried to delay these meals or to skip them altogether. She reported large episodes of binge eating every night (a typical binge including a loaf of bread, a large family-size carton of ice cream, and a packet of cookies). During the evening she would vomit up to five times. The patient described a range of rigid dietary rules about how much she should eat at each meal, and she avoided eating many foods that she regarded as fattening and likely to trigger binges.

A found her body "repulsive" and had avoided weighing herself for the past six months. She frequently used mirrors to spend lengthy periods checking her body (to see "how fat she was") and had missed important lectures as a result. At assessment she weighed 140 lbs (63.5 kg) giving her a BMI of 24.9. At the time of assessment she had a number of work deadlines to meet and her mood appeared low. She was also drinking a bottle or more of wine each night.

The patient attended her assessment appointment alone and gave a clear history of the nature of her difficulties. She was reluctant to be weighed, but understood the rationale and after some discussion agreed to being told her BMI, but not her weight. Aside from the eating difficulties, two other areas appeared to be difficulties and possible contraindications to immediate CBT-E: her apparently persistently low mood together with a range of features suggestive of a comorbid depression (reduced interest and socializing, negative thinking, hopelessness) and her alcohol intake. The assessing clinician explained how these might interfere with treatment. The patient responded by acknowledging that she was drinking too much and saying that she would like to reduce it. As she had a number of work deadlines in the following two weeks, a second appointment was arranged after these and it was agreed that she would reduce her alcohol intake. At her second appointment, the patient was more relaxed having completed her work. Her mood seemed considerably improved and she was no longer reporting other depressive symptoms. She had greatly reduced her alcohol intake, confining her drinking to two glasses of wine on weekend evenings. It was agreed that CBT-E would begin shortly. Details of her progress through treatment are integrated with the description of the treatment.

The treatment protocol

The treatment has four stages.

Stage one

The aims of the first stage are as follows: to educate patients about treatment and the disorder; to engage the patient in treatment and change; and to introduce and establish a pattern of regular eating and weekly weighing. This stage comprises approximately eight sessions, which are held twice weekly over four weeks.

Jointly creating the formulation

This is usually done in the first treatment session and is a personalized visual representation of the processes that appear to be maintaining the patient's eating problem. The therapist draws out the relevant sections of Figure 9.1 incorporating the patient's own experiences and terms. It is usually best to start with something the patient wishes to change (e.g., binge eating). This helps patients to realize both that their behavior is comprehensible and that it is maintained by a variety of self-perpetuating mechanisms that are open to change. The formulation provides a guide to what needs to be targeted in treatment if patients are to achieve a full and lasting recovery. At this early stage in treatment, the therapist should indicate that it is provisional and may need to be modified as treatment progresses.

Establishing real-time self-monitoring

This is the ongoing "in-the-moment" recording of eating and other relevant behaviors, thoughts, feelings, and events (see Figure 9.2 for an example monitoring record). Self-monitoring is initiated in the first session

Day ....Thursday ....   Date..... March 19th ....

Time	Food and drink consumed	Place	*	v/l	Context and comments
7.30	Glass water	Kitchen			Thirsty after yesterday
8:10	Half banana } Black coffee }	Cafe			Must be good and not binge today!
11:45	Smoked turkey on wheat bread } Light mayo Diet coke }	Cafe			Usual lunch
6.40 to 7.30	Piece of apple pie 1/2 gallon ice cream 4 slices of toast with peanut butter Diet coke Raisin bagel 2 slices of toast with peanut butter Diet coke Peanut butter from jar Raisin bagel Snickers bar Diet coke - large	Kitchen	* * * * * * * *	 V V	Help - I can't stop eating. I'm completely out of control. I hate myself. I am disgusting. Why do I do this? I started as soon as I got in. I've ruined another day.
9:30	Rice cake with fat-free cheese Diet coke	Kitchen			Really lonely. Feel fat and ugly. Feel like giving up.

Figure 9.2 A monitoring record (reproduced with permission from Fairburn CG. *Cognitive Behavior Therapy and Eating Disorders*. New York: Guilford Press, 2008 [24]).

and continues throughout treatment. It serves two purposes: it assists in the identification of the patient's problems and progress and, more importantly, it facilitates change by helping patients address problems as they occur. Fundamental to establishing accurate recording is going over the patient's records in detail, especially in the session when the patient brings them back for the first time. Reviewing the records should be a joint process with the patient taking the therapist through each day's record in turn. Apart from the first time when records are completed, this review should generally be brief. Therapists need to remember not to address identified problems during the review but to simply acknowledge them and put them on the session agenda. Table 9.1 summarizes how sessions are typically structured and the allocation of time.

127

Table 9.1 Typical session structure and timing

1. Weighing; updating and interpreting weight graph (5 minutes)

2. Reviewing monitoring records and assignments completed between sessions; identifying issues to cover in main body of session (10 minutes)

3. Setting session agenda collaboratively (3 minutes)

4. Working through agenda and agreeing on next steps (30 minutes)

5. Summarizing the session (2 minutes)

Establishing "weekly weighing"

The patient and therapist check the patient's weight once a week and plot it on an individualized weight graph. Patients are strongly encouraged not to weigh themselves at other times. Weekly in-session weighing has several purposes: (1) it provides patients with accurate data about their weight at a time when their eating habits are changing; (2) it provides an opportunity for the therapist to help patients interpret the numbers on the scale, which otherwise they are prone to misinterpret; and, (3) it addresses the important maintaining processes of excessive body-weight checking or its avoidance.

Providing education

From the second session onwards, an important element of treatment is education about weight and eating since many patients have misconceptions that maintain their eating disorder. The following topics need to be covered:

- body weight and its regulation: the BMI and its interpretation; natural weight fluctuations; and the effects of treatment on weight
- physical complications of binge eating, self-induced vomiting, the misuse of laxatives and diuretics, and the effect of the eating disorder on hunger and fullness
- Ineffectiveness of vomiting, laxatives, and diuretics as a means of weight control
- Adverse effects of dieting: the types of dieting that promote binge eating; dietary rules versus dietary guidelines.

To provide reliable information on these topics, patients are asked to read relevant sections from *Overcoming Binge Eating* [28] and their reading is discussed in subsequent treatment sessions.

Establishing "regular eating"

The establishment of a pattern of regular eating is fundamental to successful treatment whatever the form of the eating disorder. It addresses an important type of dieting ("delayed eating"); it displaces episodes of binge eating; and, for underweight patients, it introduces regular meals and snacks that can be subsequently increased in size. Early in treatment (usually by the third session) patients are asked to eat three planned meals each day, plus two (or if underweight three) planned snacks, and they are asked not to eat between them. Patients may choose what they eat at these times with the only conditions being that the meals and snacks are not followed by any compensatory behavior and that there should rarely be more than a four-hour interval between these occasions of eating. The new eating pattern should take precedence over other activities but should not be so inflexible as to preclude the possibility of adjusting timings to suit the patients' commitments each day.

Patients should be helped to adhere to their regular eating plan and to resist eating between the planned meals and snacks. Two rather different strategies may be used to achieve this: the first involves helping patients to identify activities that are incompatible with eating or make it less likely, and the second is to help patients to recognize that the urge to eat is a temporary phenomenon. Through using these strategies patients learn to distance themselves from the urge to eat, which they find gradually fades with time.

Involving significant others

The treatment is primarily an individual treatment for adults and hence it does not actively involve others. Despite this, it is our practice to see "significant others" with the patient if this is likely to facilitate treatment and the patient is willing for this to happen. There are two specific indications for involving others: if others could help the patient in making changes, or if others are making it difficult for the patient to change by, for example, commenting adversely on eating or appearance.

Patient A's progress through Stage one

The patient was initially very quiet during treatment sessions and appeared to simply agree to everything the therapist suggested. The therapist actively encouraged her to ask questions and express any doubts she had. The patient responded positively to the formulation as she felt it "explained" her eating disorder and she was "shocked" that her attempts to diet during the day were leading to binge eating at night. She was able to complete real-time monitoring records and responded well to the educational material.

Two difficulties were encountered at this stage: the patient was very reluctant to be weighed arguing that she would only become more preoccupied with her weight; and she did not think that she would be able to eat regular meals and snacks because she had never eaten in this way before and it would certainly lead to weight gain. Once the therapist had explained the rationale for weekly weighing, A agreed to be weighed but was nevertheless very anxious and upset when she was told her weight. However, she agreed to persist with weighing and soon discovered that she was much less anxious about her weight and her preoccupation had not increased. With regard to regular eating the therapist explained, with reference to the formulation, that adopting this pattern of eating would help to protect her from binge eating and hence to begin to overcome her eating problem. Her reluctance to eat meals and snacks for fear of weight gain was tackled by reassuring her that this rarely occurs since patients are not asked to change the amount that they eat or what they eat. Also, it was pointed out that regular eating results in a decrease in the frequency of binge eating and thereby a significant reduction in overall energy intake (since even when she vomited she was absorbing a significant amount of energy from each binge).

Stage two

Stage two is a transitional stage, which generally comprises two appointments, a week apart. While continuing with the procedures introduced in Stage one the therapist and patient conduct a joint review of progress to date, identify problems still to be addressed, revise the formulation if necessary, and design Stage three.

Stage three

The aim of this stage is to address the key mechanisms that are maintaining the patient's eating disorder. The order in which these mechanisms are addressed depends upon their relative importance in maintaining the particular patient's psychopathology. There are generally eight weekly appointments.

Addressing the overevaluation of shape and weight

The first step involves explaining the concept of self-evaluation and helping patients identify the life

domains that contribute to their judgment of themselves. The relative importance of these domains can be visually represented on a pie chart, which for most patients is dominated by a large slice representing shape and weight, and controlling eating.

The patient and therapist then identify the problems inherent in this scheme for self-evaluation. Briefly there are three related problems: (1) the overevaluation of shape and weight tends to marginalize other domains and thus self-evaluation is overly dependent on performance in one area of life; (2) the area of controlling shape and weight is one in which success is elusive, thus undermining self-esteem; and (3) the overevaluation leads to behavior that is unhelpful and that itself maintains the disorder.

The final step in educating about self-evaluation involves identifying its four main expressions or consequences and creating an extended formulation (see Figure 9.3). These are dieting, body checking and body avoidance, feeling fat, and marginalization of other areas of life. The therapist uses this extended formulation to explain how these behaviors and experiences serve to maintain and magnify the patient's concerns about shape and weight, and it is agreed therefore that they need to be addressed in treatment.

Addressing body checking and avoidance

Patients are often not aware that they are engaging in body checking and that it is maintaining their body dissatisfaction. The first step in addressing this checking involves obtaining a detailed account of the behavior by asking patients to record it. Patients are then helped to realize that body checking is not a helpful way of assessing their shape or weight as it provides unreliable and biased information. Certain forms of body checking are best stopped altogether. In the case of more normative checking such as mirror use, education should stress that, as with other forms of body checking, what one finds depends to an important extent upon how one looks (e.g., scrutiny of perceived flaws tends to magnify them). Another form of body checking that actively maintains dissatisfaction with shape involves comparing with others. The nature of these comparisons generally leads patients to conclude that their bodies are less attractive than others. This is both because the comparisons are highly selective (comparing only to those who are perceived as thin and attractive) and the appraisal of others is less harsh and critical (while self-appraisals involve scrutiny, others are judged more superficially). Patients need

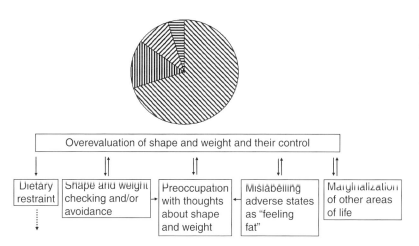

Figure 9.3 The overevaluation of control over shape and weight: an "extended formulation" (reproduced with permission from Fairburn CG. *Cognitive Behavior Therapy and Eating Disorders*. New York: Guilford Press, 2008 [24]).

to understand the inherent bias in such comparisons. For patients who avoid seeing their bodies, the therapist needs to explain that this too maintains dissatisfaction. Patients need to be encouraged to get used to the sight and feel of their body. Participation in activities that involve a degree of body exposure can be helpful, for example swimming.

Addressing "feeling fat"

"Feeling fat" is an experience reported by many women but the intensity and frequency of this feeling appears to be far greater among people with eating disorders. Feeling fat is a target for treatment since it tends to be equated with being fat (irrespective of actual shape and weight) and hence maintains body dissatisfaction. Although this topic has received little research attention, clinical observation suggests that in many patients feeling fat is a result of mislabeling certain emotions and bodily experiences. It may be addressed by helping patients appreciate that feeling fat tends to be triggered by the occurrence of certain negative mood states (e.g., feeling bored or depressed) or by physical sensations that heighten body awareness (e.g., feeling full, bloated, or sweaty). Patients can then be encouraged to question the feeling when it occurs and correctly label and address the underlying triggering state using a problem-solving approach.

Developing marginalized domains for self-evaluation

Tackling the expressions of the overevaluation of shape and weight will gradually reduce it. At the same time, it is also important to encourage the patient to increase the number and significance of other domains for self-evaluation. Although this is an

indirect means of diminishing the overevaluation of shape and weight, it is nevertheless a powerful one.

Exploring the origins of the overevaluation

Towards the end of Stage three it is often helpful to explore the origins of the patient's sensitivity to shape, weight, and eating. An historical review can help to make sense of how the problem developed and evolved, highlight how it might have served a useful function in its early stages, and help patients distance themselves from the past. If a specific event appears to have played a critical role in the development of the eating problem, the patient should be helped to re-appraise this from the vantage point of the present. This review tends to highlight that the eating disorder is beginning to resolve and helps patients to distance themselves further from the eating disorder frame of mind or "mindset."

Addressing dietary restraint

A major goal of treatment is to reduce, if not eliminate altogether, strict dieting. This dieting has two aspects: an attempt to limit eating termed "dietary restraint," and actual undereating in physiological terms termed "dietary restriction." "Regular eating" will already have addressed one form of dietary restraint (delayed eating). Patients need to recognize that their multiple extreme and rigid dietary rules lead to preoccupation with food and eating, encourage binge eating, and impose practical and social restrictions. It should therefore be agreed that dietary restraint needs to be addressed. To do this, the patient's various dietary rules should be identified together with the beliefs that underlie them. The patient should be helped to break the rules in order to test the beliefs in question and to learn that the feared consequences that maintain the dietary rule (typically sudden weight gain or binge eating) are not an inevitable result of breaking it. With patients who binge eat it is important to pay particular attention to food avoidance and to help them systematically re-introduce such foods into their diet.

Addressing event-triggered changes in eating

Among patients with eating disorders, eating habits may change in response to outside events. The change may involve eating less, stopping eating altogether, overeating, or binge eating. If these changes persist into Stage three, they should be addressed by helping patients to tackle the triggering events using a problem-solving approach and by helping patients to accept the occurrence of intense moods states and identify ways (that are not harmful) of modulating their moods.

Patient A's progress through Stage three

A review of progress conducted in Stage two with A revealed that she was eating regular meals and snacks, she was no longer anxious about weighing, nor had she become more preoccupied with her weight. There was a marked reduction in the frequency of her binge eating and vomiting. Problems that still needed addressing in Stage three included her dieting and her overevaluation of the importance of weight and shape.

The first issue tackled in Stage three was the patient's overevaluation of weight and shape. When A and the therapist completed a pie chart, she was distressed to see that controlling eating, weight, and shape filled three quarters of her chart. She was also able to see that as a result other areas in her life had become marginalized and she was immediately prepared to expand these by going swimming and joining an art class. A agreed that her weight and shape concerns were expressed in her body checking and feeling fat, and was able to understand, using the extended formulation, how these expressions were maintaining her concerns. She was much less convinced by the therapist's suggestion that dieting was also playing a role. Thus, while the patient was able to reduce her body checking (and remove all but one of the six mirrors in her room) and relabel feeling fat successfully she was very reluctant to tackle her dieting

(expressed as numerous food rules and, especially, her long list of avoided foods). She did not see it as a problem and thought that she would feel better about herself if she were to reduce her weight to the lower, rather than higher end, of the healthy weight range. The therapist addressed this difficulty in treatment by returning to the formulation and explaining how this form of dieting maintained her binge eating in just the same way as her delayed eating at the beginning of treatment had done. She also initiated a discussion about the major adverse effects of such dieting including preoccupation with food and eating, anxiety about eating generally, and an inflexible eating pattern that often makes eating socially impossible. A was eventually able to begin to break some of her dietary rules and start eating previously avoided foods. With encouragement from the therapist she was also able to reconsider the advantages and disadvantages of losing weight given that her weight was already in the healthy range.

By the time the patient and therapist conducted the historical review, A could see that the eating problem was beginning to resolve and that she was now able to distance herself from it and the eating disorder "mindset."

Stage four

The aims in Stage four are to ensure that the changes made in treatment are maintained over the following months and that the risk of relapse is minimized in the long term. There are three appointments, each two weeks apart. During this stage, as part of their preparation for the future, patients discontinue self-monitoring and transfer from in-session weighing to weighing themselves at home.

To maximize the chances that progress is maintained the therapist and patient jointly devise a specific written plan for the patient to follow over the following few months until a post-treatment review appointment. Typically this includes further work on body checking, food avoidance, and perhaps further practice at problem solving. In addition, the therapist encourages patients to continue their efforts to develop new interests and activities.

There are two elements to "relapse prevention." First, patients must have realistic expectations regarding the future. A common problem is that many hope never to experience any eating difficulties again. It needs to be explained that this makes them vulnerable to relapse since it encourages a negative reaction to even minor setbacks. Patients should be told to expect lapses, with the eating problem continuing to be their Achilles' heel. The goal is for patients to identify setbacks as early as possible, view them as a "lapse" rather than a "relapse," and use a well developed plan to deal with them. Thus, the second element of relapse prevention is the construction of such a plan. The therapist and patient should review the components of treatment with the aim of identifying the principles and procedures that were most relevant and helpful and devise a written plan for the future incorporating this information.

Patient A: ending treatment and post-treatment review

By the end of treatment, A was eating regularly and was no longer binge eating and vomiting. Her weight had remained unchanged during treatment. She identified regular eating, not avoiding certain foods, and taking up new activities as the most helpful aspects of treatment and planned to work on maintaining these changes until the post-treatment review. To prevent further problems she identified two early warning signs: starting to diet again and increasing her alcohol intake. At the review appointment she described three occasions when under stress she had experienced a "lapse." On these occasions, she was able to implement the strategies she had learned in treatment to prevent a "relapse."

Conclusion

A major challenge in developing evidence-based treatments is to balance the clinically appealing flexibility achieved by a treatment based on a functional analysis of the individual's difficulties with the more structured and specified style of empirically validated manual-based treatments. A major limitation of some manual-based treatments is that the form treatment takes is determined almost exclusively by the patient's DSM-IV diagnosis thereby ignoring the heterogeneity that exists within many of these categories. Enhanced CBT is derived from a transdiagnostic theory, and its particular form depends upon a highly personalized formulation rather than a DSM-IV-based one. Thus the treatment has much in common with functional analysis, a defining feature of behavior therapy, while also being derived from an empirically supported treatment for bulimia nervosa. By identifying the mechanisms that maintain the patient's particular eating disorder and targeting them using evidence-based treatment procedures, CBT-E attempts to integrate clinical research findings with therapist judgment [29].

Enhanced CBT has implications for psychological treatment beyond the field of eating disorders. It is consistent with emerging evidence on the role of common psychopathological processes across different diagnostic categories [30]. The transdiagnostic approach could be applied to other groups of related clinical disorders: consider, for example, Barlow and colleagues' [31, 32] unified treatment protocol for anxiety and mood disorders. The specific way that the transdiagnostic treatment for eating disorders has been operationalized might provide a model for designing treatments for other groups of functionally related conditions.

In summary, despite the considerable advances achieved in the cognitive–behavioral treatment of eating disorders in recent years, at least three important challenges remain. Two of these challenges concern the treatment itself. First, treatment needs to be made more effective. Despite its successes, CBT-E does not help everyone. There is an urgent need to understand the reasons for treatment failure in order to improve it further. The second related challenge is to better understand how treatment works. Knowledge of the active ingredients of treatment would provide the basis for further enhancing these and omitting redundant ones. It might also suggest ways to simplify treatment, more generally, or in certain cases. A third challenge concerns dissemination of the treatment. There is an urgent need to understand how this is best achieved.

Suggested readings

Fairburn CG (ed.) *Eating Disorders and Cognitive Behavioral Therapy*. New York: Guildford Press, 2008. (A comprehensive and practical guide to a leading empirically supported cognitive behavioural treatment for the full range of eating disorders.)

Grilo CM. *Eating and Weight Disorders*. NewYork: Psychology Press, 2006. (An authoritative research based overview of eating and weight disorders.)

References

1. National Institute for Health and Clinical Excellence. *Eating Disorders – Core Interventions in the Treatment and Management of Anorexia Nervosa, Bulimia Nervosa and Related Eating Disorders*. NICE Clinical Guidance No. 9. London: NICE, 2004. www.nice.org.uk

2. Wilson GT, Grilo CM, Vitousek KM. Psychological treatment of eating disorders. *Am Psychol* 2007; **62**(3): 199–216.

3. Fairburn CG, Cooper Z, Bohn K, *et al.* The severity and status of eating disorder NOS: implications for DSM-V. *Behav Res Ther* 2007; **45** (8): 1705–15.

4. Fairburn CG, Cooper Z, Doll HA, *et al.* Transdiagnostic cognitive-behavioral therapy for patients with eating disorders: a two-site trial with 60-week follow-up. *Am J Psychiatry* 2009; **166**: 311–19.

5. American Psychiatric Association. *Diagnostic and Statistical Manual of Mental Disorders, 4th edn., text revision.* Washington, DC: APA, 1994.

6. Fairburn CG, Bohn K. Eating disorder NOS (EDNOS): an example of the troublesome "not otherwise specified" (NOS) category in DSM-IV. *Behav Res Ther* 2005; **43**: 691–701.

7. Machado PP, Machado BC, Gonçalves S, *et al.* The prevalence of eating disorder not otherwise specified. *Int J Eat Disord* 2007; **40**(3): 212–17.

8. Dalle Grave R, Calugi S. Eating disorder not otherwise specified on an inpatient unit. *Eur Eat Disord Rev* 2007; **15**: 340–9.

9. Fairburn CG, Cooper Z, Bohn K, *et al.* The severity and status of eating disorder NOS: implications for DSM-V. *Behav Res Ther* 2007; **45**(8): 1705–15.

10. Fairburn CG, Harrison PJ. Eating disorders. *Lancet* 2003; **361**: 407–16.

11. Milos G, Spindler A, Schnyder U, Fairburn CG. Instability of eating disorder diagnoses: prospective study. *Br J Psychiatry* 2005; **187**: 573–8.

12. Fairburn CG, Cooper Z, Shafran R. Cognitive behavior therapy for eating disorders: a "transdiagnostic" theory and treatment. *Behav Res Ther* 2003; **41**: 509–28.

13. Fairburn CG, Cooper Z, Cooper P. The clinical features and maintenance of bulimia nervosa. In Brownwell KD, Foreyt JP, eds. *Physiology, Psychology and Treatment of Eating Disorders.* New York: Basic Books. 1986, 389–404.

14. Wilson GT, Grilo CM, Vitousek KM. Psychological treatment of eating disorders. *Am Psychol* 2007; **62**(3): 199–216.

15. National Collaborating Centre for Mental Health. *Eating Disorders: Core Interventions in the Treatment and Management of Anorexia Nervosa, Bulimia Nervosa and Related Eating Disorders.* London: British Psychological Society and Royal College of Psychiatrists, 2004.

16. Fairburn CG, Marcus MD, Wilson GT. Cognitive behaviour therapy for binge eating and bulimia nervosa: a comprehensive treatment manual. In Fairburn CG, Wilson GT, eds. *Binge Eating: Nature, Assessment and Treatment.* New York: Guildford Press. 1993, pp. 361–404.

17. Lock J, le Grange D, Agras WS, Dare C. *Treatment Manual for Anorexia Nervosa: A Family-based Approach.* New York: Guildford Press, 2001.

18. Fairburn CG. Evidence-based treatment of anorexia nervosa. *Int J Eat Disord* 2005; **37**: S26–S30.

19. Fairburn CG, Marcus MD, Wilson GT. Cognitive behaviour therapy for binge eating and bulimia nervosa: a comprehensive treatment manual. In Fairburn CG, Wilson GT, eds. *Binge Eating: Nature, Assessment and Treatment.* New York, Guildford Press. 1993, pp. 361–404.

20. Fairburn CG, Cooper Z, Shafran R, *et al.* Enhanced cognitive behavioural therapy for eating disorders: the core protocol. In Fairburn CG, *Eating Disorders and Cognitive Behavioural Therapy.* New York: Guildford Press, 2008.

21. Fairburn CG, Cooper Z, Shafran R, Bohn K, Hawker D. Clinical perfectionism, core low self-esteem and interpersonal problems. In Fairburn CG, *Eating Disorders and Cognitive Behavioural Therapy.* New York: Guildford Press, 2008.

22. Dalle Grave R, Bohn K, Hawker D, Fairburn CG. Inpatient, day patient, and two forms of out patient CBT-E. In Fairburn CG, *Eating Disorders and Cognitive Behavioural Therapy.* New York: Guildford Press, 2008.

23. Cooper Z, Stewart A. Younger patients. In Fairburn CG, *Eating Disorders and Cognitive Behavioural Therapy.* New York: Guildford Press, 2008.

24. Fairburn CG, ed. *Cognitive Behavior Therapy and Eating Disorders.* New York: Guildford Press, 2008.

25. Fairburn CG, Beglin S. Eating disorder examination questionnaire (EDE-Q6.0). In Fairburn CG, *Eating Disorders and Cognitive Behavioural Therapy.* New York: Guildford Press, 2008.

26. Bohn K, Fairburn CG. Clinical impairment assessment questionnaire (CIA 3.0). In Fairburn CG, *Eating Disorders and Cognitive Behavioural Therapy.* New York: Guildford Press, 2008.

27. Fairburn CG, Cooper Z, Waller D. *"Complex patients" and comorbidity.* In Fairburn CG, ed., *Eating Disorders and Cognitive Behavioural Therapy.* New York: Guildford Press, 2008.

28. Fairburn CG. *Overcoming Binge Eating.* New York: Guildford Press, 1995.

29. Wilson GT. Cognitive behaviour therapy for eating disorders: progress and problems. *Behav Res Ther* 1999; **37**: S79–S95.

30. Harvey A, Watkins E, Mansell W, Shafran R. *Cognitive Behavioural Processes Across Psychological Disorders: A Transdiagnostic Approach to Research and Treatment*. Oxford: Oxford University Press, 2004.

31. Barlow DH, Allen LB, Choate ML. Towards a unified treatment for emotional disorders. *Behav Ther* 2004; **35**: 205–30.

32. Allen LB, McHugh RK, Barlow DH. Emotional disorders: a unified protocol. In Barlow DH, ed., *Clinical Handbook of Psychological Disorders: A Step-by-step Treatment Manual*. New York: Guildford Press. 2008, pp. 216–49.

10 Schizophrenia and psychotic disorders

Sandra Bucci and Nicholas Tarrier

The nature of schizophrenia and psychotic disorders

Schizophrenia and psychotic disorders involve significant changes in a person's beliefs, perceptions, behaviors, and emotions. Individuals can differ in their symptoms, and the course and duration of their illness, but they are characterized by the fact that people experience a loss of contact with reality.

Schizophrenia is a serious mental illness that affects approximately one in every hundred people at some time in their life. It is characterized by *positive* symptoms (reflecting an excess of normal functioning) and *negative* symptoms (reflecting a diminution or loss of normal functioning). The positive symptoms consist of hallucinations, delusions, disorders of language and thought process (disorganized speech), and grossly disorganized behavior. Hallucinations occur in each of the sensory modalities, although auditory hallucinations are most common. These can take the form of commanding voices, voices commenting on the person's thoughts or actions, or multiple voices conversing with each other. Delusions are erroneous and often bizarre beliefs that are held with strong convictions and typically involve a misinterpretation of a perception or experience. An example of a bizarre delusion would be a person's belief that aliens have removed his/her brain. Delusions can include beliefs regarding persecution, self-reference, somatic sensations, religion, grandiosity, or control. Disorders of language and thought process manifest in the form of disorganized speech, while grossly disorganized behavior varies from difficulties carrying out activities of daily living (e.g., maintaining hygiene, dressing in an unusual manner) to unpredictable agitation or, in a few minor cases, catatonic behavior.

Negative symptoms are also frequently present and account for a substantial amount of the morbidity associated with schizophrenia. These include cognitive dysfunction, restriction in the range and intensity of emotions, in the fluency and productivity of thought and language, and in behavior initiation. Negative symptoms are often difficult to recognize because they tend to be relatively non-specific and could be accounted for by other problems such as medication side effects. These symptoms can affect a person's personal, social, occupational, and vocational functioning.

Age of onset of a first episode of psychosis (FEP) in schizophrenia is typically between 20 and 30 years, although an FEP can occur in the teenage years. The onset can be abrupt or insidious and a number of phases are recognized during which the intensity, frequency, and associated morbidity varies. The prodromal phase is characterized by attenuated psychotic symptoms (e.g., suspiciousness, ideas of reference, unusual perceptual disturbances) and a range of non-specific symptoms such as anxiety, mild depression or dysphoria, irritability, mood fluctuations, sleep disturbance, mood instability, and behavior change (e.g., withdrawal, social avoidance, abandoning hobbies/interests). As the prodrome progresses these signs and symptoms intensify and strange and bizarre behavior may be exhibited, such as being unable to care for self, becoming socially or sexually inappropriate, making accusations against others, and muttering to self. At this stage, an individual might enter the acute phase of a psychotic illness, during which time distinct positive psychotic symptoms manifest. The acute phase is followed by either a remission period or a period of residual symptoms in which symptoms persist but at a reduced intensity.

Cognitive–behavioral Therapy with Adults: A Guide to Empirically Informed Assessment and Intervention, ed. Stefan G. Hofmann and Mark A. Reinecke. © Cambridge University Press 2010.

The course of schizophrenia-spectrum disorders vary and outcome is variable despite treatment. On average, 20% of patients who experience an FEP will not go on to experience another episode; however, approximately 70% of people will experience at least two further acute episodes, the second typically occurring within five to seven years of the initial episode [1]. Some people will make a full recovery between episodes, while others are resistant to conventional treatments and recovery can be incomplete with residual symptoms often present. A small minority of patients, however, will experience a progressive worsening of symptoms with significant associated disability. Some factors that influence a patient having a better prognosis include displaying good premorbid adjustment, having an acute and late age onset of illness, insight, being female, receiving early intervention, a supportive and non-critical or hostile social environment, complying with medication, and an absence of a family history of a psychotic-related disorder.

There is evidence to suggest that genetic factors play an important role in the etiology of schizophrenia. For example, first-degree biological relatives of a person with a schizophrenia-spectrum disorder are ten times more likely to develop a related disorder than the general population. Moreover, concordance rates are elevated in monozygotic twins. However, these figures themselves do not account for the discordance rates in monozygotic twins, reflecting the importance of environmental factors such as stress, substance use, and high expressed emotion within families on the development of psychotic conditions.

Comorbid problems such as social anxiety, trauma, suicide risk, depression, suicide behavior, and substance use are common in psychotic disorders and can further impact on patients' functioning, although it is unclear whether these problems are distinct from, part of, or a consequence of, the psychotic illness. Social anxiety is common and the nature of a psychotic illness means that people find difficulty understanding their social world and the intentions of others (termed a "theory of mind deficit"). Some people develop social phobia due to fear of negative evaluation of others and the stigma associated with mental illness [2]. There is also evidence to suggest that people suffering from psychotic disorders tend to have been exposed to traumatic events. Studies such as that conducted by Mueser, Goodman, Trumbetta *et al.* [3] suggest that lifetime rates of childhood physical and sexual abuse and post-traumatic stress disorder (PTSD) in patients with severe

mental illness far exceed rates in the general population. Post-traumatic stress disorder is also associated with increased rates of self-harm, which may further increase the risk of suicide in already vulnerable schizophrenia patients [4]. Indeed, between 4% and 10% of patients with schizophrenia will complete suicide and a substantial number will attempt suicide, with suicidal ideation a common experience for many patients. Suicide risk factors include being young and male, having a chronic and often relapsing illness, high levels of symptomatology, functional impairment, and feelings of hopelessness.

Depression is also common. For example, in a study by Birchwood, Meaden, Trower *et al.* [5], over 60% of their sample with auditory hallucinations reported very high levels of depression. Furthermore, about half of all people with schizophrenia misuse substances or alcohol. These people tend to have a poorer prognosis, poorer treatment outcomes, a greater likelihood of developing chronic and disabling conditions, and more hospital admissions compared with their non-substance using counterparts. There is recent evidence showing that cognitive–behavioral therapy for psychosis (CBTp) interventions targeting comorbid substance use and psychotic disorders can improve general functioning, although much more research is needed in this area (e.g., [6, 7]).

The focus of CBTp in recent years has targeted the positive symptoms of psychosis and will be the focus of this chapter. First-line treatments for schizophrenia-spectrum disorders remain antipsychotic medication in combination with case management; however, the CBTp described in this chapter can be delivered in addition to this.

Review of cognitive models of schizophrenia

There has been considerable debate about the theoretical understanding of schizophrenia with biological explanations being dominant. However, psychological and social factors have been consistently shown to be influential, certainly in affecting the course of schizophrenia, and have been incorporated into stress-vulnerability models, which have emphasized the importance of these psychosocial factors in precipitating and maintaining psychotic episodes [8]. More recently, cognitive models of the positive symptoms of psychosis have been developed in tandem with advances in cognitive–behavioral treatments. We will briefly review three cognitive models that have been proposed, namely those by Garety and colleagues [9], Morrison [10], and Tarrier [11–13].

Garety and colleagues' [9] model focuses on various social and cognitive factors that influence the development and maintenance of symptoms such as delusions and hallucinations. The model draws on a biopsychosocial vulnerability framework thought to be triggered by stressful life events. Consistent with cognitive models targeting other psychological disorders, the authors suggest that it is not the symptoms per se that are problematic, rather the interpretation or *appraisal* of symptoms that causes significant emotional distress. Emotional changes and low self-esteem are thought to influence patients' appraisals as well as basic cognitive processes such as information processing. The authors suggest that deficits in information processing might trigger anomalous experiences, and rather than attribute such experiences as internally generated, psychotic patients tend to attribute them to external factors (e.g., a "voice"), therefore resulting in the expression of positive symptoms. These factors, in combination with reasoning biases, dysfunctional self/world schemas, and an adverse social environment are thought to play a significant role in overall symptom formation and maintenance (see [9, 14] for a detailed review).

Drawing on the components of anxiety models, Morrison [10] also offers a cognitive model in an attempt to explain the formation and development of positive psychotic symptoms. The author views symptoms such as hallucinations and delusions as intrusions that enter a person's awareness. Intrusions are misinterpreted by the psychotic patient and thus give rise to a psychotic experience. These intrusions are thought to be maintained by a combination of safety behaviors (including selective attention), plans for processing, faulty metacognitive processes and social knowledge, as well as mood and physiology. At the core of the model is the cultural unacceptability of the *interpretation* of the intrusion (e.g., a patient might interpret a self-critical thought as a malevolent voice), which is key in determining whether an individual is deemed to be psychotic or not (see [10] for a detailed account of this model).

The third model we review has been developed by the second author but bears many similarities to other models although it refers more to the maintenance of symptoms rather than their genesis. The basic tenet is the recovery model in which the patient is actively

coping with a potentially persistent illness and strange and disturbing experiences, which may well change many aspects of their lives, affect their hopes and aspirations, and be associated with comorbid disorders such as depression and anxiety. The various behavioral and cognitive coping strategies may ameliorate or exacerbate their symptoms. As applied to treatment the model emphasizes coping with symptoms rather than curing them, intervening to modify cognitive processes (such as attention) as well as cognitive content and behavior. Figure 10.1 provides a clinical heuristic of how a patient's psychotic symptoms are thought to be maintained.

This model is helpful for clinicians as it serves as a guide for directing therapy by describing the interaction between internal antecedents and external, or environmental, factors. The model assumes that the experience of hallucinations and delusions is a dynamic interaction between internal and external factors, which is important both in the origins and maintenance of symptoms. Internal factors may be either biological or psychological, can be inherited or acquired, and serve to increase an individual's vulnerability to psychosis. For example, genetic factors may influence the biochemical functioning of the brain and cognitive capacity. Alternatively, biological and psychological dysfunction may be acquired (e.g., deficits in cognitive flexibility and maladaptive attitudes). Risk is further increased through demanding environmental stressors. Defective information processing mechanisms, such as source monitoring deficits in hallucinations and probabilistic reasoning biases in delusions, in combination with dysfunctions in the regulation of the arousal system will result in perceptual and cognitive disturbances. Once a psychotic symptom is activated, there is a process of primary and secondary appraisal in which the individual attempts to interpret and give meaning to this experience and react to its consequences. Typically, the interpretation given to psychotic experiences results in feelings of threat to physical integrity or social standing and subsequent avoidant and safety behavior. The short-term consequences of appraising psychotic experiences in this way will involve emotional, behavioral, and cognitive elements. Secondary effects such as low mood, anxiety in social situations, and the effect of trauma may further compound the situation.

According to this model, and consistent with other cognitive models, a key aspect of the maintenance of psychotic phenomena is that a person's appraisal and

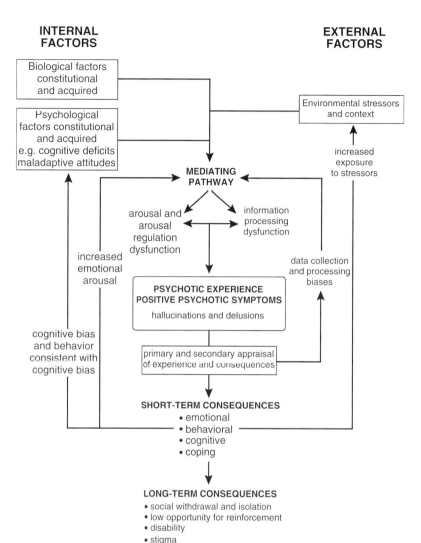

INTERNAL FACTORS

EXTERNAL FACTORS

Figure 10.1 A clinical heuristic of how a patient's psychotic symptoms are thought to be maintained.

reaction to the psychotic experience will feed back through a number of possible routes and increase the probability of the psychotic experience being maintained. For example, panicking in response to hearing a voice will result in elevated levels of autonomic arousal, which act either directly through sustained increased levels of arousal or indirectly through further disrupting information processing. Together, this will increase the likelihood of ongoing psychotic symptoms. Similarly, behavioral responses to psychotic symptoms (e.g., violent behavior, social avoidance) might increase exposure to environmental stress or increase risk of trauma, which will further maintain psychotic symptoms. For example, social avoidance

could result in confirmatory rumination and resentment with a lack of opportunity to disconfirm paranoid beliefs. Thus psychotic experiences can lead to dysfunctional beliefs that the patient acts upon, resulting in a confirmatory bias to collecting and evaluating evidence on which to base future judgments of reality. This process is termed the experience–belief–action–confirmation cycle (EBAC cycle; discussed later in this chapter) and suggests that such cycles maintain psychotic experience through reinforcement of maladaptive beliefs and behavior.

It is expected that as these cognitive models develop and are subjected to empirical test, further refinements of CBTp treatment will evolve.

Empirical support for the efficacy and effectiveness of treatment

Clinical, ethical, and economic considerations have encouraged clinical practice to be guided by an evidence base that has been produced from evaluations of treatments. Systematic reviews of studies of CBTp with schizophrenia demonstrate moderate effect sizes, which suggest that CBTp is a useful intervention for schizophrenia-related illnesses. A number of meta-analyses indicating that CBTp is effective in treating positive psychotic symptoms in psychotic patients have been published. For example, Tarrier and Wykes [15] identified 20 controlled trials of CBT for schizophrenia from which data were available from 19 studies on the effects of CBT on positive symptoms. Sixteen studies involved chronic outpatients, one included chronic inpatients, and three involved inpatients in the acute phase of illness. These studies were found to have a mean effect size of 0.37 indicating a modest effect size in improving positive symptoms compared to standard psychiatric care (treatment as usual; TAU). In an updated meta-analysis and review of 34 clinical trials of CBTp, there were significant and beneficial effects for the target symptom (effect size = 0.4; 33 studies), positive symptoms (effect size = 0.37; 32 studies), negative symptoms (effect size = 0.44; 23 studies), functioning (effect size = 0.38; 15 studies), mood (effect size = 0.36; 15 studies), and social anxiety (effect size = 0.36; 2 studies). However, there was no effect on hopelessness. Improvements in one domain were correlated with improvements in others [16].

While there is good support for CBTp in reducing chronic and persistent residual psychotic symptoms, the evidence for enhancing recovery in acute inpatients and reducing relapse in both chronic and acute patients is less compelling. For example, studies on relapse prevention strategies have only revealed reduction in relapse rates when the intervention specifically targets relapse reduction strategies [17]. There is less success in relapse rates when relapse prevention is part of a larger CBTp package [15].

Overall, CBTp has beneficial (modest) effects particularly for persistent positive symptoms. The evidence that CBTp speeds recovery in acutely ill patients is more equivocal, while only interventions targeting relapse reduction strategies have been found to produce reductions in relapse rates. In light of these findings, there is sufficient evidence for CBTp to be included in the UK's National Institute for Health and Clinical Excellence (NICE, the government body that recommends which treatments should be used in clinical practice in the National Health Service) as a preferred list of treatment for schizophrenia. Also, CBTp is recommended in the Schizophrenia Patient Outcomes Research Team guidance n the United States [18].

Introduction to a clinical case

Lauren is a 26-year-old woman who lives with her parents and works as an administrative assistant. She developed a psychotic illness when she was 21. In the six months leading up to her FEP, Lauren's family and close friends noticed a number of changes. For example, Lauren began to neglect her appearance and at times appeared unkempt. She began to withdraw from friends and family, and over time became increasingly isolated. She refused to eat meals with her parents because she believed that her mother was poisoning the food. Lauren stopped answering calls from friends and began missing days from work, saying that she was the victim of bullying and harassment. She believed that her boss was attempting to let her know that he intended to fire her through messages hidden within regular work-related emails. On a couple of occasions, Lauren's mother noticed her mumbling to herself and Lauren seemed increasingly distracted and preoccupied. The feeling that something was *"not quite right"* had been with her for some months.

During her FEP, Lauren became increasingly paranoid and accused her close friends and family of gossiping behind her back. She continued to believe that her boss was sending her covert messages. She began to panic when she started to hear voices. These auditory hallucinations were in the form of multiple voices commenting and conversing. Lauren identified three voices that made insulting and accusatory comments and told her that her close friends and family were against her. They accused her work colleagues of scheming to *"bring me down"* and warned her to be *"on guard."* The voices also made direct comments about her being *"stupid"* and *"useless."* Lauren described these voices as *"evil"* and it felt like they knew all about her thoughts and emotions. They also made commands such as *"put your hands on the hot stove"* or *"jump in front of that car."* On one occasion, Lauren's parents found her standing on the side of a busy road. When they asked her what she was doing, she said *"If I stand here then they'll leave me alone."* As well as these *"evil"* voices, Lauren described a *"good"*

139

voice warning her about potentially dangerous situations. For example, she occasionally heard a voice that warned her about *"nasty people"* who might attack her in the street. In response, she would hide in the closest store until she believed the person had passed. Lauren believed these warnings were very helpful and she was convinced that acting upon these warnings was keeping her from harm. Also, while at work, she occasionally heard a voice that warned her when her boss was going to send her a hidden message within the email system, so she printed off every email her boss sent her. Her parents would find these emails around the house with various passages heavily underlined.

Lauren's situation deteriorated very rapidly over the Christmas period and peaked on the day of her work Christmas party. Just before going out for Christmas lunch, Lauren noticed her boss and a few work colleagues in a meeting. She saw her boss look in her direction and noticed her colleagues laughing. Lauren knew *"at once"* that they were laughing about her. She felt outraged. She stormed in the meeting and shouted at her boss, accusing him of plotting to fire her because she was *"pathetic"* at her job. She became increasingly agitated and confrontational, despite a colleague's attempt at placating her. The voices grew louder in her head and she started shouting and swearing at them. It was at this point that a staff member called the ambulance and Lauren was taken to the local psychiatric unit for assessment, where she was admitted and detained under the Mental Health Act. Lauren spent four weeks in hospital and was treated with antipsychotic medication. Her care plan included counseling and her parents received psycho-education about her diagnosis and general advice on how to manage her at home. Her symptoms remitted during her admission and she was discharged with frequent outpatient appointments and home treatment from the assertive outreach team.

Over the intervening years Lauren had three further relapses during which a similar pattern of paranoia, referential ideas, auditory hallucinations, and withdrawal and isolation followed. Each relapse involved a short hospital stay and increased medication. Residual symptoms were common following each episode and in spite of pharmacological intervention, psychotic symptoms persisted. She usually avoided socializing with others and going out in general because of her symptoms. With the increasing awareness of the potential benefits of psychological treatments and as part of a multidisciplinary approach to her care and to promote recovery, she was referred to a clinical psychologist for cognitive–behavioral therapy in an attempt to treat her persistent positive symptoms.

Overview of treatment protocol

Structure of therapy

General points

The treatment described in this chapter is for individual CBTp and can be delivered in a variety of settings, including inpatient and outpatient settings and in the patient's home, no matter what the patient's stage of illness. Cognitive therapy sessions typically consist of one-hour sessions over weekly intervals; however, clinicians working with psychotic patients will need to be flexible and sessions might need to be shorter in length (25 to 30 minutes) depending on the circumstances and the patient's tolerance. It is possible to deliver treatment in a group format and some studies have revealed clinical benefits in terms of enhanced self-esteem; however, the reductions are modest when compared with individual treatments [19].

Evidence from research trials indicates that cognitive–behavioral treatments are delivered over about 20 treatment sessions. These can either be intensive, delivered over three months, or less intensive, delivered over nine months. How therapists deliver a CBTp intervention will differ depending on the nature of the patient's illness, although clinically some patients will benefit from continued but less intensive treatment, while others will benefit from booster sessions or a longer duration of treatment. For example, during an acute admission for a psychotic episode, the patient is often disturbed, distressed, and agitated. Thus therapy sessions are often brief and frequent, whereas in chronically ill patients living within the community, therapy sessions will follow the normal outpatient format. Keeping individual differences and the nature of the schizophrenia illness in mind when structuring treatment sessions is an important component of CBTp. In general, the structure of therapy involves the following stages: assessment; development of a problem-list based, case formulation; strategies and techniques targeting psychotic symptoms; schema-focused interventions; and relapse prevention.

Structure of individual sessions

Blackburn and Davidson [20] have developed guidelines for structuring individual cognitive therapy sessions. The structure of an individual session includes: (a) reviewing the patient's mental state by asking how things have been since the previous session; (b) setting an agenda in a collaborative fashion, keeping in mind that the agenda should not be too exhaustive; (c) reviewing homework – homework that was not completed between sessions can be completed in session – reasons for not completing homework can be explored at this time; (d) identifying session targets, which involves exploring patient's cognitions and how these affect emotions and behaviors so that psychotic experiences can be evaluated and alternative appraisals generated; (e) setting agreed homework based on the problem areas discussed in (d), thus enabling patients to test hypotheses and conduct behavioral experiments in vivo; and (f) eliciting feedback about the current session. This final stage gives the patient an opportunity to discuss their fears, concerns, or hopes about therapy and allows for any misinterpretations to be addressed and clarified directly. Clinicians should be led by clinical need and not rigidly adhere to a "one sign fits all" approach.

The therapeutic relationship

At the outset of therapy it is important to develop a collaborative, empathic, trusting, and warm relationship with patients. A strong therapeutic relationship is an essential element for the effective delivery of CBTp. The clinician will need the experience and the patience to be able to develop a positive relationship. Often, commencing therapy with a gentle, warm, and relaxed conversation about a general topic of interest can facilitate engagement and build rapport. At this stage, the therapist might only briefly discuss symptoms or mention them in passing. Normalizing symptoms and distress, as well as the difficulties of entering into a new relationship with the therapist, can assist patients in feeling understood and diffuse fear or angst associated with therapy. Engaging with family members and staff is also important. Maintaining engagement and the therapeutic relationship throughout treatment is essential, and important clinical decisions must always consider this point.

Lauren was initially resistant to contact with a therapist. Therefore, in order to engage Lauren in therapy, the therapist decided to visit her at home for her first appointment (home visits are common practice in the UK). Lauren refused to open the door. A short conversation ensued through the door, which ended in the clinician stating that she would return at another convenient time. One further visit resulted in Lauren again refusing to open the door. The strategy here was just to make contact to reassure Lauren that her views were perfectly valid and the psychologist requested permission to visit at another convenient time. Persistence is important but must be balanced with allowing patients space to consider treatment. In situations where the initial engagement is problematic the best strategy is to "roll with resistance" by being patient and trying to alleviate any agitation but maintaining contact and returning at another time. On the next occasion Lauren felt more relaxed and allowed the clinician into her flat. These first few sessions were kept brief and covered her general well-being and topics of interest, with the primary focus of keeping Lauren engaged.

After about four sessions, the therapist felt that she had started to develop a more open and comfortable rapport with Lauren, so she asked a few questions exploring Lauren's beliefs about her voices and delusions. The therapist asked questions such as *"I understand you have been hearing voices when no one is there. What do you make of this? Have you any idea what these voices are?"; "I also understand that you have been having difficulties with people. You mentioned you have been feeling as though some people are against you? What do you make of this?"* These questions enabled the therapist to raise the topic of the psychotic experience and gently introduce cognitive exploration of symptoms by exploring Lauren's *beliefs* about her experiences. Particularly in the early phase of therapy, when the therapeutic relationship is more vulnerable, it is important to validate the patient's experience but not necessarily agree on their cause. In Lauren's case it was important to agree that *she did hear voices* and that *she did believe that people were against her* and to validate her distress. In cases when the patient is very deluded or lacks insight into their symptoms, trying to persuade them that eliminating their symptoms, the experiences that they believe to be real, can be counter-productive and jeopardize the therapeutic relationship. However, trying to reduce distress is a more viable alternative for a collaborative goal.

To further build engagement, it is important not to dispute or argue with the patient especially at this early stage when the patient is not convinced that there is any benefit to be gained from treatment. If clinicians notice that a patient has become guarded or suspicious, exploring this shift is vital. Simply asking the question *"Have I said or done something that has upset you?"* can often diffuse the situation and allows you to nip problems in the bud.

In summary, it is important that the clinician embodies the characteristics of empathy, unconditional acceptance, warmth, and genuineness in order to engage patients and to develop and maintain a strong therapeutic relationship. Patients need to feel accepted and understood, and this is particularly true for psychotic patients who have, in most cases, been dismissed or misunderstood as a result of their illness.

Strategies and techniques

Case formulation

It is our premise that any CBTp intervention should be based upon a thorough understanding of the patient's clinical problem and its determinants; this is known as developing a case formulation [11]. Thus, interventions need to be driven by an idiosyncratic case formulation developed collaboratively with the patient. Formulations can be developed based on a heuristic model or in relation to specific symptoms. The cognitive model described here was developed by the second author and suggests that psychotic experiences can lead to dysfunctional beliefs, which are then acted upon in a way that leads to their confirmation or disconfirmation. This is termed the experience–belief–action–confirmation cycle or EBAC cycle (Figure 10.2).

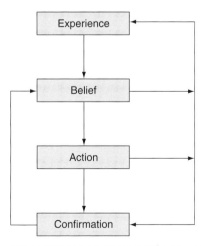

Figure 10.2 The experience–belief–action–confirmation (EBAC) cycle.

It is suggested that such cycles maintain psychotic experience through reinforcement of maladaptive beliefs and behavior. Lauren reported that she experiences *"evil"* voices but also voices she appraised as being helpful. Because Lauren occasionally heard a voice warning her about *"nasty people"* who might attack her in the street, she hid in the nearest store until her possible attacker passed. By carrying out this safety behavior, Lauren believed that she had avoided being attacked; however, this in fact confirmed her belief that the voice had saved her from danger. Here is an example of an EBAC cycle.

> **EXPERIENCE** – voice tells her that a potential attacker might be approaching
> **BELIEF** – she is in imminent danger
> **ACTION** – she hides in the nearest store
> **CONFIRMATION** – she has avoided being attacked and remained safe by listening to and acting upon what the voice tells her.

The case formulation facilitates alternative explanations of patients' psychotic experiences and enables patients to examine their beliefs and behavior in a systematic manner.

Lauren had previously been told that her psychotic symptoms are a result of a mental illness involving a chemical imbalance in her brain. She did not find this a particularly helpful explanation as it did not reflect her actual experience and was stigmatizing for her. Lauren needs to be presented with an alternative model of her experiences that allows her to collaborate in her psychological treatment. Through the EBAC cycle, patients become aware of alternative explanations and learn that unusual beliefs are reinforced and confirmed by their own behavior, and that this cycle serves to maintain their psychotic experiences.

Once a formulation is developed, cognitive and behavioral strategies can be implemented to target symptoms and associated distress. It is important to keep in mind that not all patients will be able to collaboratively work through a problem list or case formulation because they might either be too disturbed or their beliefs are too entrenched. In some cases, patients might be completely convinced of their delusional thoughts and will not accept any alternative view, in which case *coping* with distress can be advanced as a suitable goal. In these cases, pragmatic strategies can be used in an attempt to reduce high levels of distress associated with, rather than tackling, the delusional beliefs themselves.

Coping strategies

The underpinning to our approach is that coping with disturbing and distressing experiences is central to the recovery process. Thus, learning a range of coping strategies is important. To ensure that these coping strategies can be implemented, they are carried out systematically through a process of graded exposure and through over-learning, simulation, and role-play until the required procedure is internalized by the patient and under internal control. Learning such control techniques allows the patient to challenge the beliefs he or she may have had about psychotic experiences (e.g., the voice is all-knowing and powerful). Coping strategies include the following.

1. **Attention switching**. This is a process whereby a patient actively shifts the focus of their attention from one subject or experience to another. Patients are trained within the session to switch attention on cue through rehearsal. For example, there were times when Lauren became anxious when she discussed her voices in sessions, so the psychologist asked Lauren to describe a picture hanging on the wall in order to shift her attention. Alternatively, patients can focus their attention on a set of positive images. Lauren applied this strategy by recalling a time when she holidayed on a beach in Spain. She was trained to elicit a visual image of the beach by describing the scene in great detail. She was asked to remember the experience of the beach through all her senses. She then continually rehearsed this memory until she was able to elicit it at will.
2. **Awareness training**. This strategy involves teaching patients to be aware of their symptoms, especially their onset, but not react to them or become captured by their content. By monitoring when and in which situations symptoms occur, patients can use other coping strategies, such as attention switching, to reduce the emotional impact of the content. The aim here is two-fold: to assist patients in becoming *mentally disengaged* from the content of symptoms; and to use symptoms as a *cue to alternative action*.
3. **De-arousing techniques**. High levels of arousal have been implicated in the psychopathology of schizophrenia and frequently occur as both antecedents and responses to psychotic experiences. Teaching patients brief relaxation or breathing exercises can therefore help reduce arousal associated with psychotic experiences.
4. **Increased activity levels**. Psychotic patients are particularly prone to isolation and reduced physical activity, therefore standard activity scheduling exercises can be a powerful coping strategy, especially if implemented at the onset of the symptom, thus creating a dual task competing for attentional resources.
5. **Social engagement and disengagement**. Although many patients can find it difficult tolerating social interactions, teaching patients that there are *levels* of social disengagement can also be used to help develop tolerance of social stimulation. For example, following a period of recovery, Lauren gradually returned to work (two days per week). When she felt overstimulated, she left the office, walked around the block, and returned to her desk (regular breaks were agreed with her boss). Using this method can help patients feel that they have some control over their social environment and can increase their confidence to initiate social interaction as a method to reduce the impact of their symptoms.

Cognitive techniques

Once some coping strategies are in place, patients can learn to examine psychotic beliefs via cognitive methods, such as *generating alternative explanations* and *examining the evidence* for their beliefs. Many patients do this to some extent already, but the level of arousal experienced or the level of isolation and avoidance can make these attempts unsuccessful. These methods are very similar to those used in traditional cognitive therapy, except that the patient may need more prompting and the goal is to incorporate the skills of belief modification into a self-regulatory process. Patients may find it helpful to write down their beliefs so that the patient and therapist can collaboratively investigate the evidence for and against these beliefs.

Generating alternative explanations

The goals here are to help patients consider as many explanations (not just the delusional interpretation) as possible for situations or experiences, and help them view thoughts as beliefs and not consider them fact. People with delusions show information processing biases, so considering alternatives is important in broadening patients' thinking. Patients are encouraged to question their beliefs as they occur, such as; *"Why do I think that man is looking at me when I've never seen him before?"* Similarly, patients can be encouraged to look for inconsistencies and to use these to make challenges. In Lauren's case, she did not have an alternative explanation for the voices other than they represented some, albeit vague and poorly defined, powerful entity or that they were the manifestation of a chemical imbalance in her brain. Following a series of questions, the therapist suggested to Lauren that the voices might be her own thoughts or a leakage from memory into awareness that she wasn't able to identify as self-generated. This was why the voices often reflected her fears or concerns or perhaps aspects of her past.

Examining the evidence

Patients can learn to examine evidence to challenge their beliefs about their symptoms so that disconfirmatory evidence can be collected. Where voices are seen as omnipotent and truthful, evidence can be examined to see if they have been wrong or incorrect in the past. For example, Lauren's voices told her that she was *"stupid"* and *"useless."* She concluded that the voices must be true given that she believed she was on the verge of being sacked at work. However, when the evidence was examined, Lauren had not been sacked after all and in fact her boss had been extremely concerned about her. This helped her challenge her own idea that she was "stupid" by creating doubt about the truthfulness of her voices. In combination with this strategy, patients can rehearse statements to question their psychotic experience. Statements such as *"It may seem like a real voice but it's just my own thoughts"* can help reattribute patients' experiences. Verbalizing such statements in session is important and can gradually be reduced until they are internalized.

Sometimes a patient's delusions persist in spite of evidence to contradict them. To weaken these delusional explanations, the therapist can use *guided discovery* and *Socratic questioning* techniques to help the patient reappraise the evidence for their explanation of events with the goal of weakening delusions. Pointing out the contradictory evidence in a quizzical and puzzled manner, often known as the *"Columbo technique,"* is advised, so the patient has to account for contradictions and review his or her explanation in light of this new and contradictory evidence.

Behavioral techniques

Probably the strongest way of evaluating beliefs is to test them out in reality via behavioral experiments. Behavioral experiments can also be used to disprove delusional and inappropriate beliefs. Particular attention is paid to identifying avoidance and safety behaviors that reinforce inappropriate beliefs. Changing these behaviors is a powerful method of changing beliefs and delusions. Patients will sometimes test out their beliefs naturally, although a tendency to bias interpretation and for hypothesis protection will lead them to erroneous conclusions. Patients may be assisted in their attempts at behavior change by means of self-instruction and coping strategies that decrease arousal (such as breathing exercises, brief relaxation, and guided imagery).

Changes in behavior and cognition complement each other. Changes in behavior should always be used to examine and potentially challenge maladaptive thoughts and beliefs, or as a learning experience. Similarly, changes in cognition should be used as an opportunity to change behavior and establish new behaviors. The therapist should always look for opportunities to prompt the patient to reappraise their beliefs. In some refractory cases, the patient's conviction that his or her delusional beliefs are true is unshakable and they are unwilling to examine the veracity of this subjective experience. In these cases, the clinician must negotiate treatment goals aimed at reducing distress rather than focusing on the symptoms themselves.

Enhancing coping strategies

Coping methods have developed over time and vary in their complexity from simple and direct attempts to control cognitive processes to more complex self-directed methods that modify cognitive content and inference. Frequently, combinations of different coping strategies are built up, for example the use of attention switching and de-arousing techniques helps to dull the strength of a delusion so that reality testing can be implemented. Without these initial coping methods the patient might not be able to undergo reality testing or consider carrying out behavioral experiments. Initial coping strategies can be used to challenge the strength of symptoms. Questions can be asked such as *"You've used these attention switching methods to cope effectively with your voices, what does that tell you about them having total power and control over you and you being helpless?"* The patient may well make statements that indicate the voices have been demonstrated as fallible, which can then be used as self-statements to further enhance self-efficacy and coping.

Low self-esteem

Patients suffering from schizophrenia frequently have low self-esteem. Emphasis has been placed upon improving the patient's self-esteem and techniques have been developed to enhance the patient's self-esteem [13, 21]. In Lauren's case, low self-esteem was addressed by asking her to produce a list of ten positive qualities or statements (two per session) about herself and to rate her belief that she had these qualities on a scale of 0 to 100. The psychologist asked her to produce as many specific examples of evidence of each positive quality as she could. She was then asked to mentally rehearse the events so as to strengthen the positive memories and then re-rate the strength of her belief that she possessed the qualities she identified. For homework, Lauren monitored her behavior over the following week and recorded any evidence to support the contention that she possessed these qualities. During the next session, Lauren provided feedback on examples of positive attributes and the therapist prompted her for further examples. Again, Lauren was asked to re-rate the belief that she did possess these positive qualities. By working through this process, Lauren became aware that keeping her weaknesses in balance with her strengths (attentional focus) greatly affected her mood and self-esteem.

Relapse prevention

Identification of early signs of relapse

Schizophrenia is in many cases a relapsing condition. Thus an important part of any CBTp intervention is to plan for the future as it is a very real possibility that relapse will occur. The aim of any relapse prevention intervention is to *minimize* the impact of a relapse rather than avoid the possibility of further relapses occurring. Furthermore, normalizing a lapse, and differentiating this from a relapse, is important in instilling a sense of hope for the future.

Relapses rarely occur without any forewarning. They are usually preceded by prodromal symptoms that can last days, weeks, or months, although the typical prodrome period is about four weeks [22]. Common prodromal signs and symptoms were described earlier, although no one single trigger or symptom will result in a relapse. Rather, identifying patients' early warning signs can reduce the time it takes for patients to access necessary treatment. This can be achieved by asking patients to recall the signs and symptoms that preceded previous psychotic episodes or relapses. The case formulation, and

information gathered from family members or carers, can help patients identify warning signs and potential triggers of further relapse. Care must be taken to differentiate between normal mood fluctuations and signs of illness development.

In Lauren's case, the psychologist spent time with both Lauren and her parents discussing in detail when changes in her mood or behavior were first noticed, what these changes were, how they progressed, and in what sequence. Her case formulation was also reviewed. Each sign or symptom was then written on a card and Lauren was asked to arrange them in temporal order of occurrence. In this way, Lauren and the therapist were able to devise a *relapse signature;* that is, the individual set of signs and symptoms that characterized her prodrome and its time course leading to relapse. Lauren identified that withdrawing from her parents and close friends, not showering, regularly taking time off work, and not eating family meals could be signs of a possible relapse. To differentiate between possible signs of a relapse and normal mood fluctuations, the therapist encouraged Lauren to keep a diary of her mood and experiences over a number of weeks, a process called *"discrimination training."* The goal is to help the patient learn to distinguish a real prodrome from a "false alarm" of normal mood fluctuations.

The final step is to develop a plan of action should a prodrome ensue. Coping strategies and behavioral responses can be formulated and rehearsed, the help of others such as family members can be elicited, and seeking assistance of mental health services can be requested, which may involve altering medication doses. By focusing on relapse prevention strategies, patients are able to identify and have a record of their early warning signs of a relapse and the "window of opportunity" to intervene is more likely to occur at the optimal time. Now that email and short message service (sms) mobile phone messages are mainstream forms of communication, maintaining contact with, and monitoring, patients is more likely to be effective in reducing the interval between patients seeking assistance and the potential onset of an acute episode.

Difficulties encountered during treatment

Thought disorder

Thought disorder, typically characterized by disruption to language and classified largely by its effects on speech and writing, makes it difficult to comprehend the flow of a patient's dialogue and the meaning he or she is imparting. However, with experience and patience, it is possible to follow some internal logic in the patient's speech. This can be accomplished by asking the patient to explain the meaning, by the therapist reflecting back their understanding, and then the therapist rephrasing their meaning in more coherent language.

Suicide and self-harm

The risk of suicide in patients suffering from schizophrenia is significant and will likely be a problem clinicians encounter at some stage when working with psychotic patients. Risk factors in patients include being young and male, chronic illness with numerous exacerbations, having high levels of symptomatology and functional impairment, feelings of hopelessness in association with depression, fear of further mental deterioration, and excessive dependence on treatment or loss of faith in treatment.

It is important to be aware that suicide attempts are a very real possibility while treating someone suffering from schizophrenia. Unfortunately, patients with schizophrenia often commit suicide impulsively and use lethal methods, such as jumping from heights, immolation, or firearms. The presence of suicidal ideation needs to be assessed and the patient needs to be asked whether any specific plans have been made or actions have been taken. It is necessary to be aware of factors that can elevate risk including low self-esteem; increased sense of hopelessness and despair especially related to the perception of the patient's illness and recovery; disruptive family or social relationships; any changes in social circumstances or loss of supportive relationships (e.g., changes in mental health staff or staff holidays or leave). Furthermore, the occurrence of life events, loss, or shameful experiences can lead to despondency.

Some factors that can increase risk for suicide are quite unique to the psychotic disorders, such as the experience of command hallucinations telling patients to self-harm. In the case of Lauren, she experienced a voice commanding her to *"Jump in front of that car."* In some cases, patients will develop appeasement strategies whereby patients resist serious commands by enacting less serious behaviors such as complying with the voice in their imagination or expressing intent to comply. For example, Lauren appeased her commanding voice by standing on the side of a busy

road. Behavioral experiments, together with strategies focused on promoting the patient's sense of power and control over their voice, can be implemented as a way of challenging such commanding voices [23].

The clinician needs to be aware of all these factors, to know his or her patients well, and to monitor changes in their circumstances or mood that may be problematic. It is important to be aware of predictable changes and plan for them, to establish good communication with other mental health workers, and to address low mood and hopelessness in an open manner. When risk is high, emergency psychiatric services should be called upon. Specific strategies for reducing suicide behavior have been developed (see [24]).

Comorbid substance use and psychosis

Comorbid substance use is common in patients with psychotic-related disorders and is associated with poorer clinical outcome, higher levels of aggression and violence, and greater risk of suicide and self-harm. Motivational interviewing (MI) combined with CBTp has shown promising results in improving functioning in schizophrenia patients with associated drug or alcohol misuse [7, 25]. The potentially important interaction between alcohol or substance use and psychotic symptoms requires this dual treatment approach. Many patients do not consider their alcohol or substance use a problem. The aim during the initial sessions is to elicit change or motivational statements from the patient. The therapist uses the MI skills of reflective listening, empathy, developing discrepancy, rolling with resistance, and selective reinforcement to elicit such statements. Once the patient identifies substance or alcohol use as a problem and expresses a desire to change, therapy can then progress to using CBT-based strategies to achieve this goal.

Conclusion

Cognitive–behavioral therapy for psychosis does have significant benefits for patients suffering from schizophrenia and psychosis. It should be carried out as part of a comprehensive care plan. It is unlikely to "cure" patients but may assist them in coping and recovering from their illness. Intervention is based upon a detailed assessment and formulation. It does require considerable skill, experience, and knowledge of CBT and psychosis, and does not lend itself easily to simple protocol format. Further research on theoretical aspects of understanding psychosis from a psychological perspective is important to further inform and develop cognitive–behavioral treatment procedures. Research into dissemination and on how new psychological treatments penetrate into mental health services and become accessible to patients is required. Although the cost of well qualified and experienced clinicians delivering CBTp is thought to be high, this is offset by the economic gains in reducing the personal, social, and economic burden of persistent psychosis.

Suggested readings

Books

Barrowclough C, Tarrier N. *Families of Schizophrenic Patients: A Cognitive-behavioural Intervention*. London: Chapman & Hall, 1992. (Reprinted in 1997; Cheltenham: Stanley Thornes.)

Tarrier N. A cognitive-behavioural case formulation approach to the treatment of schizophrenia. In Tarrier N, ed. *Case Formulation in Cognitive Behaviour Therapy: The Treatment of Challenging and Complex Cases*. London: Routledge. 2006, pp. 167–87.

Tarrier N. Cognitive-behavior therapy for schizophrenia and psychotic disorders. In Barlow DH, ed. *Clinical Handbook of Psychological Disorders: A Step-by-step Treatment Manual*, 4th edn. New York: Guilford Press, 2007.

Morrison AP. Cognitive behaviour therapy for psychotic symptoms in schizophrenia. In Tarrier N, Wells A, Haddock G, eds. *Treating Complex Cases: The Cognitive Behaviour Therapy Approach*. Chichester: John Wiley & Sons. 1998, pp. 195–216.

Online resources

Rethink: the National Schizophrenia Fellowship www.rethink.org

The National Institute of Mental Health www.nimh.nih.gov

References

1. National Institute of Health and Clinical Excellence. Schizophrenia: core interventions in the treatment and management of schizophrenia in primary and secondary care. Clinical guidelines CG1. UK: NICE, 2002.

2. Bogels SM, Tarrier N. Unexplored issues and future directions in social phobia research. *Clin Psychol Rev* 2004; **24**(7): 731–6.

3. Mueser KT, Goodman LB, Trumbetta SL, *et al*. Trauma and posttraumatic stress disorder in severe mental illness. *J Consult Clin Psychol* 1998; **66**(3): 493–9.

4. Tarrier N, Barrowclough C, Andrews B, Gregg L. Risk of non-fatal suicide ideation and behaviour in recent onset schizophrenia: the influence of clinical, social, self-esteem and demographic factors. *Soc Psychiatry Psychiatr Epidemiol* 2004; **39**(11): 927–37.

5. Birchwood M, Meaden A, Trower P, Gilbert P, Plaistow J. The power and omnipotence of voices: subordination and entrapment by voices and significant others. *Psychol Med* 2000; **30**(2): 337–44.

6. Barrowclough C, Haddock G, Lowens I, *et al*. Psychosis and drug and alcohol problems. In Baker A, Velleman R, eds., *Mental Health and Drug and Alcohol Problems*. London: Routledge. 2007, pp. 218–40.

7. Barrowclough C, Haddock G, Tarrier N, *et al*. Randomized controlled trial of motivational interviewing, cognitive behavior therapy, and family intervention for patients with comorbid schizophrenia and substance use disorders. *Am J Psychiatry* 2001; **158**(10): 1706–13.

8. Nuechterlein KH. Vulnerability models for schizophrenia. State of the art. In Hafner H, Gattaz WF, Janzarik W, eds., *Search for the Cause of Schizophrenia*. Heidelberg: Springer-Verlag. 1987, pp. 297–316.

9. Garety PA, Kuipers E, Fowler D, Freeman D, Bebbington PE. A cognitive model of the positive symptoms of psychosis. *Psychol Med* 2001; **31**(2): 189–95.

10. Morrison AP. The interpretation of intrusions in psychosis: an integrative cognitive approach to hallucinations and delusions. *Behav Cogn Psychother* 2001; **29**(3): 257–76.

11. Tarrier N, Calam R. New developments in cognitive-behavioural case formulation. Epidemiological, systemic and social context: an integrative approach. *Cogn Behav Psychother* 2002; **30**: 311–28.

12. Tarrier N. A cognitive-behavioural case formulation approach to the treatment of schizophrenia. In Tarrier N, ed., *Case Formulation in Cognitive Behavior Therapy: The Treatment of Challenging and Complex Cases*. New York: Routledge. 2006, pp. 167–87.

13. Tarrier N. Cognitive-behavior therapy for schizophrenia and psychotic disorders. In Barlow DH, ed., *Clinical Handbook of Psychological Disorders: A Step-by-step Treatment Manual, 4th edn*. New York: Guilford Press, 2007.

14. Kuipers E, Garety P, Fowler D, *et al*. Cognitive, emotional, and social processes in psychosis: refining cognitive behavioral therapy for persistent positive symptoms. *Schizophr Bull* 2006; **32** Suppl 1: S24–31.

15. Tarrier N, Wykes T. Is there evidence that cognitive behaviour therapy is an effective treatment for schizophrenia? A cautious or cautionary tale? *Behav Res Ther* 2004; **42**(12): 1377–401.

16. Wykes T, Steel C, Everitt B, Tarrier N. Cognitive behavior therapy for schizophrenia: effect sizes, clinical models, and methodological rigor. *Schizophr Bull* 2008; **34**(3): 523–37.

17. Tarrier N. Cognitive-behaviour therapy for schizophrenia: a review of development, evidence and implementation. *Psychother Psychosom* 2005; **74**: 136–44.

18. Lehman AF, Kreyenbuhl J, Buchanan RW, *et al*. The Schizophrenia Patient Outcomes Research Team (PORT): updated treatment recommendations 2003. *Schizophr Bull* 2004; **30**(2): 193–217.

19. Barrowclough C, Haddock G, Lobban F, *et al*. Group cognitive-behavioural therapy for schizophrenia. Randomised controlled trial. *Br J Psychiatry* 2006; **189**: 527–32.

20. Blackburn IM, Davidson K. *Cognitive Therapy for Depression and Anxiety*. Cambridge: Cambridge University Press, 1995.

21. Hall PH, Tarrier N. The cognitive-behavioural treatment of low self-esteem in psychotic patients: a pilot study. *Behav Res Ther* 2003; **41**: 317–32.

22. Birchwood MJ, MacMillan F. Early intervention. In Birchwood MJ, Tarrier N, eds., *Psychological Management of Schizophrenia*. Chichester: Wiley. 1994, p. 77–108.

23. Byrne S, Birchwood M, Trower P, Meaden A. *A Casebook of Cognitive Behaviour Therapy for Command Hallucinations: A Social Rank Theory Approach*. New York: Routledge, 2006.

24. Johnson J, Gooding P, Tarrier N. Suicide risk in schizophrenia: explanatory models and clinical implications: the Schematic Appraisal Model of Suicide (SAMS). *Psychol Psychother* 2008; **81**: 55–77.

25. Baker A, Bucci S, Lewin TJ, *et al*. Cognitive-behavioural therapy for substance use disorders in people with psychotic disorders: randomised controlled trial. *Br J Psychiatry* 2006; **188**(5): 439–48.

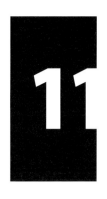

11 Body dysmorphic disorder

Jennifer Ragan, Jennifer L. Greenberg, Elise Beeger, Madeline Sedovic, and Sabine Wilhelm

Nature of the disorder

Diagnostic criteria

Body dysmorphic disorder (BDD) is defined as a preoccupation with an imagined or slight defect in appearance that results in significant distress or impairment in functioning and cannot be accounted for by another psychological condition (e.g., dissatisfaction with weight or shape in anorexia nervosa) [1]. If a slight physical anomaly is present the concern must be excessive [1]. Some individuals with BDD are so convinced about the existence of their perceived flaw that they are unable to consider that their appearance concerns might be exaggerated or exist only in their imagination. While insight is often poor in individuals with BDD, approximately 35 to 40% of patients qualify for an additional diagnosis of delusional disorder, somatic subtype [2, 3]. Two-thirds of patients with BDD have delusional ideas of reference, in that they are completely convinced that others are taking special notice of (e.g., laughing about or staring at) their perceived flaw [2]. Of note, insight often varies over the course of the disorder, and individuals with delusional and non-delusional BDD are largely similar in demographics and clinical features. Moreover, both non-delusional and delusional variants respond favorably to treatment with serotonin reuptake inhibitors (SRIs). Thus, given the fluctuations in insight that occur throughout the course of the disorder and the comparable treatment response, it has been suggested that delusional and non-delusional forms of BDD reflect a single disorder with a continuum of insight [4].

Symptoms

Appearance concerns may focus on any body area, but most commonly involve the face and head [5]. For example, individuals may be preoccupied with imagined or minimal flaws involving their skin (e.g., acne, marks, pores, wrinkles, scars), nose (e.g., worries that their nose is too large, wide, uneven, disproportionate), or hair (e.g., thinning, balding, hair loss, excessive body hair, texture, symmetry). Most individuals are concerned with multiple body parts. Over time, the number of preoccupations often progresses and may shift from one body area to another [5, 6]. A recent study of 200 individuals with BDD found that, on average, individuals were preoccupied with six to seven body areas over the course of their illness [3].

Some BDD patients worry that their perceived flaws or general appearance are "unattractive" or "not normal," whereas others describe their appearance as "hideous," "deformed," "ugly," or "monstrous." Thoughts and images about the perceived flaw are obsessive in nature in that they are time consuming (e.g., occurring on average three to eight hours a day), difficult to resist, and hard to control. Intrusive and time-consuming appearance-related thoughts can cause significant emotional distress, poor self-esteem, and difficulty concentrating. More than 90% of BDD patients perform repetitive, compulsive behaviors in an effort to alleviate or prevent distress associated with appearance-related preoccupations.

Common rituals include comparing their appearance with that of others, frequent checking in mirrors and other reflective surfaces (e.g., store windows), camouflaging the perceived flaw with clothing, makeup, or body positioning (e.g., wearing a hat to hide perceived hair loss or applying concealer to hide perceived acne or scars), excessive grooming (e.g., hair combing, makeup application, shaving), tanning, reassurance seeking, and skin picking. Excessive exercise, particularly weightlifting, dieting, use of prohormones/supplements/anabolic steroids,

Cognitive–behavioral Therapy with Adults: A Guide to Empirically Informed Assessment and Intervention,
ed. Stefan G. Hofmann and Mark A. Reinecke. © Cambridge University Press 2010.

and camouflaging with extra layers are particularly common in men with muscle dysmorphia, whose pre-occupation focuses on being too small or having inadequate musculature [7, 8]. All of these behaviors are conceptualized as compulsive in that patients feel driven to perform them repeatedly, and find them hard to resist or control. However, the behaviors provide only temporary relief and ultimately play a role in maintaining distress.

Some rituals can actually worsen the preoccupation with the perceived defect. For example, skin picking, a ritual about one-third of BDD patients engage in to try to "fix" perceived or minor blemishes, may involve the use of sharp implements (e.g., razor blades) and can cause noticeable skin damage [9, 10], which in turn may increase feelings of shame and anxiety. In a desperate attempt to reduce distress, some individuals resort to "do it yourself" procedures, such as breaking one's own nose [5, 11]. Individuals may also obtain costly medical or non-medical cosmetic procedures with typically poor outcomes. Clinical reports and retrospective studies of BDD patients who received cosmetic procedures [12, 13] found that patients often experience no change in BDD symptoms or an exacerbation of BDD symptoms; it is not uncommon for patients to experience a shift in the focus of the concern from one feature to another following cosmetic procedures. Of the small percentage of people who may experience an improvement in BDD symptoms, the benefits tend to be short term, and some patients worry about how long the improvement will last [12]. Extreme dissatisfaction resulting from cosmetic procedures can also result in violence against the self or treating physician. It may increase suicidality in an already vulnerable population, and there are documented cases of extremely dissatisfied BDD patients who threatened or executed lawsuits and homicides against their physicians [14].

Fear of negative evaluation by others also contributes to avoidance of daily activities, including school and work, and peer interactions (e.g., dating, social events) [6, 15]. Body dysmorphic disorder patients often go to great lengths to avoid situations that might exacerbate their appearance concerns. For instance, some patients find themselves avoiding mirrors, although many patients alternate between checking and avoiding mirrors and reflective surfaces. Some patients may go so far as to remove mirrors from their homes. Patients may avoid activities that require showing off or viewing body parts they are ashamed of, such as shopping (i.e., where they may be forced to look at themselves in a dressing room), swimming, or going to the beach. Individuals with BDD may avoid having sex because they are too embarrassed to be seen naked. Patients often avoid social situations such as work or school, and may stop going to work or school completely. They stop attending social engagements that they feel would bring attention to their flaws and lead to ridicule, such as dating or parties. They may also avoid bright lighting as they believe that it would accentuate their flaws, and may only choose certain restaurants with softer lighting when daring to venture out. When symptoms are severe, BDD patients can sometimes become socially isolated, including being housebound [15].

Course and epidemiology

Body dysmorphic disorder appears to be a relatively common disorder that usually begins in late childhood or early adolescence and has a chronic course if left untreated. In the largest epidemiological study to date [16], a nationwide survey in Germany ($n = 2,552$), the prevalence of BDD was 1.7% (95% CI = 1.2–2.1%). Prevalence rates have ranged from 0.7 to 3% in smaller community studies [17, 18] and 2.3 to 13% in non-clinical student samples [5]. Differences in obtained prevalence rates may be due to methodological differences between studies. For example, use of self-report measures, inclusion of subclinical cases, or studying groups in which higher base rates may be expected, may increase base rates. In addition, studies attempting to assess the prevalence of a disorder with a relatively low base rate are at risk for being underpowered with a sample of less than 1,000 participants [16]. Thus, it is possible that these rates underestimate the true prevalence of BDD.

During adolescence, when symptoms typically emerge, BDD may be overlooked or mistaken for normal developmental concerns about appearance. In an examination of adult and adolescent inpatients, Grant et al. [19] found that 13% ($n = 16$) of 122 patients met DSM-IV criteria for BDD; however, none of the patients had been diagnosed with BDD by their treating physician. Of note, all of these patients reported that they would not volunteer information about their BDD symptoms to their physician unless specifically asked. Subsequently, Conroy and colleagues found 16% of 100 adult psychiatric inpatients met criteria for past or current BDD, and had disclosed BDD symptoms to only a small percentage of current or previous providers [20]. Of those seeking mental healthcare, individuals usually present with secondary symptoms, such as depression and anxiety.

The comorbidity of BDD and depression has been well documented in the literature. A recent study by Phillips, Didie, and Menard [21] found a 38% current and 74% lifetime prevalence of major depression in individuals with BDD, and found poorer functioning and quality of life and higher rates of suicidality among BDD patients with comorbid depression. Nierenberg et al. [22] reported 28 (8%) lifetime and 23 (6.6%) current BDD diagnoses among 350 outpatients with typical and atypical depression; patients with BDD had an earlier age of onset of depression and were more likely to have atypical depression. Although they appear to be at increased risk for suicidality and poorer quality of life and functioning, individuals with comorbid BDD and depression may present or receive treatment solely for depressive symptomatology unless they are asked about BDD symptoms. This underscores the importance of careful and specific assessment of appearance-related concerns. Similarly, individuals with BDD may be diagnosed based on a comorbid anxiety disorder. For example, the prevalence of BDD among outpatients seeking treatment for anxiety has been shown to be in the range of 12% of patients with social phobia and 7.5% of patients with obsessive–compulsive disorder (OCD) [23]. Lastly, higher prevalence rates in dermatology and reconstructive surgery settings support clinical observations that individuals with BDD are more likely to consult dermatologists, plastic surgeons, or dentists rather than psychologists because they are ashamed and embarrassed of their symptoms, or because they are convinced that the flaw is physically rather than psychologically related [24, 25]. A number of studies have examined the rate of BDD among individuals presenting for medical and non-medical cosmetic procedures. In the United States, the rates of BDD range from 7 to 8% in cosmetic surgery populations [26, 25] and 8.5 to 15% in dermatology populations [24, 14].

Studies of gender differences in BDD show more similarities than differences between genders, and the gender ratio for BDD is approximately 1:1 [27, 7]. However, some differences emerge with respect to demographic and clinical features. Differences between the genders typically pertain to the body area of concern; however, males are more likely than females to be single and living alone [27, 7]. Men are more likely to be preoccupied by their genitals, musculature, and hair (i.e., thinning/balding), and to engage in excessive weightlifting. Women are more likely to be concerned with their skin, stomach, weight, breasts/chest, buttocks, thighs, legs, hips, toes, and excessive body/facial hair. Women also endorse more areas of excessive concern and are more likely to engage in regular safety and compulsive behaviors, including camouflaging techniques, mirror checking, changing clothes, and skin picking [27, 7].

Comorbidity

Due to its frequent comorbidity with other disorders, the diagnosis of BDD is often overlooked in clinical settings. Depression, social anxiety disorder, OCD and substance abuse disorders are among the most common comorbid Axis I disorders [28, 3]. Personality disorders, particularly avoidant, obsessive–compulsive, paranoid, and dependent are also common among adults with BDD [29, 11]. More than 60% of patients with BDD have comorbid depression and suicide is common [28, 15]. Available data suggest that 80% of individuals with BDD experience lifetime suicidal ideation and 24 to 28% have attempted suicide [30]. Rates of suicidal ideation and attempts in BDD patients are markedly high compared to US population norms and other psychological disorders, including major depressive disorder, bipolar disorder, and eating disorders [31, 15]. Suicide risk factors, including high rates of psychiatric hospitalization, being single or divorced, psychiatric comorbidity (including anxiety, depression, and impulsive aggression), and poor social supports have all been associated with BDD [30, 31, 3]. Not surprisingly, the level of functioning varies in BDD but is generally poor. Individuals with BDD tend to have poor self-esteem and a markedly poor quality of life when compared with US general population norms and individuals with depression, diabetes, or a recent myocardial infarction [32]. Notably, individuals with delusional BDD tend to report more impairment and poorer quality of life than those with the non-delusional variant [4, 32].

However, shame about symptoms and lack of insight can make individuals with BDD reluctant to seek treatment from mental health providers or to volunteer appearance-related concerns unless specifically queried. Thus, providers need to ask specifically about BDD. Body dysmorphic disorder is commonly misdiagnosed due to similar and comorbid disorders, including depression, OCD, social phobia, trichotillomania, eating disorders, and psychotic disorders. If BDD is misdiagnosed individuals may not be treated or may receive ineffective treatments.

Review of cognitive models of the condition

The etiology and maintenance of BDD involve an interaction of cognitive, affective, behavioral, biological, and sociocultural factors. Cognitive–behavioral models hypothesize a diathesis–stress model [33] by which individuals with a biological predisposition to BDD develop symptoms in response to a stressor (e.g., socioenvironmental, hormonal, psychological). The precipitous psychological, physical, and social changes that occur in the context of heightened emphasis on physical appearance may explain the onset of symptoms during adolescence.

Sociocultural factors, including mass-media messages purporting a thin, young ideal, have been implicated in the rising rate of body image dissatisfaction in the United States. Evidence from prospective and experimental studies largely support a moderate negative effect of the media on body image. A recent meta-analysis of 25 studies that randomly assigned women to view images of thin models versus normal or plus-size models or inanimate objects found a medium negative overall effect (d = −0.31) on body satisfaction [34]. In addition to ubiquitous media messages related to physical appearance, excessive appearance-based reinforcement, including teasing or praise, can contribute to the development and maintenance of body dissatisfaction and BDD [35]. Sociocultural theorists have highlighted the role of spreading Western values in the rising rate of body image dissatisfaction and disorders across cultures [36]. Given the omnipresence of sociocultural messages and the relatively low incidence of BDD, it is unlikely these factors play a direct causal role in its etiology. Indeed, although general body dissatisfaction is more prevalent in cultures where physical attractiveness is highly valued, such as the United States, the prevalence of clinically significant BDD does not appear to vary cross-culturally. In the only cross-cultural study of BDD, Bohne *et al.* compared its prevalence in non-clinical samples of American (*n* = 101) and German (*n* = 133) students, and found similar rates in both groups (4.0%

of Americans and 5.3% of Germans) [37]. Variants of BDD, including muscle dysmorphia and shubo-kyofu (a variant of a Japanese phobia, taijin kyofusho, in which individuals are afraid of offending others by their "deformed body") have also been described in case reports from Western and non-Western cultures. Body dysmorphic disorder has been reported in the United States, the United Kingdom, Africa [38], Asia [39, 40], Australia, Europe [37, 41, 42, 43], and South America [44]. Although no cross-cultural studies have examined clinical features in clinical or community samples, case reports suggest that culture may influence the body part of concern as well as patients' access to and attitude toward mental health treatment.

As noted, the most common areas of concern in BDD involve the face, nose, hair, and skin; however, the significance or meanings of these body areas may vary cross-culturally. For example, studies of ethnic minorities both within and outside of the United States have found that Latino women report a preference for dark hair, eyes, and skin, and larger breasts [45]; African Americans, particularly women, use hairstyle and skin tone/color as important determinants of physical appearance; and cosmetic surgeries are common in Asian cultures to obtain "Western" features, such as the double eyelid (i.e., eyefold) and sculpted nose [46]. Concern that one's appearance may cause others distress may also be more common in non-Western cultures. For example, koro, a relatively common culturally related syndrome occurring primarily in Southeast Asia is characterized by a preoccupation with penile (labia, nipples, or breasts in women) shrinking or retraction into the body resulting in death [1, 47]. Koro is similar to genital retraction syndromes reported in other cultures, such as suo yang in China, and some have questioned its relationship to BDD. As with BDD, individuals with koro are preoccupied with some aspect of physical appearance and often go to extreme measures to prevent associated negative consequences (e.g., the use of weights, needles, hooks, and fishing line to prevent retraction); however, koro differs from BDD in its typically brief duration, associated features (e.g., acute anxiety and fear of death), response to reassurance, and occasional collective development as an epidemic [48].

Examining stages of acculturation (e.g., such as time spent in residence, socioeconomic status, ethnic group identification and relatedness, and language) with a patient may be helpful in ensuring a culturally-sensitive treatment. For example, studies of body dissatisfaction among Latino minorities in the United States, have found an inverse relationship between level of acculturation (e.g., time spent in residence, socioeconomic status, ethnic group identification and relatedness, and language) and body satisfaction [49]. However, findings have been largely mixed regarding the relationship between level of acculturation and body image among ethnic minorities. It is possible that ethnic identity development and conflicts may engender negative psychological sequelae, including body image dissatisfaction. While these studies have examined body dissatisfaction, and not clinical BDD, they underscore the importance of considering the developmental and psychological impact of the acculturation process.

Individuals with BDD place an excessive value on sociocultural ideals of physical attractiveness in determining their sense of self. In addition, they are more likely to underestimate their own physical attractiveness and overestimate others' attractiveness [50]. Body dysmorphic disorder patients also tend to determine their body image and self-esteem based exclusively on their area(s) of concern. In other words, they pay attention only to the aspects of their appearance with which they are dissatisfied. Subsequently, individuals may develop maladaptive beliefs about their appearance and the importance of their appearance. For instance, "People are judging me based on my appearance"; "In order to be accepted or loved, I must be attractive"; or "I have acne, therefore I am hideous." Situations that trigger these negative thoughts leave individuals feeling shamed, depressed, disgusted, and anxious; therefore they come to avoid anxiety-provoking situations whenever possible. In addition, selective attention to the perceived flaw and compulsive behaviors (e.g., checking) increase the frequency and distress associated with intrusive appearance-related cognitions and prevent habituation.

Selective attention and overimportance of appearance contribute to the maintenance of BDD symptoms by increasing feelings of distress and negative, appearance-related thoughts, making the individual with BDD more likely to engage in compulsive or avoidant behavior in order to try to reduce their distress. This phenomenon is consistent with neuropsychological findings [51, 52, 53] that patients with BDD overfocus on the small details in lieu of seeing the big picture. In other words, BDD patients who do engage in anxiety-provoking situations will often use rituals or safety behaviors to cope with the anxiety-provoking

event (e.g., spending hours concealing perceived blemishes and seeking reassurance around the appearance of their face). If they can get through the situation, they may be left thinking, "I was able to cover my acne successfully this time" or "No one was looking at me." Based on the principle of negative reinforcement, the next time an occasion occurs that triggers the same appearance-related thoughts and distress, the BDD patient will rely on the same strategies that seemingly worked the last time to reduce distress and prevent perceived negative consequences. Similarly, by avoiding or escaping situations, the BDD patient does not allow for disconfirming evidence or experiences. This maintains a vicious cycle in which the BDD patient constantly faces anxiety upon encountering similar stimuli without learning that another outcome or experience may be possible (e.g., "Maybe I would be able to tolerate the party even without concealer"), including the gradual decline of distress and anxiety with repeated exposure over time.

Empirical support for efficacy and effectiveness of treatment

Effective treatments are available for BDD. Pharmacotherapy with SRIs and cognitive–behavioral therapy (CBT) are considered the first-line treatments for BDD. Medication studies have primarily examined SRIs and have found clomipramine [54], fluvoxamine [55, 56], fluoxetine [57], citalopram [58], and escitalopram [59] to be effective, reporting response rates from 53 to 73%. Notably, SRIs tend to be more effective for BDD symptoms than other antidepressants.

It is recommended that SRIs be tried at their optimal dose for at least 12 weeks before other medications are tried or added to a patient's regimen. Although evidence for the effectiveness of non-SRI antidepressants (e.g., tricyclic antidepressants) or neuroleptics in treating BDD symptoms has not been adequately demonstrated, treaters can consider augmentation strategies if patients do not have an adequate response on an SRI [29, 60]. Successful treatment with SRIs can lead to improvement in BDD symptoms, such as reduced preoccupation with appearance and related ritualistic and avoidant behaviors; insight, depressive symptoms, and overall quality of life may also improve over the course of treatment. After successful pharmacotherapy, many patients report that, although they think they look the same, they are less distressed and anxious about their appearance. Some patients do report a belief that their appearance has improved over the course of treatment.

Cognitive–behavioral therapy, cognitive therapy (CT; cognitive restructuring techniques alone), and behavior therapy (BT; exposure-response prevention alone) have also been shown to be effective in treating BDD. These therapies are the psychological treatments that have been systematically studied in the treatment of BDD, and they have been delivered effectively in both individual [61, 62] and group formats [63, 64]. The number of sessions and length of treatment have varied widely across studies. Some treatments were delivered weekly over the course of eight to twelve weeks and others were delivered daily over the course of four to six weeks. Currently, there are no data regarding the optimal length or frequency of treatment.

Veale and colleagues [62] reported significantly greater reductions in mean Yale–Brown Obsessive–Compulsive Scale – modified for body dysmorphic disorder (BDD-YBOCS) scores for treated patients in comparison to wait-list patients. Seven of nine treated patients were rated as either having absent or subclinical BDD at the end of the trial, whereas all patients on the wait list were rated as having clinical BDD at the end of the trial. Wilhelm and colleagues reported similar reductions in mean BDD-YBOCS scores to those reported by Veale for treated patients [63]. Rosen [64] reported response rates as high as 82% in BDD patients assigned to a CBT group treatment. Similarly to medication, not only did patients report symptoms of BDD improved as a result of CBT, they also often reported reductions in depressive symptoms.

A meta-analysis comparing medications to CBT, BT, and CT [65] found that all treatments led to improvements in BDD symptoms and depression. They also found large effect sizes that supported the effectiveness of these treatments, both for case series and randomized controlled trials (RCTs). When psychotherapies were subdivided into CBT and BT interventions, CBT yielded larger effect sizes than pharmacotherapy. No differences were revealed between CBT and BT, or between BT and pharmacotherapy. Future research is needed to further elucidate the relationship between CBT and pharmacotherapy interventions, both as monotherapies and in combination, in order to determine the most effective treatment package for patients with BDD.

Introduction to clinical case

Sarah is a 31-year-old single Caucasian female who came to treatment with excessive concerns about the appearance of her skin (NB: the patient's name has been changed to protect her anonymity). Sarah's skin concerns had surfaced at age 29 and worsened over time. Although others often complimented her on the appearance of her skin, she nonetheless worried about its color and smoothness for up to eight hours a day. She described her skin as bumpy with acne and believed others noticed her flaws and judged her for them. She desperately wanted to feel attractive, but she considered herself to be "ugly."

Sarah spent up to two hours a day checking her appearance in a hand-held mirror, her car rear-view mirror, her cell phone, and in store windows. On "bad" days, she checked her appearance every five minutes. She spent three to five hours a day on the internet looking for pictures of celebrities to compare herself to, and for skin products she hoped would improve the appearance of her skin. She bought these products weekly, tried them once, and then threw them away for fear they would worsen, rather than improve, her appearance. Thus, she spent hundreds of dollars and countless hours in the pursuit of the perfect skincare product.

She avoided foods (dairy, etc.) she believed produced acne, took cold showers, and drove without heat in her car during the winter because she believed heat worsened her acne. She washed her pillowcase daily to avoid having any dirt or foreign substance come in contact with her face. She was often late to work or appointments and would avoid going out with friends to social engagements for fear of being judged and humiliated in public. At work, she often got "stuck" in the bathroom looking at her face and could not leave because coworkers might notice that she had been crying. She frequently asked people close to her for reassurance about the appearance of her skin, but was unable to accept or be soothed by this reassurance.

Sarah had been to the dermatologist several times seeking treatments for acne and rosacea, and had purchased a prescription acne treatment (Accutane) over the internet in order to treat her "skin problems." She took this medication without the supervision of a doctor and it had severe side effects (i.e., damage of the intestines), which resulted in surgery and led her to seek psychiatric treatment. Around the same time, her boyfriend had also become extremely concerned about her. Based on her extreme appearance preoccupations and costly and dangerous behaviors to "correct" her appearance, he urged her to consider that she might have BDD, and convinced her to seek treatment at a BDD specialty clinic. The program they found offered CBT and pharmacotherapy. Sarah chose to start with CBT because she was somewhat reluctant to take medications. At the beginning of treatment Sarah was skeptical that she had a psychological problem. She reported, "I hate that I can't stop thinking about my skin, but I can't believe what people tell me . . . I know I look ugly!" The therapist refrained from trying to convince Sarah of her BDD diagnosis. Instead, she explained that therapy would focus on relieving Sarah's distress about her appearance and on improving her quality of life. Sarah was able to acknowledge that her appearance concerns had significantly impacted her life, and was therefore willing to engage in treatment.

Before starting treatment, a structured diagnostic interview [66] was used to assess Sarah's symptoms. She was diagnosed with BDD and major depression. Additional information was gathered regarding the severity of Sarah's concurrent depression in order to help predict safety concerns and poor treatment adherence that might arise during the course of treatment.

The BDD-YBOCS was administered in order to establish BDD baseline symptom severity [67]. The BDD-YBOCS is a clinician-administered scale that measures the severity of BDD symptoms. It assesses time spent occupied by thoughts and behaviors related to the perceived defect; distress and interference caused by these thoughts and behaviors; resistance against and control over these thoughts and behaviors; avoidance; and insight level. Sarah received a score of 32, which was in the moderately severe range. Additionally, Sarah completed the Beck Depression Inventory-II (BDI-II) [68], which assesses for symptoms of depression, including suicidal ideation (SI). Due to its brief, self-report nature, the BDI-II can be administered at every session to help monitor SI. This is important given the high rates of SI and attempts in BDD patients compared to patients with other psychological disorders. Sarah received a 25 on the BDI-II, which was in the moderate range.

During their initial session, Sarah's therapist also asked about symptoms of depression and suicidal thoughts, plans, means, and past attempts. Sarah provided an emergency contact (e.g., a person close to the patient whom the therapist could contact in the event that Sarah's safety came into question). She denied SI at the onset of treatment, but did continue to have urges to use Accutane, which had caused serious physical damage in the past. Therefore, the therapist and Sarah monitored Sarah's urge to buy and use Accutane at each session.

Overview of treatment protocol

Sarah's treatment followed the protocol outlined in Wilhelm, Phillips, and Steketee's (2008) CBT manual for BDD [69]. The first step in CBT for BDD is to gather information about the presenting problem, with specific attention being paid to areas of concern, automatic thoughts, avoidance strategies, and ritualistic behaviors that maintain and exacerbate BDD symptoms. Patients often feel ashamed and may not volunteer details of their symptoms on their own. Therefore it is important to ask them directly about specific body parts that may be of concern and any associated ritualistic and avoidant behaviors.

Sarah divulged that when she was younger, her appearance concerns focused solely on her hair. However, over time, this concern diminished and was replaced by anxiety about her facial skin. Sarah was not only worried about the current state of her skin, but also worried about it worsening over time. "Even though my face has never exploded with acne, I worry one pimple could turn into one hundred some day. I'm always thinking what if this is the time it actually happens?"

Her concerns about her appearance led her to engage in several compulsive rituals in an attempt to ameliorate her anxiety. The frequency and length of time that Sarah engaged in each of these behaviors was assessed at baseline. Patients are often embarrassed by the length of time they spend in these activities, so therapists should be aware of potential underreporting and should allow for a wide range of responses (e.g., seconds, minutes, an hour, multiple hours). For example, Sarah described spending "a little bit of time in the morning and night" on the internet; however, when her therapist asked Sarah how many minutes or hours that she was spending on the internet, Sarah disclosed that she actually spent three to five hours per day online comparing herself to celebrities she admired and looking for new skincare products.

Finally, BDD patients often avoid situations that cause them anxiety about their appearance. It is important to elicit details about these behaviors so they can be incorporated into the treatment. Sometimes patients have engaged in avoidance for so long that they no longer recognize their behavior as a maladaptive avoidance strategy. In these cases, asking what the patient would do if their appearance concerns were eliminated can help patients identify what they are missing in their lives. In Sarah's case, she found that she had lost contact with several friends. She also described lost opportunities at work to move into leadership roles that would require more contact with coworkers and clients.

Psychoeducation

The next few sessions were spent educating Sarah about the potential causes of BDD, including biological, psychological, and sociocultural causes of BDD. She learned how biological factors, such as a genetic predisposition to BDD, neurotransmitters in the brain, and personality factors such as being shy or perfectionistic may put a person at risk for developing BDD. She also came to understand how environmental and psychological factors, such as being teased by family members or classmates, and importance placed on one's appearance by family and society, could trigger the manifestation of a biological vulnerability for BDD. Finally, her therapist outlined how other factors such as stressful life events, including loss of a job or the loss of an important relationship, can trigger or worsen BDD symptoms over the course of the disorder.

After explaining the potential causes and factors involved in maintaining BDD, Sarah and her therapist discussed how these applied to her. Sarah identified perfectionistic tendencies, a biological vulnerability for anxiety and body image concerns (history of OCD and anorexia), and stressors in her life that contributed to her BDD symptoms. In addition, Sarah's family regularly impressed upon her the importance of looking good in order to be accepted by others in her life and by society at large. Sarah completed a personalized model [33] of how these factors interacted with negative automatic thoughts, feelings, and rituals/avoidance to maintain her symptoms, so that it became clear how CBT would target each of these factors.

Therapeutic relationship

The next session focused on treatment rationale, and therapist and patient roles. For example, Sarah learned

about the short-term nature of CBT and its focus on the thoughts and behaviors that maintained and exacerbated her BDD symptoms. The therapist described how Sarah would learn skills aimed at identifying and changing these thoughts and behaviors and would complete homework assignments to help her master these skills outside of the sessions. Her therapist would act as her coach, teaching Sarah the skills she needed to learn in order to overcome her symptoms and ultimately become her own therapist over the course of six months.

Structure of session

Weekly therapy sessions were structured to include a mood and symptom check, a review of completed homework, an introduction and review of new skills, assignment of homework for the upcoming week, and a summary of the session. The mood and symptom check alerted the therapist to significant changes or safety issues that should be addressed, and helped Sarah and the therapist to keep track of her progress in therapy. Reviewing homework helped Sarah and her therapist to assess Sarah's use of skills, including successes and challenges, since the previous session; challenges, including difficulty adhering to homework assignments, were addressed using problem-solving strategies in session. Setting the agenda collaboratively allowed time for Sarah's concerns to be addressed and for new skills to be taught. Assigning homework for the following week helped underscore the importance of practice outside the session. Summarizing the major points from the session helped Sarah to recapitulate what she had learned; summarizing also highlighted and allowed for her therapist to correct any misunderstandings or misinterpretations that Sarah may have had about what occurred in session. Sarah was encouraged to take notes during sessions so that she could review them while completing homework assignments and when therapy was completed.

Strategies and techniques: cognitive restructuring

The next three to four sessions addressed cognitive restructuring. Cognitive restructuring involves identifying and evaluating negative automatic thoughts and cognitive errors a patient holds regarding his or her appearance. The goal of cognitive restructuring is to generate more accurate and helpful beliefs by reviewing the evidence for, or utility of, negative, distorted beliefs. Sarah learned how to use thought records to identify automatic thoughts, evaluate the validity of her thoughts, and generate more balanced responses.

The therapist also taught her about common cognitive errors that individuals often make, so she could identify when she was making an error in thinking. Cognitive errors for patients with BDD include black-and-white thinking ("Any flaw means I'm completely ugly"), mind reading ("I know others are laughing at how I look"), fortune telling or catastrophizing ("My face is going to explode with acne if I do one thing wrong to my skin"), emotional reasoning ("I know I'm ugly because I feel ugly"), labeling ("My nose looks like a pig nose"), discounting the positive ("People only compliment me because they feel bad for me"), personalization ("When my friends were talking about people they feel sorry for, I know they were referring to me"), and overgeneralization ("That one guy told me once that he didn't like my hair, and now I know that everyone must be thinking the same thing!").

After Sarah learned to recognize cognitive errors, she practiced identifying the negative beliefs she held with regard to her appearance. Once Sarah identified her appearance-related distortions, she was instructed to use a detective/scientist approach to gather evidence for and against her beliefs. After weighing the evidence for and against her beliefs, Sarah was encouraged to generate an alternative belief that would be more accurate and helpful to her.

Sarah was also taught how to identify intermediate ("My skin is ugly, therefore no one will love me") and core beliefs ("I am unlovable and defective"). Sarah believed that if her physical flaws were corrected, she would feel like a happy, loveable, and worthwhile human being. She believed her family and friends would love her more if she perfected her appearance. Through cognitive restructuring, Sarah was reminded that going to extremes to change one's appearance (e.g., cosmetic dermatologic procedures) rarely has positive effects on one's self-worth and could lead to a worsening of symptoms. Sarah also learned to find healthier ways of defining herself and what made her loveable. Her therapist used strategies such as the "self-esteem pie" to help Sarah determine which traits were of value to her in determining her identity and to elicit non-appearance related components of her self-worth. This helped Sarah to recognize how much emphasis she put on her appearance in comparison to other areas of her life. Subsequently, she devoted more time to developing new friendships, expressing her creativity through writing and playing the piano, and finding a new job that made better use of her talents and helped her to develop a sense of mastery.

Strategies and techniques: exposure and response prevention

Sarah's avoidant behaviors were targeted through exposure. Sarah learned that her avoidance strategies, which reduced anxiety in the short term, only served to exacerbate and reinforce her anxiety in the long term. The therapist and Sarah developed a hierarchy of situations that Sarah would confront gradually. They started with situations that were moderately difficult (50 on a 0 to 100 subjective units of distress [SUD] scale) and worked up to more difficult situations. Sarah's hierarchy included going to social events, going on dates in restaurants with "harsh lighting," using heat in her car, exercising enough to break a sweat, allowing her boyfriend to kiss and touch her face, eating "off-limit" foods, and using tap water to wash her face instead of bottled water. Before practicing an exposure, Sarah filled out a behavioral experiment record that helped prepare her for the exposure. For example, Sarah was encouraged to think about and record subtle avoidance or ritual behaviors that she should look out for during the exercise, specific predictions about the outcome, and specific goals she hoped to accomplish during the exercise. Sarah was encouraged to use exposure tasks as behavioral experiments to help test the validity of her negative beliefs.

Sarah and her therapist also reviewed the role of rituals in reinforcing BDD symptoms; namely, that by engaging in rituals Sarah never allowed herself to experience disconfirming evidence (e.g., that she could go to a party without spending two hours camouflaging her "acne" with concealer) or tolerate distress. They reviewed the list of rituals Sarah reported during the assessment, including her extensive face cleansing routine, internet searches (e.g., for skin products and browsing dermatology sites), purchasing skincare products, reassurance seeking, mirror checking, and visits to the dermatologist. Sarah's therapist reminded her that they would gradually reduce rituals using a variety of strategies, including ritual delay, decreasing time spent doing rituals, engaging in competing responses, and increasing healthy behaviors to replace the rituals.

During sessions focused on exposure and response prevention, it can be helpful to involve family members and significant others. Sarah chose to have her boyfriend come to two sessions. Having her boyfriend in the session allowed for Sarah and her therapist to provide him with information about the CBT model of BDD; moreover, it paved the way for him to become part of the treatment team. Sarah and her therapist were able to enlist her boyfriend's help when they started working on reducing reassurance seeking. Sarah's boyfriend learned about the tendency for significant others to often inadvertently become involved in this and other rituals, believing they are helping patients. Sarah and her boyfriend were encouraged to abstain from seeking or providing reassurance, and Sarah agreed to engage in an activity that would be more beneficial, such as completing a thought record.

Strategies and techniques: mirror retraining

Patients with BDD have often come to view themselves in mirrors in unhelpful ways. They may stand too close to mirrors or spend large amounts of time inspecting their perceived "flaw" rather than looking at their entire face or body. Indeed, anyone who focused that much attention on one area of their body would begin to see themselves in a distorted way. Mirror retraining was introduced as a means to correct these behaviors. The therapist first demonstrated how to do this by describing her whole face in neutral terms ("I have short, light-brown hair. My face has an oval shape. I have a scar under my chin that is ½ inch long."). Then she asked Sarah to do the same. Sarah practiced mirror retraining in session in order to learn how to view herself in the mirror from an appropriate distance, to "take in the big picture," and to describe herself in non-judgmental, neutral terms [70]. This exercise is often very difficult for patients, but can be powerful as well. Sarah was encouraged to do these exercises every day in different lighting and with a variety of mirrors; concurrently, Sarah was asked to generally reduce the amount of time she spent examining her "flaws" in the mirror.

Relapse prevention

Finally, Sarah and the therapist discussed relapse prevention. They reviewed her gains in therapy and which techniques helped her make those gains. In preparation for ending treatment, Sarah began weekly self-sessions, which mirrored what she did with the therapist. They discussed her fear and excitement about ending treatment, and how she would know whether or not she needed to return to therapy in the future. Sarah then gradually ended treatment by attending booster sessions every three weeks for two months after the termination session. Her final BDD-YBOCS score was an 8 and her BDI-II score was a 9. In addition to reduced BDD symptomatology, these scores reflected Sarah's increased mood and quality of life. Sarah was able to go through a day without crying or getting stuck in the bathroom at work. She was able to go out with friends and engage others in conversation because she felt confident. She was able to let her boyfriend touch her face and could make it to work on time because her morning routine had been significantly shortened. She could exercise again without fearing a breakout, enjoyed looking in the mirror, and accepted compliments about her looks.

Difficulties encountered during treatment

While many patients benefit greatly from CBT, others do not. Level of delusionality may affect treatment process or outcome in CBT for BDD. When patients hold a fixed belief that their problems would be solved by a change in their appearance rather than a change in their perception of themselves, engaging in CBT can be a difficult process. Therapists may have to move more slowly in teaching skills with these patients, and spend more time focusing on issues of motivation. Notably, since SRIs have been found to be effective in treating both delusional and non-delusional variants of BDD, concurrent or sequential pharmacotherapy with CBT may be indicated for patients with delusionality.

Motivation for change and ambivalence about treatment and treatment goals can also present a challenge to treatment. As noted, issues around motivation may stem in part from a patient's level of insight (delusionality) into the disorder. However, ambivalence may also be evoked by the level of difficulty and discomfort associated with the treatment. Cognitive–behavioral therapy can be difficult for patients because it asks them to intentionally face situations they may have previously avoided. Cognitive–behavioral therapy requires that patients take risks and experience a certain level of anxiety at the beginning of treatment with the understanding that distress and anxiety will abate over the course of the treatment. Thus, patients may feel more anxious and distressed before they experience relief, making it difficult for some patients to maintain motivation. Generally, therapists should try to move at a pace that is comfortable for patients. Gradual exposure, starting with less anxiety-provoking situations, allows for patients to experience early success and mastery, thereby building confidence and motivation for subsequent exposure tasks. When patients express ambivalence about treatment or change, MI strategies can help patients move forward [69]. Through MI, Sarah described how exhausted she felt in her quest to perform all of her rituals. She realized that letting go of these behaviors would lead to a perceived loss of control for her in the short term, but in the long run would allow her more time, energy, and confidence to do things she had avoided for a long time.

Comorbid depression is common and could interfere with treatment. Depression can make it difficult for patients to engage in therapy; for example, lack of energy, concentration, and motivation can make it difficult for patients to complete homework and attend sessions. When depression seems primary, or if it is interfering with the patient's ability to effectively engage in CBT for BDD, the therapist may target the depression (e.g., by using cognitive restructuring and behavioral activation focused on depressive symptoms). Pharmacotherapy may also be considered. When patients become acutely suicidal, a higher level of care may be indicated. Decisions about the focus of treatment and treatment options should be discussed and made jointly between the therapist and patient [69].

Finally, treatment occurs within a context, and life stressors should be addressed as necessary throughout the treatment. Patients with BDD, particularly severe BDD, may have limited financial, occupational, and social resources. Patients may be housebound or without a job. They may have limited contact with friends or family, and may have spent so much time thinking about or engaged in rituals related to their appearance they have given up other daily activities or hobbies. Therefore, restoring activity across these dimensions becomes an integral part of a successful treatment.

Clinical decision making: integrating science and practice

When designing a treatment plan for an individual patient, therapists must integrate available research, clinical expertise, and the individual needs of the patient. The variab conditions that occu modular approach, suc Phillips, and Steketee [6

A modular manual a ized approach to treatmen et al. [69] manual offers sp who engage in excessive ski concerns about weight/shape dysmorphia), or desires to hav ...en may be present in some, but ...ents with BDD. Therapists should admin .cr measures that assess for these specific symptoms and use the available modules as appropriate [69].

A flexible and modular approach also allows for more clinical decision making around time spent on particular topics and strategies. For example, some BDD patients struggle with frequent mirror checking and have to be persuaded to reduce their checking. Other patients have become so avoidant of mirrors that they have removed all mirrors from their homes. For these patients, mirror exposure and retraining may constitute a larger part of therapy than for patients who spend more time engaging in other rituals.

Some patients may be limited in terms of their ability to engage in cognitive restructuring. They may have difficulty identifying their thoughts, generating alternative beliefs, and being able to think abstractly about their cognitive processes. In these cases, it can be helpful to do the minimal amount of cognitive restructuring and then move on to mostly behavioral strategies that may have a greater chance of impacting symptoms.

Conversely, for BDD patients who are afraid of, or unwilling to do, behavioral work, more time can be spent on cognitive restructuring. Sometimes patients make significant gains through cognitive strategies alone. Although behavioral interventions can be quite powerful adjuncts to cognitive work, if patients cannot tolerate behavioral work, CT can be a useful way to make progress while lowering the risk that the patient will drop out of treatment.

Finally, anecdotal data suggest that BDD patients from minority origin might also report difficulties with ethnic identity development, which in turn might account for some of their BDD symptoms. As such, it would behove clinicians to inquire about ethnic identity development as part of their assessment and address this in treatment [71].

morphic disorder is a common, underdiagnosed, and often debilitating disorder. Many people with the disorder live with shame and despair. Although they may seek treatment for comorbid psychiatric disorders, they often do not disclose their struggles with BDD to their therapists, and therapists often do not think to ask about symptoms of BDD; therefore their symptoms frequently go unnoticed and untreated. This chapter is intended to alert clinicians to the presence of this disorder and to offer some useful tools for the detection, assessment, and treatment of BDD. Studies thus far have shown promise for CBT and pharmacotherapy in the treatment of adult BDD, and more research is being done in an effort to improve the quality of care for these patients.

References

1. American Psychiatric Association. *Diagnostic and Statistical Manual of Mental Disorders*, 4th edn., text revision. Washington, DC: APA, 2000.

2. Phillips KA. Psychosis in body dysmorphic disorder. *J Psychiatr Res* 2004; **38**: 63–72.

3. Phillips KA, Menard W, Fay C, Weisberg R. Demographic characteristics, phenomenology, comorbidity, and family history in 200 individuals with body dysmorphic disorder. *Psychosomatics* 2005; **46**: 317–25.

4. Phillips KA, McElroy SL, Keck PE, *et al.* A comparison of delusional and nondelusional body dysmorphic disorder in 100 cases. *Psychopharmacol Bull* 1994; **30**: 179–86.

5. Phillips KA. *The Broken Mirror: Understanding and Treating Body Dysmorphic Disorder* (revised and expanded edition). Oxford: Oxford University Press, 2005.

6. Phillips KA, McElroy SL, Keck PE Jr, Pope HG, Hudson JI. Body dysmorphic disorder: 30 cases of imagined ugliness. *Am J Psychiatry* 1993; **150**: 302–8.

7. Phillips KA, Menard W, Fay C. Gender similarities and differences in 200 individuals with body dysmorphic disorder. *Compr Psychiatr* 2006; **47**: 77–87.

8. Pope CG, Pope HG, Menard W, *et al.* Clinical features of muscle dysmorphia among males with body dysmorphic disorder. *Body Image* 2005; **2**: 395–400.

9. Grant JE, Menard W, Phillips KA. Pathological skin picking in individuals with body dysmorphic disorder. *Gen Psychiatry* 2006; **28**: 487–93.

10. Phillips KA, Taub SL. Skin picking as a symptom of body dysmorphic disorder. *Psychopharmacol Bull* 1995; **31**: 279–88.

11. Veale D, Boocock A, Gournay K, *et al.* Body dysmorphic disorder: a survey of fifty cases. *Br J Psychiatry* 1996; **169**: 196–201.

12. Crerand CE, Phillips KA, Menard W, Fay C. Non-psychiatric medical treatment of body dysmorphic disorder. *Psychosomatics* 2005; **46**: 549–55.

13. Phillips KA, Grant J, Siniscalchi J, Albertini RS. Surgical and nonpsychiatric medical treatment of patients with body dysmorphic disorder. *Psychosomatics* 2001; **42**: 504–10.

14. Sarwer DB, Crerand CE. Body dysmorphic disorder and appearance enhancing medical treatments. *Body Image* 2008; **5**: 50–8.

15. Phillips KA, Menard W. Suicidality in body dysmorphic disorder: a prospective study. *Am J Psychiatry* 2006; **163**: 1280–2.

16. Rief W, Buhlmann U, Wilhelm S, *et al.* The prevalence of body dysmorphic disorder: a population-based survey. *Psychol Med* 2006; **36**: 877–85.

17. Bienvenu OJ, Samuels JF, Riddle MA, *et al.* The relationship of obsessive–compulsive disorder to possible spectrum disorders: results from a family study. *Biol Psychiatry* 2000; **48**: 287–93.

18. Otto MW, Wilhelm S, Cohen LS, Harlow BL. Prevalence of body dysmorphic disorder in a community sample of women. *Am J Psychiatry* 2001; **158**: 2061–3.

19. Grant JE, Kim SW, Crow SJ. Prevalence and clinical features of body dysmorphic disorder in adolescent and adult psychiatric inpatients. *J Clin Psychiatry* 2001; **62**: 517–22.

20. Conroy M, Menard W, Fleming-Ives K, Modha P, Phillips KA. Prevalence and clinical characteristics of body dysmorphic disorder in an adult inpatient setting. *Gen Hosp Psychiatry* 2008; **30**: 67–72.

21. Phillips KA, Didie ER, Menard W. Clinical features and correlates of major depressive disorder in individuals with body dysmorphic disorder. *J Affect Disord* 2007; **97**: 129–35.

22. Nierenberg AA, Phillips KA, Peterson TJ, Kelly, *et al.* Body dysmorphic disorder in outpatients with major depression. *J Affect Disord* 2002; **69**: 141–8.

23. Wilhelm S, Otto MW, Zucker BG, Pollack MH. Prevalence of body dysmorphic disorder in patients with anxiety disorders. *J Anxiety Disord* 1997; **11**: 499–502.

24. Phillips KA, Dufresne RG, Wilkel C, Vittorio C. Rate of body dysmorphic disorder in dermatology patients. *J Am Acad Dermatol* 2000; **42**: 436–41.

25. Sarwer DB, Wadden TA, Pertschuk MJ, Whitaker LA. The psychology of cosmetic surgery: a review and reconceptualization. *Clin Psychol Rev* 1998; **18**: 1–22.

26. Crerand CE, Sarwer DB, Magee L, *et al.* Rate of body dysmorphic disorder among patients seeking facial cosmetic procedures. *Psychiat Ann* 2004; **34**: 958–65.

27. Phillips KA, Diaz SF. Gender differences in body dysmorphic disorder. *J Nerv Ment Dis* 1997; **185**: 570–7.

28. Gunstad J, Phillips KA. Axis I comorbidity in body dysmorphic disorder. *Compr Psychiatr* 2003; **44**: 270–6.

29. Neziroglu F, McKay D, Todaro J, Yaryura-Tobias JA. Effects of cognitive behavior therapy on persons with body dysmorphic disorder and comorbid axis II diagnoses. *Behav Ther* 1996; **27**: 67–77.

30. Phillips KA. Suicidality in body dysmorphic disorder. *Prim Psychiatry* 2007; **14**: 58–66.

31. Phillips KA, Coles ME, Menard W, *et al.* Suicidal ideation and suicide attempts in body dysmorphic disorder. *J Clin Psychiatry* 2005; **66**: 717–25.

32. Phillips KA. Quality of life for patients with body dysmorphic disorder. *J Nerv Ment Dis* 2000; **188**: 170–5.

33. Wilhelm S. *Feeling Good about the Way You Look: A Program for Overcoming Body Image Problems.* New York: Guilford Press, 2006.

34. Groesz LM, Levine MP, Murnen SK. The effect of experimental presentation of thin media images on body satisfaction: a meta-analytic review. *Int J Eat Disord* 2002; **31**: 1–16.

35. Buhlmann U, Cook LM, Fama JM, Wilhelm S. Perceived teasing experiences in body dysmorphic disorder. *Body Image* 2007; **4**: 381–5.

36. Warren CS, Gleaves DH, Cepeda-Benito A, del Carmen Fernandez M, Rodriguez-Ruiz S. Ethnicity as a protective factor against internalization of a thin ideal and body dissatisfaction. *Int J Eat Disord* 2005; **37**: 241–9.

37. Bohne A, Keuthen NJ, Wilhelm S, Deckersbach T, Jenike MA. Prevalence of symptoms of body dysmorphic disorder and its correlates: a cross-cultural comparison. *Psychosomatics* 2002; **43**: 486–90.

38. Hitzeroth V, Wessels C, Zungu-Dirwayi N, Oosthuizen P, Stein DJ. Muscle dysmorphia: a South African sample. *Psychiatry Clin Neurosci* 2001; **55**: 521–3.

39. Suzuki K, Takei N, Kawai M, Minabe Y, Mori N. Is taijin kyofusho a culture-bound syndrome? *Am J Psychiatry* 2003; **160**: 1358.

40. Ung EK, Fones CS, Ang AW. Muscle dysmorphia in a young Chinese male. *Ann Acad Med Singapore* 2000; **29**: 135–7.

41. Cansever A, Uzun O, Donmez E, Ozsahin A. The prevalence and clinical features of body dysmorphic disorder in college students: a study in a Turkish sample. *Compr Psychiatry* 2003; **44**: 60–4.

42. Faravelli C, Salvatori S, Galassi F, *et al.* Epidemiology of somatoform disorders: a community survey in Florence. *Soc Psychiatry Psychiatr Epidemiol* 1997; **32**: 24–9.

43. Tignol J, Biraben-Gotzamanis L, Martin-Guehl C, Grabot D, Aouizerate B. Body dysmorphic disorder and cosmetic surgery: evolution of 24 subjects with a minimal defect in appearance 5 years after their request for cosmetic surgery. *Eur Psychiatry* 2007; **22**: 520–4.

44. Fontenelle LF, Telles LL, Nazar BP, *et al.* A sociodemographic, phenomenological, and long-term follow-up study of patients with body dysmorphic disorder in Brazil. *Int J Psychiatry Med* 2006; **36**: 243–59.

45. Altabe MN. Issues in the assessment and treatment of body image disturbance in culturally diverse populations. In Thompson JK, ed., *Body Image, Eating Disorders, and Obesity: An Integrative Guide for Assessment and Treatment.* Washington, DC: American Psychological Association. 2001, pp. 129–47.

46. Kawamura KY. Asian American body images. In Cash TF, Pruzinsky T, eds., *Body Image: A Handbook of Theory, Research and Clinical Practice.* New York: Guilford Press. 2002, pp. 243–9.

47. Chowdhury AN. The definition and classification of koro. *Cult Med Psychiatry* 1996; **20**: 41–65.

48. Phillips KA. Body dysmorphic disorder: recognizing and treating imagined ugliness. *World Psychiatry* 2004; **3**: 12–17.

49. Altabe M, O'Garo KN. Hispanic body images. In Cash TF, Pruzinsky T, eds., *Body Image: A Handbook of Theory, Research and Clinical Practice.* New York: Guilford Press. 2002, pp. 250–6.

50. Buhlmann U, Etcoff NL, Wilhelm S. Facial attractiveness ratings and perfectionism in body dysmorphic disorder and obsessive–compulsive disorder. *J Anxiety Disord* 2008; **22**: 540–7.

51. Deckersbach T, Savage CR, Phillips KA, *et al.* Characteristics of memory dysfunction in body dysmorphic disorder. *J Int Neuropsych Soc* 2000; **6**: 673–81.

52. Feusner JD, Townsend J, Bystritsky A, Bookheimer S. Visual information processing of faces in body dysmorphic disorder. *Arch Gen Psychiatry* 2007; **64**: 1417–25.

53. Saxena S, Feusner JD. Toward a neurobiology of body dysmorphic disorder. *Prim Psychiatry* 2006; **13**: 41–8.

54. Hollander E, Allen A, Kwon J, *et al.* Clomipramine vs desipramine crossover trial in body dysmorphic disorder: selective efficacy of a serotonin reuptake inhibitor in imagined ugliness. *Arch Gen Psychiatry* 1999; **56**: 1033–9.

55. Perugi G, Giannotti D, Di Vaio S, *et al.* Fluvoxamine in the treatment of body dysmorphic disorder (dysmorphophobia). *Int Clin Psychopharmacol* 1996; **11**: 247–54.

56. Phillips KA, Dwight MM, McElroy SL. Efficacy and safety of fluvoxamine in body dysmorphic disorder. *J Clin Psychiatry* 1998; **59**: 165–71.

57. Phillips KA, Albertini RS, Rasmussen SA. A randomized placebo-controlled trial of fluoxetine in body dysmorphic disorder. *Arch Gen Psychiatry* 2002; **59**: 381–8.

58. Phillips KA, Najjar F. An open-label study of citalopram in body dysmorphic disorder. *J Clin Psychiatry* 2003; **64**: 715–20.

59. Phillips KA. An open-label study of escitalopram in body dysmorphic disorder. *Int Clin Psychopharmacol* 2006; **21**: 177–9.

60. Phillips KA, Hollander E. Treating body dysmorphic disorder with medication: evidence, misconceptions, and a suggested approach. Body Image. *Int Journal Res* 2008; **5**: 13–27.

61. McKay D, Todaro J, Neziroglu F, *et al.* Body dysmorphic disorder: a preliminary evaluation of treatment and maintenance using exposure with response prevention. *Behav Res Ther* 1997; **35**: 67–70.

62. Veale D, Gournay K, Dryden W, *et al.* Body dysmorphic disorder: a cognitive behavioural model and pilot randomized controlled trial. *Behav Res Ther* 1996; **34**: 717–29.

63. Wilhelm S, Otto MW, Lohr B, Deckersbach T. Cognitive behavior group therapy for body dysmorphic disorder: a case series. *Behav Res Ther* 1999; **37**: 71–5.

64. Rosen JC, Reiter J, Orosan P. Cognitive–behavioral body image therapy for body dysmorphic disorder. *J Consult Clin Psych* 1995; **63**: 263–9.

65. Williams J, Hadjistavropoulos T, Sharpe D. A meta-analysis of psychological and pharmacological treatments for body dysmorphic disorder. *Behav Res Ther* 2006; **44**: 99–111.

66. First MB, Spitzer RL, Gibbon M, Williams JB. *Structured Clinical Interview for DSM-IV-TR Axis I Disorders, Research Version, Patient Edition.* (SCID-I/P). New York: Biometrics Research, New York State Psychiatric Institute, 2002.

67. Phillips KA, Hollander E, Rasmussen SA, *et al.* A severity rating scale for body dysmorphic disorder: development, reliability, and validity of a modified version of the Yale–Brown Obsessive Compulsive Scale. *Psychopharmacol Bull* 1997; **33**: 17–22.

68. Beck AT, Steer RA, Brown GK. *Manual for the Beck Depression Inventory-II.* San Antonio, TX: Psychological Corporation, 1996.

69. Wilhelm S, Phillips KA, Steketee G. *A Cognitive Behavioral Treatment Manual for Body Dysmorphic Disorder.* New York: Guilford Press, in press.

70. Rosen JC. Cognitive–behavioral body image therapy. In Garner DM, Garfinkel PE, eds. *Handbook of Treatment for Eating Disorders*, 2nd edn. New York: Guilford Press. 2007, p. 188.

71. Marques L, Greenberg JL, Wilhelm S. *Adapting CBT for Ethnic Minorities, Children and Adolescents with BDD.* Proceedings of the 15th Annual OCF Conference; 2008 Aug 1–3; Boston, MA.

Mindfulness in cognitive–behavioral therapy

Lawrence D. Needleman and Cynthia Cushman[1]

Introduction

Mindfulness is a simple concept. Kabat-Zinn defined it simply as the process of "paying attention in a particular way: on purpose, in the present moment, and nonjudgmentally" [1: 4]. Lau *et al.* invoked mindfulness with this simple instruction: "For the next 15 minutes, please pay attention to your breathing and anything [else] that might arise during your experience" [2: 1450].

There are two sides to this simplicity. Richelle commented that "simple devices (as well as simple concepts) in science often seem to give better access to complex realities than complicated ones" [3: 26]. But sometimes simple concepts are merely simplistic; given the recent surge in popularity of mindfulness there is reason for caution. Too often, popularity brings hyperbole.

Our aim in writing this chapter is to provide a straightforward guide to the emerging work on mindfulness in cognitive–behavioral science, based both on our experience with mindfulness practices and on the rapidly-evolving empirical literature on mindfulness. We will look at general principles and also at three specific interventions: mindfulness-based cognitive therapy (MBCT), dialectical behavior therapy (DBT), and acceptance and commitment therapy (ACT). We will explore basic questions: What is the phenomenon of mindfulness? How is it defined? How is it applied in the clinic? What is the evidence for its efficacy?

The phenomenon of mindfulness

From our perspective, the key function of mindfulness is to discriminate between "direct" and "constructed" experience. Direct experience is simple, and close to immediate sensory experience. It has a "here and now" quality and often is described as "observing," "noticing," "paying attention to," "being aware of," or "watching." In contrast, constructed experience is

complex and involves higher (cortical) cognitive processing, such as verbalizing, interpreting, comparing, analyzing, judging, visualizing, imagining, predicting, planning, and remembering.

To say it differently, mindfulness points out the gap between what we think things are and what our senses tell us things are. Being mindful does not create the gap, or eliminate or change the gap. Mindfulness just brings it to light. Much of what we have to say about mindfulness derives from this simple view of the function of mindfulness. We believe it is useful to think about mindfulness as consisting of two components: noticing the direct experience of how things are, and noticing ideas about how things are as distinct from the things themselves.

Mindfulness of direct experience

A paradox that pervades the study of mindfulness hampers us in this discussion: every word we write is an idea, and not the experience itself. We hope, therefore, to begin with your direct experience of mindfulness before considering ideas about what mindfulness is. However, we cannot do so without your active engagement. If you would pay attention to your own current thoughts and feelings as you read, then your direct experience may provide living instances of what our words by themselves can merely point to. If you are willing to play along with this, please bring to mind one specific, brief moment in your life that fully engaged your interest. This might have been during a big event such as a wedding or a birth, or during a more ordinary moment while working, playing with your dog, singing,

---

1 The order of authorship does not reflect the degree of contribution. Both authors fully participated in all intellectual and technical facets of the chapter.

Cognitive–behavioral Therapy with Adults: A Guide to Empirically Informed Assessment and Intervention, ed. Stefan G. Hofmann and Mark A. Reinecke. © Cambridge University Press 2010.

walking in the woods – any activity that you naturally find deeply absorbing and intrinsically rewarding.

Now, rather than using words to describe the experience, please visualize that moment in your mind's eye. If you really linger in the details of the visualization, you may possibly experience the interested, engaged quality of that moment to some degree at this time.

We would like to highlight one aspect of that interested state of mind: the sense of being in direct sensory contact with the experiences of the moment – of really seeing, hearing, and feeling. During the interesting activity, one is *here*, rather than thinking about being here. It is not that thoughts are suppressed. One is simply completely engaged in vivid awareness of experience from one's own current perspective. Later on, one may tell stories about this event, but in the moment the mind is silent. This is an instance of spontaneous mindfulness of "direct" experience. Note that experiencing an event directly is not the same as experiencing the absolute truth of the event. Experience is always filtered by the perceptual apparatus and biased by the time and location of one's perspective. Direct experience simply means that it is as direct as it can be.

Mindfulness of direct experience occurs spontaneously and fully during those rare times in life when there is no perceived threat or perceived deprivation. It happens when one is quite interested, or when one is in a state of relaxed alertness. Such moments are uncommon even for long-time practitioners of mindfulness techniques. However, one can choose to deliberately increase one's mindful attention during ordinary life under any conditions. This relative independence from internal and external conditions sets mindfulness apart from states of flow and relaxation. One can be mindful of boredom, mindful of anxiety, and so on.

Mindfulness is not an all-or-nothing phenomenon. With practice, one can increase the probability of becoming more mindful than one might naturally be in a given situation. Thus, the dissociating client who deliberately feels the temperature of her fingertips, notes that she still is somewhat dissociated, and worries that she is not doing the exercise right, is engaged in mindfulness practice. Over time, she may begin to observe the worries themselves simply as transient events that do not have to capture her full attention. She might begin to notice other thoughts and sounds and sights, so that her contact with experience becomes wider and richer. All of this is mindfulness. Mindfulness is sometimes compared to a light that illuminates whatever object it happens to shine on, without changing that object in any way. With practice, one learns to shine the light on a wider range of experiences and to notice what is illuminated in greater detail.

Direct experience only reveals the world in this moment, from one first-person perspective. It does not invoke the past, the future, or places or perspectives other than here, which are all ideas. Thus, there is a directionless or purposeless quality to it. It exists for its own sake and is complete in itself. Mindfulness does not solve problems or accomplish anything. (It is rather like basic science, or love.)

Mindfulness of direct experience seamlessly blends into other purposeless and intrinsically rewarding states such as curiosity, interest, discovery, acceptance, and compassion – all of which invite an affiliative relationship with other people and the world. In theory and as part of scientific inquiry, mindfulness may be separated out from these other states, but in practice they usually occur together.

Mindfulness of constructed experience

The well known Stroop effect sheds light on the relationship between direct experience and constructed verbal experience. The Stroop task presents a list of color names written in incongruently colored letters (e.g., the word "red" written in green) and asks subjects to name the colors of the words rather than to read the words. The Stroop effect is the delay and error rate of this task compared with simply reading the words. Once we are literate, reading is so automatic that we usually are not aware of the actual symbols on the page.

More generally, initial appraisal of a situation can obscure accurate perception of that situation. Thought impersonates reality with relentless automaticity, as illustrated by the fact that one is more likely to salivate over the words "fresh-baked chocolate chip cookie" than over the words "beady-eyed rat." What the observer *directly* sees above are sets of black shapes against a white background. The mind tends to respond with learned associated mental images that have enough verisimilitude to trigger affective and autonomic responses.

The automaticity and verisimilitude of thought makes it difficult to detect. People typically do not know how much they think, or how much the process of thinking distorts awareness of direct experience. One illustration comes from a study of "attentional blindness" [4]. In one part of the study, subjects watched a short video of a basketball-tossing game and counted the number of passes made. During the video, a person in a gorilla suit ambled through the middle of the game, faced the camera, and did some chest-thumping before strolling away. When asked later if they had seen this, approximately half of the subjects said they had not.

Cognitive constructs mimic and obscure reality so constantly and so successfully that people generally do not even know that this is happening. Yet, this is most often not a problem but rather a way to solve problems. Recall that direct experience has a direction-less or purposeless quality to it. In contrast, the con-structed domain has been called the "doing" mode of mind [5:70]. It is essential for solving problems, making progress, understanding complexities, plan-ning for the future, remembering facts, exerting con-trol, and changing circumstances. In the doing mode, the mind compares an *idea* of how things are with an *idea* of how they should be. The gap between the two ideas generates urges and emotions that motivate purpose-driven action.

The ubiquitous, rapid, and automatic nature of this doing-mode process, and the fact that it emerges most potently when there is a perceived threat or deprivation, suggests that it may have been selected evolutionarily for survival. In times of actual threat, this driven, narrowly focused, escape-oriented action can be life saving. However, since verbal processes are disconnected from direct experience they are capable of generating a sense of urgency in any setting, even when there is no actual danger. Thus, it is not just actual risk of violence that one feels compelled to escape but memories of long-past victimization and anything that by remotest association begins to stir those memories.

Since mindfulness sheds light on internal processes without changing them, it leaves the content of thought undisturbed but changes one's perspective on thinking. Hayes (2002) commented that the

> "illusion of language is that one is dealing with the world through thought. In fact, one is actively structuring the world through thought ... It is language and cognition that accomplish this feat, but the process is automatic and transparent. It appears to the thinker that one is simply dealing with the structured world, not that one is struc-turing as an ongoing process. Mindfulness and acceptance catch this bird in flight, and like an audience that learns how a magic trick is

accomplished, they can profoundly change the effects of the language illusion" [6: 104].

Clinical applications of mindfulness

The fact that mindfulness occurs intermittently, partially, and in company with other affiliative states allows it to weave into daily life and into clinical practice. Rather than an extra thing to do, mindful-ness is a way of doing ordinary things simply and without verbal elaboration. In clinical practice, being mindful means slowing down and investigating all current experiences without immediately attempting to improve one's circumstances or to reduce symp-toms. The MBCT manual terms this relationship to experience "decentering" and states: "The stance of the mindful approach is one of welcoming and allowing. It is invitational. It encourages 'opening' to the difficult and adopting an attitude of gentleness to all experience" [5:58]. During the fifth session of MBCT the therapist reads to the group these lines from Rumi's poem *The Guest House*, as translated by Coleman Barks:

> The dark thought, the shame, the malice.
> Meet them at the door laughing,
> and invite them in. [5: p. 222]

This counterintuitive approach to symptoms requires courage and strong motivation on the part of the client. It is justified when past attempts at symptom reduction have not worked and future attempts are likely to fail. From a mindfulness perspective, it appears that reason-able, universal, and necessary verbal change and control strategies can sometimes backfire when applied to inner experiences. Acceptance and commitment therapy, MBCT, and DBT all rest on theories suggesting that counterproductive attempts to reduce intense symp-toms are a driving force behind refractory conditions such as addiction, borderline personality disorder, and recurrent major depression. These theories portray mindfulness as an effective stance to take at times. Knowing how to take this stance opens up the freedom to choose between fixing circumstances and letting them be as they are, depending on what works best in a given context and for a particular purpose.

These theories also suggest that excessive and automatic attempts to reduce distress actually fixate attention on dysfunction and away from what ACT calls "values" [7] and DBT describes as building "a life worth living" [8: 118]. Generally speaking, what makes life worth living for a person is contact with certain subjectively valued, unquantifiable experiences: the sense of discovery, of intimacy, of creativity, of belonging, of vitality, or of meaning in one's life. One detects the presence of these experiences directly, not cognitively. One *feels* "interested," "alive," "connected," or "moved" in certain situations more readily than others, regardless of whether one *thinks* one should. Helping the client to identify these types of situations and orienting therapy around them is central to ACT and DBT and is implicit in MBCT. Value orientation provides motivation and meaning for the often-painful work of mindfulness-based therapies. It also provides an important way to evaluate the progress of treatment. If the client is subjectively experiencing life as richer and more worth living, then therapy is serving its essential purpose regardless of the presence or absence of symptoms.

As an illustration, a patient admitted to the hospital following a near-lethal suicide attempt remained actively suicidal for several weeks. During a family meeting, his normally-stoic mother began to weep as she imagined out loud what it would be like for her if he died by suicide. He flushed, his expression softened, and a single tear rolled down his cheek as he watched her face. His therapist gently invited him to notice what was happening, and to let it happen. Later on, still crying, he said, "This is very strange . . . I'm in agony, and I feel alive, and I feel completely committed to staying alive." Long after this session, he continued to cry readily as he rebuilt his life. When reflecting on process he commented, "As long as I can cry, I'm OK."

Just as the mindfulness approach does not attempt to remove symptoms related to emotional content, it also does not attempt to change the content of thought. Segal *et al.* suggest that through mindfulness practice "we may eventually come to realize deep 'in our bones' *that all thoughts are only mental events* (including thoughts that say they are not), that *thoughts are not facts*, and that *we are not our thoughts*" [5: 262] (emphasis in original). This change in perspective on thinking is a form of decentering from experience. In ACT theory, this is termed "defusion," which is considered to be one of the core processes of mindfulness [7].

Learning to take a mindful and accepting stance as a therapist is difficult. Human beings naturally seek to solve problems. Not doing so can be challenging. Working with mindfulness in the clinic requires a subtle but fundamental shift in perspective. This shift does not come from reading ideas about mindfulness but from directly practicing it. Dialectical behavior therapy, ACT, and MBCT all offer experiential training workshops and require therapists to have some first-person experience with mindfulness practices prior to using their interventions with clients [5, 7, 9].

There are two general types of mindfulness training. Informal practices simply involve deliberately bringing awareness to ordinary events. For instance, one might carefully attend to the cadence and pitch of speech during conversation. Formal mindfulness practices involve pausing and refraining from ordinary activities to practice mindfulness meditation or another type of mindfulness exercise. For example, a therapist might ask a client to pause and notice what part of the left hand is the coolest. Mindfulness-based cognitive therapy, ACT, and DBT all teach both formal and informal mindfulness techniques, but only MBCT builds the daily practice of formal mindfulness meditation into its protocol [5].

The most important way to bring mindfulness into clinical practice is through the clinician's own in-session mindfulness. Awareness and acceptance may be common to all effective therapies whether or not they are called "mindfulness based." Expanding one's capacity for awareness is worth deliberate and persistent practice. Potential benefits of clinician mindfulness include strengthened therapeutic relationships and heightened awareness of subtle therapeutic processes.

Although all therapy probably works best when clinicians are mindful during sessions, training clients in mindfulness is only warranted in some circumstances. The decision to offer mindfulness training – or any other intervention – should be the result of a clear case conceptualization that indicates that mindfulness is likely the most effective approach given the situation. There is some evidence that employing mindfulness interventions when they are not indicated may be harmful [10].

Also, leading clients in effective mindfulness exercises is vastly more difficult than it seems. Without extensive practice in a setting in which one can receive comprehensive feedback, putative mindfulness exercises can inadvertently take on the function of relaxation or cognitive restructuring exercises. Indeed, we have repeatedly observed researchers and clinicians unknowingly lead ineffective mindfulness exercises.

Of even greater concern is the fact that clients frequently initially misinterpret the therapist's "mindfulness" instructions as a criticism of their cognitive content, which can set off shame, ruminations, and vigorous attempts at thought suppression. Therapists who have inadequate mindfulness skills training typically do not recognize that this is happening and do not know how to move the exercise back into the intended direction.

We suggest learning to lead mindfulness exercises by studying one of the recommended reference books and trying mindfulness exercises yourself. Then practice implementing mindfulness exercises by recording yourself and listening to those recordings. Finally, guide colleagues in brief mindfulness exercises and ask for their honest feedback. What they hear you say may be surprisingly different from what you intend to convey. We cannot overemphasize how important it is to seek this supervision, particularly from peers who are themselves familiar with the mindfulness paradigm. Another way to become proficient at engaging mindfulness in the clinic is to learn one of the mindfulness and acceptance-based therapies. These combine mindfulness with change-oriented strategies in complex therapeutic packages. We review three of these in this chapter.

Acceptance and commitment therapy (ACT)

Acceptance and commitment therapy is a behavioral intervention rooted in basic research on language and cognition [7]. The applied theoretical model derived from that research attributes both frank psychopathology and ordinary human unhappiness to universal and normal language-based processes. Acceptance and commitment therapy aims to decrease the avoidance of unwanted cognitive content and feelings and to increase "psychological flexibility – the ability to contact the present moment more fully as a conscious human being and to change or persist in behavior when doing so serves valued ends" [11: 7]. Acceptance and commitment therapy targets six processes related to mindfulness and behavioral change: (1) contact with the present moment; (2) acceptance; (3) cognitive defusion (observing thoughts as thoughts vs. believing them literally); (4) self as context ("a sense of self as a locus or perspective" rather than over-identification with *ideas* about the self [11: 9]); (5) values (that which gives meaning to one's life) and; (6) committed action.

Since ACT processes are regarded as universal, interventions are not limited to specific populations or conditions. Instead, ACT trains clinicians to have a strong practical understanding of ACT theory so they can work flexibly within the model, adapting or creating techniques based on what is needed. (Researchers have of course created protocols, which are essential for research and helpful for novice therapists.) Techniques include using metaphors and a wide range of brief experiential mindfulness exercises, values clarification tasks, and standard behavioral interventions. The following excerpt from an ACT session demonstrates several ACT processes. Rosita presented with chronic anxiety. Early in therapy, she identified "being emotionally present" with her family as a value that matters to her more than anything else does, and she identified spending more time with her son Pablo as a committed action that would serve this value. However, when asked to imagine sitting on the floor playing blocks with him, she became visibly tremulous.

THERAPIST: Are you willing to stay with this image, to open to this . . . ? [acceptance process]
ROSITA: Yes
THERAPIST: OK, try not to change or slow what you're experiencing . . . try to allow yourself to feel and think whatever you're feeling and thinking without defense [present moment awareness and acceptance processes] . . . (pauses for a few minutes). What do you notice?

The therapist then encouraged the client to observe carefully and without judgment her moment-to-moment, ever-changing experiences. He invited her to explore and describe bodily sensations, emotions, cognitions, and urges to escape or change her experiences. Then he continued:

THERAPIST: What is your mind saying about this? [cognitive defusion processes]
ROSITA: "This is silly, I shouldn't feel anxious about relaxing, there's nothing to fear, try harder to relax, it's really important!"
THERAPIST: So, let's notice that your mind is trying to help you have a happier life, and it seems wholly reasonable in what it's saying, doesn't it? [cognitive defusion process]
ROSITA: Yes.
THERAPIST: However, let's look at what your experience tells you about whether this in fact helps you engage and connect better with Pablo. [cognitive defusion and values processes].
ROSITA: Well . . . I get so preoccupied with getting rid of the anxious thoughts and feelings that even if I stay with my boy, I'm not with him.

THERAPIST: Hmmm, that sounds important. So, even though your mind says this is helpful, perhaps it doesn't work, it only makes it worse [cognitive defusion process] . . . Would you be willing to experiment with this and explore it some more? [committed action process]

ROSITA: Yes.

THERAPIST: What ways might you like to try this? [committed action process]

ROSITA: I'd like to play with Pablo and see if I can let the feelings be there without trying to get rid of them and see what happens and see if I can have those feelings and still be there with him.

THERAPIST: Emotionally?

ROSITA: Yes, emotionally.

It is important to note that this intervention involves intentional exposure to avoided thoughts and feelings, but the goal was not to reduce symptoms (habituation). Rather, it was to increase acceptance of these experiences in the service of pursuing an activity that is highly important to her.

Criticisms of ACT

Unfortunately, over the past several decades, literally hundreds of individuals have developed what they claim are new and effective psychotherapies, and many of these claims are false or at least empirically unproven. When such a claim is made, it is important not only to determine whether and for what populations the new therapy is effective, but also to determine whether it is indeed new in meaningful ways. Does it use meaningfully different procedures, or work by different mechanism than empirically established treatments?[2]

Consistent with the above concerns about new therapies making unsubstantiated claims of uniqueness, some researchers have questioned whether ACT is novel. On the one hand, Arch and Craske suggested that on the surface traditional CBT and ACT are quite different[3] [13]. For example, the goal of traditional CBT is to reduce symptoms, whereas, the goal of ACT is valued living irrespective of symptoms. These

differing goals are reflected in apparently different interventions. A primary intervention in traditional CBT is cognitive restructuring of unpleasant cognitive content. Also, traditional CBT clients are often taught relaxation or breathing techniques to decrease symptoms. In contrast, ACT interventions typically involve deliteralizing (i.e., "defusing") cognitive content without trying to change it and involve accepting unwanted feelings.

On the other hand, Arch and Craske suspected that some of the same underlying processes – such as exposure, reducing avoidance of thoughts and feelings, and defusion – are common to the two types of treatment. They suggested that much research on mediators is needed to determine which processes are common to both therapies and which are not. The authors suggest many thoughtful research questions for helping to clarify the similarities and differences.

Hofmann and Asmundson also acknowledged a number of differences between ACT and traditional CBT but believe that they are more similar than different [14]. They suggested that CBT uses antecedent-focused emotional regulatory strategies, such as teaching clients to reappraise external or internal emotion cues and that ACT uses consequence-focused strategies, such as discouraging thought suppression. However, these researchers emphasized that both ACT and CBT help clients adaptively regulate emotion. They also indicated that both are collaborative, use behavioral interventions, and are problem focused. Hofmann and Asmundson view ACT and CBT strategies as compatible and believe each might provide advantages in particular circumstances.

In a separate article Hofmann suggested that ACT interventions are not specific to ACT theory and philosophy [15]. To illustrate this proposition, he highlighted parallels between ACT and a holistic Eastern type of therapy entitled Morita therapy.

Hayes acknowledges that many ACT techniques overlap with CBT or were adapted from other therapies and traditions [16]. However, these techniques are embedded within an explicitly stated philosophy and testable basic theory, which is being examined through a growing body of basic research. This reflects a commitment to a deliberate model of scientific development of clinical interventions. For example, the ACT intervention of cognitive defusion emerged from ACT's basic theory of cognition and language, relational frame theory. In addition, the handful of studies that have compared ACT with

---

2 Regrettably, the criteria for Empirically Supported Treatments adopted by the American Psychological Association's Committee on Science and Practice do not include evidence for uniqueness [12].

3 It should be noted that the term "traditional" CBT is misleading because CBT is continually evolving. However, calling it simply "CBT" is confusing for our purposes here because ACT considers itself a CBT approach.

traditional CBT (described below) found that the two therapies exhibited different processes of change, suggesting that ACT might turn out to be a novel intervention. Because of ACT's commitment to component and mediational analysis, over time it should be able to address convincingly the questions of uniqueness and which procedures are effective.

From our perspective, the debate between traditional CBT proponents and ACT is becoming increasingly fruitful. We hope it will continue to stimulate interest, energy, insight, and important research questions in both fields.

Mindfulness-based cognitive therapy

Mindfulness-based cognitive therapy is an eight-week group experiential education program designed to prevent relapse in patients with recurrent depression [5]. It is based on cognitive theory and data suggesting that learning to "decenter" from thoughts, emotions, and body sensations is key to preventing relapse. The program is a hybrid in that the theory and problem formulation are rooted in the cognitive therapy (CT) perspective while the techniques are a blend of CT exercises and the mindfulness-based stress reduction (MBSR) program's secularized Buddhist practices. The highly structured weekly classes generally begin with a lengthy guided meditation. For example: "feel your breath moving in your abdomen . . . tuning in to sensation and feeling the full length of the inbreath . . . the full length of the outbreath . . . bringing a gentle curiosity to your experience in this moment, as it is . . . however it is . . . and as you notice the mind being distracted by thoughts or images, bringing the same gentle curiosity to seeing whatever it is that has distracted the mind . . . noticing it, and then gently bringing attention back to the breath, the simple movement of breath in the body." The meditation is followed by discussion of participants' observations, homework review, brief experiential exercises with themes such as "thoughts are not facts," and the assignment of an hour of nightly meditation homework. Classes are instructed by cognitive therapists who have their own daily mindfulness meditation practices and who attempt to embody the stance of "opening to the difficult" with friendly curiosity and kindly interest.

Dialectical behavior therapy

In its original form, DBT is a year-long outpatient program for the treatment of borderline personality disorder [9]. It has also been adapted for other populations and conditions. Dialectical behavior therapy is rooted in behavioral science, dialectical philosophy, and Zen Buddhism's mindfulness practice. The goal of DBT is to decrease reactive behaviors, including suicide, that are associated with dysregulated emotions, and to establish a life that is worth living. The therapeutic stance synthesizes complete acceptance and validation of the client just as he or she is in this moment with a relentless dedication to effective behavioral change. Irreverent humor, warmth, and a strong therapeutic alliance are hallmarks of this approach. The standard DBT protocol provides for weekly individual therapy with homework assignments, skills-coaching phone calls between sessions, and a weekly skills-training group. The group follows a structured manual with four modules: (1) interpersonal effectiveness; (2) emotion regulation; (3) distress tolerance; and (4) mindfulness. The mindfulness module is central and is taught all year. It involves the development of "wise mind" (a synthesis of reason and emotion), and the development of three "what" skills – observing, describing, and participating – and three "how" skills that specify how to practice the "what" skills – non-judgmentally, one-mindfully, and effectively.

The following excerpt from Welch, Rizvi, and Dimidjian illustrates mindfulness work with Hannah, a woman with borderline personality disorder, who commented early in therapy "'I just feel like other people have these souls and I just have this blank, it's like white space inside me . . . it's like I can't even tell what I'll do, one moment to the next'" [8: 127]. When she later asked her therapist for advice on whether to accept money from her mother, the therapist suggested she address the question through wise mind. Hannah had concerns that she would be incapable of experiencing wise mind and that wise mind might violate her religious beliefs. The therapist explored these concerns with her until she seemed willing to proceed.

> T: Well, let's just breathe together for a moment and focus, so just focus on your breath for the next few minutes . . . [moments pass] Okay, now just ask yourself this question, and then just wait and listen and see what you get. What should I do? Should I take the money? Don't force anything, just observe and see what happens . . .
>
> H: [looks up, tearful] Oh . . .
>
> T: What did you notice?
>
> H: I have to let her help, this isn't about me.

T: That's what you got?

H: Yes . . .

T: Do you think it was your wise mind?

H: I still don't know if it's listening to the Holy Spirit or to wise mind or whatever, but I see what you're talking about. It's the strangest thing, I guess I just felt like I knew . . . [8: 129]

The interface of mindfulness and science

Hayes and Wilson suggested that

> mindfulness [and related states] are not just a different way of treating traditionally conceptualized problems of depression or anxiety. They imply a redefinition of the problem, the solution, and how both should be measured. The problem is not the presence of particular thoughts, emotions, sensations, or urges; it is the constriction of a human life. The solution is not removal of difficult private events; it is living a valued life." [17: 165]

While most studies of mindfulness-based interventions currently report outcomes in terms of symptom reduction, this misses the potential contribution of the mindfulness component of those interventions. The conundrum for the science of mindfulness is how to define and measure the essentially non-verbal and unquantifiable experiences that make people's lives worth living. More generally, we believe that psychotherapy studies should undertake this challenge and develop increasingly effective means of measuring valued activities and quality of life.

A second challenge for the field of mindfulness is how to define "mindfulness." Mindfulness is a non-verbal phenomenon. To discuss mindfulness scientifically, it is necessary to bring it into the verbal realm through the construction of verbal proxies. In a sense, when we state "A is B," we are creating a kind of metaphor, which can transform psychological functions from A to B for the listener. Effective and widely used metaphors readily become invisible, automatic, and convincingly equivalent to actual phenomena. Thus, there is the very real risk that scientific definitions of mindfulness will obscure what they are designed to clarify, particularly when taken literally. On the other hand, if one reads about, thinks about, and discusses mindfulness mindfully – returning again and again to awareness of the discrimination between the experience itself and ideas about the experience – then one will anticipate that there are many useful ways to define

mindfulness. None of them are the thing itself, but each may be useful in a particular context and for a specific purpose.

Operationalizing and analyzing mindfulness as a construct: scientific definitions of mindfulness

We have discussed mindfulness as a non-verbal phenomenon that is without purpose and yet relates to subjectively valued qualities that give meaning to suffering and bring a sense of interconnection with the world. The difficult fact is that mindfulness is linked to phenomena that people usually think of as "spiritual." Creating a science of mindfulness thus entails addressing two historically awkward companions. Kabat-Zinn was among the first to secularize mindfulness training and study. He initially developed mindfulness-based stress reduction (MBSR), a flexible multicomponent educational intervention, to address the impact of chronic pain and other refractory medical conditions. Numerous outcomes studies have found that MBSR tends to produce medium-sized, positive outcomes in a wide range of clinical and non-clinical populations [18]. However, the early research had important shortcomings in terms of scientific rigor. It is also open to criticism from a spiritual perspective since it defined outcomes in terms of symptom reduction.

Some researchers called for a consensus definition of mindfulness in order to develop conceptual frameworks for understanding it and instruments for measuring its effects on clinical populations [19, 20]. Several independent research groups operationalized the mindfulness construct and developed psychometrically-sound mindfulness scales [2, 21–25]. Each scale showed expected patterns of relationships with other psychological constructs. They tended to relate positively with measures of psychological well-being and health, and negatively with symptoms measures. Although in the very early stages of research, in some studies that used these scales, mindfulness scores were shown to relate to other clinically-relevant processes and outcomes – such as meditation experience, personality-disorder status, and outcome of mindfulness training or treatment.

The medium-sized intercorrelation between mindfulness scales suggests that they overlap but also are measuring quite different phenomena. This is probably because when developing their mindfulness instruments, the different research groups had unique perspectives and different aims, and they studied different populations.

For instance, Brown and colleagues were particularly interested in advancing the study of consciousness. They considered mindfulness to be "fundamentally a quality of consciousness" [26: 212] defined as *a receptive attention to and awareness of present events and experience*" [26: 212] (emphasis in original). They explicitly distinguished mindfulness from psychological processes or skills that lead to the development of mindfulness including a general attitude of non-judging or acceptance, as well as specific skills such as labeling thoughts or emotions. They began their extensive and careful development of what would become the widely used Mindfulness Attention Awareness Scale (MAAS) with only items that they believed were congruent with these qualities of attention and awareness. Factor analyses revealed that a unidimensional model best fit the data [21].

In marked contrast, Baer *et al.* approached mindfulness from a clinical behavioral perspective rooted specifically in DBT. They described it as "a set of skills that can be learned and practiced in order to reduce psychological symptoms and increase health and well-being" [27: 27]. They developed the Kentucky Inventory of Mindfulness Skills (KIMS) as a multi-dimensional scale reflecting five component skills: (1) observing; (2) describing; (3) acting with awareness; (4) non-judging of inner experience; and (5) non-reactivity to inner experience. Factor analyses found that five factors corresponding to these skills represented the best fit of the data [27].

Lau and colleagues viewed mindfulness from a cognitive viewpoint, seeing it not as a skill set but as "a state of curious, decentered awareness of one's experience" [2: 1462]. They found their Toronto Mindfulness Scale (TMS) to consist of two factors. One factor was curiosity, defined as "an attitude of wanting to learn more about one's experiences." The second was decentering, "a shift from identifying personally with thoughts and feelings to relating to one's experiences in a wider field of awareness" [2: 1460–1].

Cardaciotto *et al.* were interested in contributing to a more detailed understanding of the components of mindfulness primarily for theoretical rather than applied purposes [25]. They developed the Philadelphia Mindfulness Scale (PMS) to measure what they considered to be the two separable but interacting facets of mindfulness: awareness and acceptance. According to Cardaciotto *et al.*, awareness is "the continuous monitoring of experience with a focus on current experience" [25: 205]. They explicitly differentiate awareness from attention. They define acceptance as a stance in which "one lets go of judgment, interpretation, and/or elaboration of internal events and makes no attempt to change, avoid or escape from the internal experience" [25: 205]. Factor analyses suggest that the two-factor solution best fits the data, and the factors showed the expected patterns of relationships with other psychological constructs and differentiated clinical from non-clinical populations.

Kabat-Zinn's famous colloquial definition of mindfulness opened this chapter: "paying attention in a particular way: on purpose, in the present moment, and nonjudgmentally." Currently, there is no agreement on whether attention and non-judgmental acceptance should be considered components of mindfulness. There is no agreement on whether mindfulness is a set of skills or a quality of consciousness. In short, there is no consensus definition of mindfulness. Moreover, while there are still calls for such a consensus definition [26], we believe it is unlikely that a meaningful consensus can ever be possible. Familiarity with the phenomenon of mindfulness leads to a friendly defusion from the belief that any of these definitions can be final or comprehensive, combined with an appreciation of just how well each definition brings some of the authentic flavor of mindfulness into scientific discourse.

Empirical studies of mindfulness therapies

In this section, we will discuss empirical studies of ACT, MBCT, and DBT.

Acceptance and commitment therapy (ACT) studies

The approach ACT researchers are using to develop the ACT model is unique in the psychotherapy field, and we believe it should be a model for research in all applied fields. Acceptance and commitment therapy alternates between induction and deduction to advance its theoretical model and interventions [11]. By way of history, behavioral analytic methods were shown to be highly effective for populations without well developed language skills (e.g., very young, developmentally disabled) but ineffective with other populations (e.g., adult outpatients). To broaden the applicability of behavioral analytic methods, ACT researchers spent many years conducting basic research on cognition and language. The result of this work was their relational frame theory (RFT) [7]. From the theory, ACT researchers derived treatment components, which they tested individually in the laboratory with non-clinical and clinical samples. This approach is in contrast to traditional CBT that has demonstrated the effectiveness of large treatment packages. But typically, only years after initially demonstrating efficacy – after widely disseminating treatment packages – do traditional CBT researchers attempt to dismantle the treatment packages to determine which components are effective. Unfortunately, by the time large-scale dismantling studies are performed, when a component is found to not add benefit or even to be associated with poorer outcomes, it often is too late to change the established practices of clinicians in the field. In addition to ongoing component analysis studies, ACT researchers have shown a strong commitment to understanding key processes that influence psychological dysfunction, psychological health, and response to treatment. They have worked at developing measures of key processes and often performed rigorous mediational analyses to test and refine the theoretical model and to determine whether ACT intervention components influence theoretically-consistent processes.

Component analysis studies: cognitive defusion

Rather than attempting to change the content or frequency of a person's thoughts, cognitive defusion techniques are designed to change the context in which thoughts occur, by helping people stop taking their thoughts to be literally true – to be believed, disputed, or followed. Two studies examined the effects of cognitive defusion. Masuda *et al.* compared a defusion condition – in which participants rapidly repeated a personally-relevant disturbing word – with distraction and thought control conditions [28]. In Healy *et al.* [29], participants were presented with negative self-statements on a computer screen in a defused format, consisting of the sentence stem: "I am having the thought that . . . " followed by a self-statement, or they were exposed to one of two non-defused formats. Both studies found that the defused condition resulted in significantly less distress than the other conditions. Masuda *et al.* found that defusion resulted in a reduction in believability of thoughts versus the control conditions, whereas the believability findings in Healy *et al.* were ambiguous.

Component analysis studies: acceptance versus control

To date, most component analysis studies were experimental analog studies that compared acceptance to control, suppression or distraction. Among studies of laboratory-based anxiety or pain challenges, several compared acceptance versus control strategies in clinical and non-clinical samples. In some of these studies, acceptance and control rationales and instructions were combined with an emphasis on valued life directions and activities, whereas in others, the focus was exclusively acceptance versus control. Studies of acceptance versus control predominantly suggest that acceptance strategies are superior to control or suppression conditions.

We found only three published studies in clinical settings in which acceptance and control rationales/instructions were compared. In two of these studies, patients with panic disorder [30] or anxiety and mood disorders [31] were exposed to distress-provoking laboratory challenges (panic patients inhaling carbon dioxide, anxious and depressed patients viewing a disturbing film). In the third, Vowles *et al.* studied low-back pain patients in a treatment setting [32]. In each of these studies, the acceptance conditions outperformed the control conditions.

In laboratory-based experiments of non-clinical samples challenged with acute pain, those in acceptance conditions endured the pain longer, experienced less distress, and/or recovered more quickly than those in control conditions [33–36]. In an analog experiment of coping with food cravings, Forman *et al.* found that whether participants benefited from acceptance- versus control-based strategies depended on whether they had a particular vulnerability at baseline (i.e., high baseline level of psychological sensitivity to food environment) [37]. Forman *et al.*'s findings suggest that tailoring coping strategy interventions to patients with different characteristics can be important. In another analog study, Marcks and Woods studied the role of acceptance versus thought suppression in the escalation of intrusive thoughts following a procedure designed to elicit OCD-like thinking (i.e., "thought–action fusion") [38]. Results of this study were mixed. As predicted, participants randomly assigned to an acceptance group had a larger decrease in frequency of intrusion thoughts over time than the suppression group. In addition, compared to the thought suppression group, the acceptance-based group exhibited greater willingness to re-experience the intrusive thoughts at the later time point. However, contrary to predictions, the two groups exhibited similar decreases in anxiety over time and did not significantly differ on several other variables.

Studies of ACT processes and mediational analysis

The best developed and most widely used measure of ACT process is the Acceptance and Action Questionnaire (AAQ), which is a measure of psychological flexibility or acceptance versus avoidance of thoughts and feelings. Hayes *et al.* cited a large number of studies (32 studies, $n = 6,628$, 74 correlations) that examined the correlations between the AAQ and measures of psychopathology and quality of life [11]. All of the correlations were in the expected direction, indicating that the AAQ was associated with less psychopathology and better quality of life, and, on average, these correlations were in the medium range. Longitudinal studies suggest that AAQ psychological flexibility predicted mental health but not vice versa. Several versions of the AAQ and several AAQ-like, population-specific measures have been developed.

Mediational analysis attempts to determine whether a hypothesized mediating variable affects the relationship between a predictor and a criteria variable. Some mediational studies test models of psychopathology and health by clarifying the relationships between hypothesized variables. Other mediational studies explore what factors account for the relationship between treatment and outcome. To convincingly demonstrate mediation, formal and rigorous statistical methods are necessary. Mediation is demonstrated when, after statistically removing the effects of potential mediator variables, the relationship between predictor and criteria is significantly *reduced* (though not necessarily or typically reduced to zero).

A clear strength of the ACT outcome literature is that in nearly every study, researchers have included process measures, and many studies included formal mediational analyses. In nearly every ACT mediational study – both outcome studies and studies of the ACT model – the hypothesized mediator evidenced mediation between the predictor and criteria variables. The hypothesized mediator in most of the studies was psychological flexibility as measured by the AAQ or population-specific versions thereof. However, in some studies, other hypothesized ACT mediators were examined. For example, values attainment [39], persistence in the face of barriers or committed action [39], degree of belief in depressive thoughts [11], and degree of belief in hallucinations [40, 41] were examined.

Acceptance and commitment therapy studies used a variety of formal mediational statistical methods to determine mediation: Baron and Kenny's regression equations [42–45], Preacher and Hayes' bootstrapped multivariate extension of the Sobel test [39, 46, 47], and MacKinnon's cross-product of the coefficients approach [11]. Ideally, mediational studies also use experimental designs that address temporal precedence, whether early changes in the hypothesized mediator are related to later changes in outcome. Many ACT studies [39–42, 48, 49] used such designs.

Below we review the seven ACT outcome studies that also included mediational analyses. The first six used designs that permitted determining whether there was a temporal relationship between mediators and outcome [39–42, 48, 49]. In each study that assessed the temporal relationship, temporal precedence was in fact established. Three studies targeted psychological problems [40, 48, 49], and the rest targeted behavioral medicine conditions: diabetes, weight management, smoking cessation, and epilepsy [39, 42, 46, 47]. All but one were randomized controlled trials.

Acceptance and commitment therapy outcome studies with formal mediational analysis including determination of temporal precedence

Dalrymple and Herbert conducted an uncontrolled, preliminary investigation with patients diagnosed with general social anxiety disorder [48]. Patients received a 12-week ACT-plus-exposure treatment. Results indicated that using stringent analyses, this treatment was effective. From pre-treatment to post-treatment, the mean effect size across all measures of social anxiety, quality of life, and functioning was large and maintained at three-month follow up. In addition, formal analyses supported mediation. Specifically, early changes in experiential avoidance (mediator) significantly predicted changes from midtreatment to follow up on social anxiety symptoms (outcome) after controlling for early changes in social anxiety symptoms and perceived control over emotions.

Gaudiano and Herbert randomly assigned inpatients with psychosis and high rates of comorbid substance misuse ($n = 40$) to either an enhanced-treatment-as-usual (ETAU-alone) intervention or to a brief ACT-plus-ETAU intervention [40]. On most variables in this study, trends favored ACT-plus-ETAU over

ETAU-alone, although, often – presumably due to low statistical power – these differences did not reach statistical significance. Among the most notable findings was that 50% of ACT-plus-ETAU participants were classified as responders (i.e., 2 + S.D. symptom reduction) versus only 7% of the ETAU-alone participants. In addition, the rehospitalization rates over four months tended to be lower in the ACT-plus-ETAU group (28% rehospitalized) as compared to the ETAU-alone group (45% rehospitalized). Regarding mediational analysis, pre-treatment believability of hallucinations significantly reduced the relationship between pre-treatment frequency of hallucinations and post-treatment distress associated with hallucinations, as predicted. These findings suggest that believability mediated the relationship between hallucination frequency and distress. (In contrast, and also as predicted, pre-treatment frequency of hallucinations did not mediate the relationship between pre-treatment believability and later distress.)

Zettle and Hayes found that depressed patients ($n = 18$) randomly assigned to an early version of ACT improved reliably more than those receiving cognitive therapy (CT), with large effect sizes (post-treatment ES = 1.23 and follow-up ES = 0.92 at two months) [49]. A weakness of the study was that the first author conducted all the therapy in both conditions and – although a well trained cognitive therapist – had allegiance to ACT. Notwithstanding this shortcoming, a subsequent reanalysis of the data using formal mediational analyses suggested that improvement was due to a hypothesized ACT process. The relationship between treatment condition and post-treatment and follow-up outcomes (measured by well-established depression measures) were significantly mediated by mid-treatment believability of depressogenic thoughts (measured by a modified version of the Automatic Thought Questionnaire, ATQ-B).

Gifford et al. randomly assigned nicotine-dependent smokers ($n = 76$) to a seven-week treatment of either ACT or nicotine replacement therapy (NRT) [42]. At post-treatment and at six-month follow up, quit rates were similar for ACT and NRT participants. However, at one-year follow up, ACT participants exhibited markedly higher quit rates than the NRT participants. The relationship between treatment condition (ACT vs. NRT) and outcome (smoking abstinence) was mediated by score on the Avoidance and Inflexibility Scale (AIS).

Lundgren et al. randomly assigned poor, South African epileptics with drug refractory seizures ($n = 27$) to an ACT (including seizure management

training) or a supportive control treatment, consisting of only nine hours of treatment over four weeks [50]. At post-treatment, six-month and twelve-month follow ups, the ACT protocol resulted in an enormous reduction in epileptic seizure index (frequency × duration) compared to baseline and to the control treatment. Also, the ACT participants experienced significant improvements on quality-of-life measures compared to the supportive control participants. Mediational analyses demonstrated that pre to follow-up changes in seizures, quality of life, and well-being were partially mediated by post-treatment ACT process measures, including acceptance, defusion, values attainment, and persistence in the face of barriers.

Acceptance and commitment therapy outcome studies with formal mediational analysis not including determination of temporal precedence

Gregg et al. studied Type-2 diabetes patients ($n = 81$) who participated in a one-day workshop on medical management of diabetes [47]. Patients were randomly assigned to education-alone or to ACT-plus-education conditions. Compared with patients who received education-alone, after three months, those in the ACT-plus-education condition were significantly more likely to use trained coping strategies, to report better diabetes self-care, and tended to have lower glycosylated hemoglobin levels (a well established measure of glycemic control) in the target range. The relationship between treatment condition (ACT-plus-education vs. education-alone) and glycosylated hemoglobin levels was significantly reduced when acceptance of diabetes-related thoughts and feelings (measured by the Acceptance and Action Diabetes Questionnaire) were statistically removed. This suggests that acceptance significantly contributed to (i.e., mediated) ACT's positive effect on diabetic management.

Lillis et al. randomly assigned patients who had completed six or more months in a weight-loss program ($n = 84$) to either an ACT (one-day ACT workshop plus workbook) or a wait-list condition [46]. Results indicated that at a three-month follow up, the ACT group showed significantly greater improvements in body mass index (i.e., weight/height), obesity-related stigma, quality of life, psychological distress, and distress tolerance; the magnitude of these effects were in the medium or large range. Mediational analyses indicated that weight-specific ACT processes mediated the relationships between treatment condition and all outcome variables.

In addition to the above outcome studies that included formal mediational analyses, several recent non-intervention studies used formal mediational analyses to test the ACT model [38, 43–45]. Most of these examined clinical populations. Unfortunately, none of the studies attempted to determine temporal precedence, as data were collected in a single session. Three of the four studies clearly demonstrated that statistically removing the effects of the ACT-hypothesized mediator reduced the relationship between the independent and dependent variable, suggesting mediation.

Other ACT outcome studies

Two meta-analyses of ACT outcome studies produced nearly identical mean effect sizes, showing that on average ACT interventions resulted in medium to large effects [11, 51]. (When compared to other active treatments, ES = ~0.5; when compared to wait-list controls, ~1.0.) Cognitive–behavioral therapy is the standard of effective psychotherapy. Thus far, five published studies directly compared ACT and traditional CBT. In three of these, ACT outperformed traditional CBT (among heterogeneous, psychotherapy outpatients [52], and among depressed recruits [53, 54]). In one, the treatments were not significantly different (among anxious and depressed outpatients [55]), and in one systematic desensitization outperformed ACT (for math anxiety [56]).

Öst quantitatively analyzed the quality of ACT versus traditional CBT and concluded that on average ACT studies were less methodologically rigorous [51]. Studies were matched – based on journal and year – and then rated on background and methodological variables. Based on his rating scheme, Öst found that, although traditional CBT and ACT were not significantly different on any background factor, traditional CBT was superior on eight of twenty-two methodological variables.

Rigorous research methodology is essential to the advancement of behavioral science. Moreover, although mindfulness researchers should carefully consider Öst's suggestions for improving quality, we believe his methodology and perspectives have important shortcomings and ignore important issues. First, studies were not matched on populations. All 13 selected traditional CBT studies targeted anxiety disorders (11 studies) or major depression (2 studies),

syndromes for which CBT demonstrated efficacy for decades [57]. In contrast, the ACT studies were preliminary investigations covering a broad range of difficult-to-treat problems that are relatively underrepresented in the overarching CBT field (e.g., drug-refractory epileptics, pain, personality disorders). Second, regarding funding, although the ACT studies and the traditional CBT studies selected by Öst did not significantly differ in terms of the number of studies that were funded, there was a significant difference in the size of the grants, favoring traditional CBT. This suggests that the ACT studies were at a large resource disadvantage in the types of designs and the level of rigor they could employ. A third limitation of the Öst study was that it did not include many recent ACT outcome studies. Finally, what we believe was the most serious limitation was that Öst did not recognize the importance of mediational and component analyses, research strategies that we believe result in more definitive findings and more rapid progress. It should be noted that none of the 13 CBT studies used in Öst included mediational analyses. Conversely, 7 out of 13 ACT studies have published (positive) mediational analyses [11, 39, 41, 42, 47, 58, 59]. (For a related discussion of controversies regarding empirically supported treatment criteria, the interested reader should see a special issue on this subject, *Behavior Modification*, Vol. 27 No. 3, July 2003 [60].)

Summary of ACT research literature

Although the number of ACT studies recently has increased dramatically, the total number of studies is relatively small. Therefore, much remains unknown about ACT. However, collectively, component analysis studies, mediational analyses, outcome studies including those that compare ACT to traditional CBT, and meta-analyses all suggest that ACT is a promising approach that is likely to be beneficial with many populations in many settings. An interesting and theory-consistent finding in several ACT outcome studies is that ACT had a significant effect on behavior and quality of life regardless of whether it reduced symptoms. For example, in studies comparing interventions for chronic pain there were often no differences between ACT and control conditions on pain measures, but ACT patients exhibited superior functioning or lower rates of disability [61, 62]. Also, control patients with psychosis reported a significantly greater reduction is psychotic symptoms than those in the ACT condition; however, those in the ACT condition had significantly and markedly lower rates of rehospitalization [63].

Mindfulness-based cognitive therapy

Of all the outcome studies involving mindfulness treatments to date, Teasdale and colleagues' MBCT studies were among the best designed and most methodologically rigorous [64, 65]. The studies compared MBCT plus treatment-as-usual (MBCT+TAU) versus TAU-alone on relapse rates among patients with recurrent depression with at least two prior episodes. The studies had similar results. They found that, as compared to TAU-alone, MBCT+TAU protected patients from recurrence/remission. Moreover, they found evidence of a positive relationship between the number of previous depressive episodes and the effectiveness of MBCT+TAU relative to TAU-alone. As the number of prior episodes increased, MBCT protected patients more from relapses than TAU-alone. Among patients with only two previous episodes, there was a non-significant but concerning trend in the opposite direction, more patients in the MBCT+TAU group had relapses than the TAU-alone group (56% vs. 31% in Teasdale *et al.*; 50% vs. 20% in Ma and Teasdale). Ma and Teasdale also compared differential relapses in those with three and four or more prior episodes. Among those with three prior episodes, 33% in MBCT+TAU relapsed versus 60% in TAU-alone, and among patients with four or more episodes, only 38% of MBCT+TAU and 100% of the TAU-alone relapsed. What seemed to account for the relationship between the number of prior episodes and the degree of protection from MBCT is that MBCT protected against autonomous episodes (which were much more likely to occur in those with more prior episodes), but did not protect against episodes triggered by negative life events. Other research groups replicated Teasdale and colleagues' findings with other depressed patient populations, for example, in a controlled study of patients with three or more prior episodes of depression who had residual symptoms [66], in an uncontrolled study of treatment-resistant depression [67], and in an uncontrolled study of a heterogeneous sample of depressed and anxious outpatients [68]. All three showed that MBCT had positive, medium to large effects. These findings suggest that MBCT can be an effective treatment for individuals with depression, especially those with the most chronic courses.

Dialectical behavior therapy

Dialectical behavior therapy has been used with patients having parasuicidal behavior and borderline personality disorder, and more recently with other treatment-refractory populations. Several outcome studies have found that DBT is a promising approach, and no other therapy has demonstrated superiority to DBT [69].

One recent DBT study stands out among the others with respect to demonstrating excellent quality. In a one-year, randomized controlled trial plus a one-year follow up, Linehan *et al.* compared DBT to (non-behavioral) community treatment by experts (CTBE) for women who engaged in recent suicidal and self-injurious behavior and who met DSM-IV criteria for borderline personality [70].

Results indicated that during both the one-year treatment and a one-year follow-up period, DBT was superior to CTBE on most outcomes. For example, compared to those in the non-behavioral community treatment, those participants receiving DBT were half as likely to make a suicide attempt, required significantly less hospitalization for suicidal ideation, and were significantly more likely to remain in treatment. The findings in this study suggest that DBT as it is typically practiced is efficacious, and its efficacy is likely the result of specific aspects of the DBT intervention and not the result of general factors associated with expert psychotherapy.

Conclusions

The treatments that include mindfulness as an important component show much promise. However, at this point in time, each of these treatments require additional, high-quality research to better understand basic processes (mediators) and to establish treatment parameters, including how to best tailor them to specific populations and conditions. A review of the efficacy of mindfulness-based treatments has been recently provided by Hofmann and colleagues [71].

References

1. Kabat-Zinn J. *Wherever You Go, There You are.* New York: Hyperion, 1994.

2. Lau MA, Bishop SR, Segal ZV, *et al.* The Toronto Mindfulness Scale: development and validation. *J Clin Psychol* 2006; **62**: 1445–67.

3. Richelle MN. *B.F. Skinner: A Reappraisal.* London: Psychology Press, 1995.

4. Simons DJ, Chabris CF. Gorillas in our midst: sustained inattentional blindness for dynamic events. *Perception* 1999; **28**: 1059–74.

5. Segal ZV, Williams JMG, Teasdale JD. *Mindfulness-Based Cognitive Therapy for Depression: A New Approach to Preventing Relapse.* New York: Guilford Press, 2002.

6. Hayes SC. Acceptance, mindfulness and science. *Clin Psychol (New York)* 2002; **9**: 101–6.

7. Hayes SC, Strosahl K, Wilson KG. *Acceptance and Commitment Therapy: An Experiential Approach to Behavior Change.* New York: Guilford Press, 1999.

8. Welch SS, Rizvi S, Dimidjian S. Mindfulness in dialectical behavior therapy (DBT) for borderline personality disorder. In Baer RA, ed. *Mindfulness-Based Treatment Approaches: Clinician's Guide to Evidence Base and Applications.* Burlington: Academic Press. 2006; pp. 117–39.

9. Linehan MM. *Cognitive–Behavioral Treatment of Borderline Personality Disorder.* New York: Guilford Press, 1993.

10. Teasdale JD, Segal VS, Williams JMG. Mindfulness training and problem formulation. *Clin Psychol Sci Prac* 2003; **10**: 157–60.

11. Hayes SC, Luoma J, Bond F, Masuda A, Lillis J. Acceptance and commitment therapy: model, processes, and outcomes. *Behav Res Ther* 2006; **44**: 1–25.

12. Chambless DL, Ollendick TH. Empirically supported psychological interventions: controversies and evidence. *Ann Rev of Psychol* 2001; **52**: 685–716.

13. Arch JJ, Craske MG. Acceptance and commitment therapy and cognitive behavioral therapy for anxiety disorders: different treatments, similar mechanisms? *Clin Psychol Sci Prac* 2008; **15**: 263–79.

14. Hofmann S, Asmundson GJ. Acceptance and mindfulness-based therapy: new wave or old hat? *Clin Psychol Rev* 2008; **28**: 1–16.

15. Hofmann S. Acceptance and commitment therapy: new wave or morita therapy? *Clin Psychol Sci Prac* 2008; **15**: 263–79,

16. Hayes S. Climbing our hills: a beginning conversation on the comparison of acceptance and commitment therapy and traditional cognitive behavioral therapy. *Clin Psychol Sci Prac* 2008; **15**: 263–79.

17. Hayes SC, Wilson KG. Mindfulness: method and process. *Clin Psychol (New York)* 2003; **10**: 161–5.

18. Grossman P, Niemann L, Schmidt S, Walach H. Mindfulness-based stress reduction and health benefits: a meta-analysis. *J Psychosom Res* 2004; **57**: 35–43.

19. Dimidjian S, Linehan MM. Defining an agenda for future research on the clinical application of mindfulness practice. *Clin Psychol (New York)* 2003; **10**: 166–71.

20. Bishop, Lau M, Shapiro S, *et al.* Mindfulness: a proposed operational definition. *Clin Psychol (New York)* 2004; **11**: 230–41.

21. Brown KW, Ryan RM. The benefits of being present: mindfulness and its role in psychological well-being. *J Pers Soc Psychol* 2003; **84**: 822–48.

22. Baer RA, Smith GT, Allen KB. Assessment of mindfulness by self-report: the Kentucky Inventory of Mindfulness Skills. *Assessment* 2004; **11**: 191–206.

23. Walach H, Buchheld N, Buttenmuller V, Kleinknecht N, Schmidt S. Measuring mindfulness: the Freiburg Mindfulness Inventory (FMI). *Pers Individ Dif* 2006; **40**: 1543–55.

24. Feldman G, Hayes A, Kumar S, Greeson J, Laurenceau J. Mindfulness and emotion regulation: the development and initial validation of the Cognitive and Affective Mindfulness Scale-Revised (CAMS-R). *J Psychopathol Behav Assess* 2007; **29**: 177–90.

25. Cardaciotto L, Herbert JD, Forman EM, Moltra E, Farrow V. The assessment of present-moment awareness and acceptance: the Philadelphia Mindfulness Scale. *Assessment* 2008; **15**: 204–23.

26. Brown KW, Ryan RM, Creswell JD. Mindfulness: theoretical foundations and evidence for its salutary Effects. *Psychol Inq* 2007; **18**: 211–37.

27. Baer RA, Smith GT, Hopkins J, Krietemeyer J, Toney L. Using self-report assessment methods to explore facets of mindfulness. *Assessment* 2006; **13**: 27–45.

28. Masuda A, Hayes SC, Sackett CF, Twohig MP. Cognitive defusion and self-relevant negative thoughts: examining the impact of a ninety year old technique. *Behav Res Ther* 2004; **42**: 477–85.

29. Healy H, Barnes-Holmes Y, Barnes-Holmes D, *et al.* An experimental test of a cognitive defusion exercise: coping with negative and positive self-statements. *Psychol Rec* 2008; **58**: 623–40.

30. Levitt JT, Brown TA, Orsillo SM, Barlow DH. The effects of acceptance versus suppression of emotion on subjective and psychophysiological response to carbon dioxide challenge in patients with panic disorder. *Behav Ther* 2004; **35**: 747–66.

31. Campbell-Sills L, Barlow DH, Brown TA, Hofmann SG. Effects of suppression and acceptance on emotional responses of individuals with anxiety and mood disorders. *Behav Res Ther* 2006; **44**: 1251–63.

32. Vowles KE, McNeil DW, Gross RT, *et al.* Effects of pain acceptance and pain control strategies on physical impairment in individuals with chronic low back pain. *Behav Ther* 2007 **38**: 412–25.

177

33. Feldner MT, Zvolensky MJ, Eifert GH, Spira AP. Emotional avoidance: an experimental test of individual differences and response suppression using biological challenge. *Behav Res Ther* 2003; **41**: 403–11.

34. Masedo AI, Rosa Esteve M. Effects of suppression, acceptance and spontaneous coping on pain tolerance, pain intensity and distress. *Behav Res Ther* 2007; **45**: 199–209.

35. McMullen J, Barnes-Holmes D, Barnes-Holmes Y, *et al.* Acceptance versus distraction: brief instructions, metaphors and exercises in increasing tolerance for self-delivered electric shocks. *Behav Res Ther* 2008; **46**: 122–9.

36. Páez-Blarrina M, Luciano C, Gutierrez-Martinez O, *et al.* The role of values with personal examples in altering the functions of pain: comparison between acceptance-based and cognitive-control-based protocols. *Behav Res Ther* 2008; **46**: 84–97.

37. Forman EM, Hoffman KL, McGrath KB, *et al.* A comparison of acceptance- and control-based strategies for coping with food cravings: an analog study. *Behav Res Ther* 2007; **45**: 2372–86.

38. Marcks BA, Woods DW. Role of thought-related beliefs and coping strategies in the escalation of intrusive thoughts: an analog to obsessive–compulsive disorder. *Behav Res Ther* 2007; **45**: 2640–51.

39. Lundgren T, Dahl J, Hayes SC. Evaluation of mediators of change in the treatment of epilepsy with acceptance and commitment therapy. *J Behav Med* 2008; **31**: 221–35.

40. Gaudiano BA, Herbert JD. Acute treatment of inpatients with psychotic symptoms using acceptance and commitment therapy: pilot results. *Behav Res Ther* 2006; **44**: 415–37.

41. Gaudiano BA, Herbert JD. Believability of hallucinations as a potential mediator of their frequency and associated distress in psychotic inpatients. *Behav Cog Psychother* 2006; **34**: 497–502.

42. Gifford E, Kohlenberg BS, Hayes SC, *et al.* Acceptance-based treatment for smoking cessation. *Behav Ther* 2004; **35**: 689–705.

43. Gratz KL, Tull MT, Gunderson JG. Preliminary data on the relationship between anxiety sensitivity and borderline personality disorder: the role of experiential avoidance. *J Psychiatr Res* 2008; **42**: 550–9.

44. Norberg MM, Wetterneck CT, Woods DW, Conelea CA. Experiential avoidance as a mediator of relationships between cognitions and hair-pulling severity. *Behav Modif* 2007; **31**: 367–81. Unlinked

45. Tull MT, Jakupcak M, Paulson A. The role of emotional inexpressivity and experiential avoidance in the relationship between posttraumatic stress disorder symptom severity and aggressive behavior among men exposed to interpersonal violence. *Anxiety Stress Coping* 2007; **20**: 337–51.

46. Lillis J, Hayes SC, Bunting K, Masuda A. Teaching acceptance and mindfulness to improve the lives of the obese: a preliminary test of a theoretical model. *Ann Behav Med* 2009; **37**(1): 58–69.

47. Gregg JA Callaghan GM, Hayes SC, Glenn-Lawson JL. Improving diabetes self-management through acceptance, mindfulness, and values: a randomized controlled trial. *J Consult Clin Psychol* 2007; **75**: 336–43.

48. Dalrymple KL, Herbert JD. Acceptance and commitment therapy for generalized social anxiety disorder: a pilot study. *Behav Modif* 2007; **31**: 543–68.

49. Zettle RD, Hayes SC. Dysfunctional control by client verbal behavior: the context of reason giving. *Anal Verbal Behav* 1986; **4**: 30–8.

50. Lundgren T, Dahl J, Melin L, Kies B. Evaluation of acceptance and commitment therapy for drug refractory epilepsy: a randomized controlled trial in South Africa – a pilot study. *Epilepsia* 2006; **47**: 2173–9.

51. Öst LG. Efficacy of the third wave of behavioral therapies: a systematic review and meta-analysis. *Behav Res Ther* 2008; **46**: 296–321.

52. Lappalainen R, Lehtonin T, Skarp E, *et al.* The impact of CBT and ACT models using psychology trainee therapists: a preliminary controlled effectiveness trial. *Behav Modif* 2007; **31**: 488–511.

53. Zettle RD, Hayes SC. Component and process analysis of cognitive therapy. *Psychol Rep* 1987; **61**: 939–53.

54. Zettle RD, Rains JC. Group cognitive and contextual therapies in treatment of depression. *J Clin Psychol* 1989; **45**: 438–45.

55. Forman EM, Herbert JD, Moitra E, Yeomans PD, Geller PA. A randomized controlled effectiveness trial of Acceptance and Commitment Therapy and Cognitive Therapy for anxiety and depression. *Behav Modif* 2007; **31**: 772–99.

56. Zettle RD. Acceptance and commitment therapy vs. systematic desensitization in treatment of mathematics anxiety. *Psychol Rec* 2003; **53**: 197–215.

57. Butler AC, Jason E, Chapman B, *et al.* The empirical status of cognitive–behavioral therapy: a review of meta-analyses. *Clin Psychol Rev* 2006; **26**: 17–31.

58. Bond FW, Bunce D. Mediators of change in emotion-focused and problem-focused worksite stress management interventions. *J Occup Health Psychol* 2000; **5**: 156–63.

59. Hayes SC, Bissett R, Roget N, *et al.* The impact of acceptance and commitment training and multicultural training on the stigmatizing attitudes and professional burnout of substance abuse counselors. *Behav Ther* 2004; **35**: 821–35.

60. Herbert JD (ed.) Special issue on empirically supported treatments. *Behav Modif* 2003; **27**: 287–430.

61. Dahl J, Wilson KG, Nilsson A. Acceptance and Commitment Therapy and the treatment of persons at risk for long-term disability resulting from stress and pain symptoms: a preliminary randomized trial. *Behav Ther* 2004; **35**: 785–801.

62. McCracken L, MacKichan F, Eccleston C. Contextual cognitive-behavioral therapy for severely disabled chronic pain sufferers: effectiveness and clinically significant change. *Eur J Pain* 2007; **11**: 314–22.

63. Bach P, Hayes SC. The use of acceptance and commitment therapy to prevent the rehospitalization of psychotic patients: a randomized controlled trial. *J Consult Clin Psychol* 2002; **70**: 1129–39.

64. Teasdale JD, Segal ZV, Williams JMG, *et al.* Reducing risk of recurrence of major depression using mindfulness-based cognitive therapy. *J Consult Clin Psychol* 2000; **68**: 615–23.

65. Ma SH, Teasdale JD. Mindfulness-based cognitive therapy for depression: replication and exploration of differential relapse prevention effects. *J Consult Clin Psychol* 2004; **72**: 31–40.

66. Kingston T, Dooley B, Bates A, Lawlor E, Malone, K. Mindfulness-based cognitive therapy for residual depressive symptoms. *Psychol Psychother* 2007; **80**: 193–203.

67. Kenny MA, Williams JM. Treatment-resistant depressed patients show a good response to mindfulness-based cognitive therapy. *Behav Res Ther* 2007; **45**: 617–25.

68. Ree MJ, Craigie MA. Outcomes following mindfulness-based cognitive therapy in a heterogeneous sample of adult outpatients. *Behav Change* 2007; **24**: 70–86.

69. Lynch TR, William TT, Salsman N, Linehan MM. Dialectical behavior therapy for borderline personality disorder. *Annu Rev Clin Psychol* 2007; **3**: 181–205.

70. Linehan MM, Comtois KA, Murray AM, *et al.* Two-year randomized controlled trial and follow-up of dialectical behavior therapy vs therapy by experts for suicidal behaviors and borderline personality disorder. *Arch Gen Psychiatry* 2006; **63**: 757–66.

71. Hofmann SG, Sawyer AT, Witt AA, Oh D. The effect of mindfulness-based therapy on anxiety and depression: a meta-analytic review. *J Consult Clin Psychol* 2010; **78**(2): 169–83.

Index